The Art of Asylum-Kee

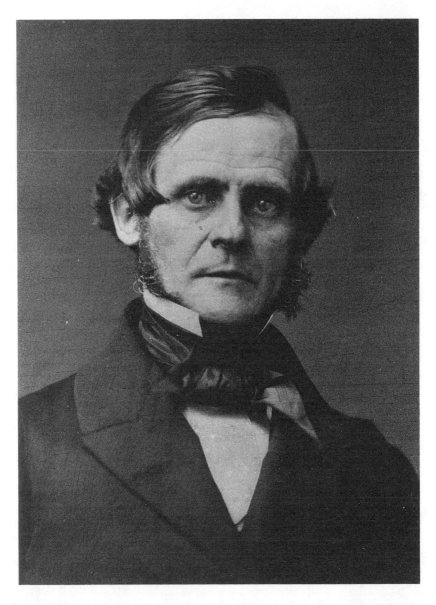

Thomas Story Kirkbride, superintendent of the Pennsylvania Hospital for the Insane, 1840-83. Photograph taken in the mid-1850s. (Courtesy of the Historic Archives, Institute of the Pennsylvania Hospital.)

The Art of Asylum-Keeping
Thomas Story Kirkbride and the Origins of American Psychiatry

Nancy Tomes

UNIVERSITY OF PENNSYLVANIA PRESS
PHILADELPHIA

University of Pennsylvania Press
STUDIES IN HEALTH, ILLNESS, AND CAREGIVING
Joan E. Lynaugh, General Editor

A complete list of books in this series
appears at the back of this volume.

Originally published in 1984 by Cambridge University Press
Paperback reprint edition copyright © 1994 by Nancy Tomes
Printed in the United States of America

Library of Congress Cataloging-in-Publication Data

Tomes, Nancy, 1952–
    [A generous confidence]
    The art of asylum-keeping: Thomas Story Kirkbride and the origins of
American psychiatry / Nancy Tomes [with new introduction].
        p.   cm. — (Studies in health, illness, and caregiving)
    Originally published by Cambridge University Press, 1984, under title:
A generous confidence.
    Includes bibliographical references and index.
    ISBN 0-8122-1539-7 (pbk.)
    1. Pennsylvania Hospital for the Insane.   2. Kirkbride, Thomas Story,
1809–1883.   3. Mentally ill—Institutional care—United States—History—
19th century.   I. Title.   II. Series.
RC445.P4P685   1994
362.2'1'0974811—dc20   93-49742
                                                                CIP

CONTENTS

TABLES AND FIGURES

Tables

Figures

INTRODUCTION TO THE PAPERBACK EDITION

In May 1994, the American Psychiatric Association marks the 150th anniversary of its founding. During that month, thousands of psychiatrists from all over the country will converge on Philadelphia to participate in the sesquicentennial celebrations. Their choice of meeting site reflects that city's rich historical associations with the psychiatric specialty. Philadelphia was the first city in the original thirteen colonies to provide hospital care for the mentally ill, at the venerable Pennsylvania Hospital (founded 1751); it was home to Benjamin Rush, the first American physician to make an original contribution to psychiatric thinking; and perhaps most significantly, it played host to the first meeting, in October 1844, of the professional group that later became known as the American Psychiatric Association.

The 150th anniversary of the APA's founding seems a particularly appropriate time to publish a paperback edition of *The Art of Asylum-Keeping: Thomas Story Kirkbride and the Origins of American Psychiatry*, which first appeared in 1984 under the title *A Generous Confidence*. The book chronicles the career of Kirkbride, one of the original thirteen founders of the American Psychiatric Association. Although not as well known today as his predecessor at the Pennsylvania Hospital, Benjamin Rush, Kirkbride in his own time was equally celebrated as an exemplary American practitioner of psychiatry. For more than forty years, he headed what was considered one of the finest mental hospitals in the country, the Pennsylvania Hospital for the Insane (now called the Institute of the Pennsylvania Hospital). As a long-time officer of the Association — he served more years as president than any of his contemporaries — Kirkbride advised governors, legislators, and presidents about the proper care of the mentally ill. His most enduring legacy to the specialty was the "Kirkbride plan," a style of hospital design and management that shaped the first major wave of asylum construction in the mid-1800s. At a more personal level, Kirkbride's career testified to the singular drama of life in the early asylum: He was shot in the head by one former patient, prosecuted in a much publicized court case by another, and, late in life, married yet a third. Both professionally and personally, the narrative of Thomas Story Kirkbride's life reflects the unique institution that was the nineteenth-century mental hospital.

Given how dramatically psychiatry has changed in the last 150 years, one might well ask whether Kirkbride's story, however colorful, has any contemporary interest or relevance. After all, the age of the asylum, when psychiatry was so closely associated with this distinctive institution, is long gone and little lamented. Even before Kirkbride's death in 1883, the optimistic faith the APA's founding generation had in the curative powers of the asylum had already begun to waver. Although the mental hospital continued to dominate the mental health care system for another three-quarters of a century, its continued existence was regarded more as a necessary evil than a symbol of professional progress. Psychiatry's romance with the asylum was over long before the number of patients resident in mental hospitals began to decline in the 1950s.

The post–World War II deinstitutionalization movement resulted from changes that Kirkbride's generation could hardly have imagined: a pharmaceutical revolution that produced drugs capable of ameliorating the worst symptoms of mental disease; a patients' rights movement that challenged the ethics of involuntary commitment; and a relentless drive to cut health care costs that effectively eliminated lengthy hospital stays for any disease, psychiatric or otherwise. These combined forces have fundamentally and probably irreversibly changed the place of the mental hospital in psychiatric practice. What was originally the specialty's raison d'être, the keystone of its professional identity, has become but one of a range of therapeutic options, and among the least desirable at that. Whereas psychiatrists in the mid-nineteenth century regarded commitment to a mental hospital as the best hope for the mentally ill, their modern descendants regard it as a last resort to be used only when other curative and palliative measures have failed.

But if American psychiatry today seems to have little in common with the vision of its founders, there is still insight to be gained in contemplating the specialty's unique historical relationship to the mental hospital. Examining the psychiatry of Thomas Story Kirkbride's day in relation to its contemporary counterpart highlights exactly what has changed and what has stayed the same in the treatment of mental illness. Read as an exercise in comparison and contrast, *The Art of Asylum-Keeping* will reward the reader with a better understanding not only of the far-reaching transformations in psychiatric theory and practice that have occurred over the last 150 years, but also of the significant continuities that remain.

For those who come to this book with little historical knowledge of psychiatry, the institution that it describes will seem simultaneously strange and familiar. If the nineteenth-century medical theories and practices described here are quite alien, the social dynamics and conflicts surrounding the treatment of mental illness are not. In particular, the social history of the nineteenth-century asylum underlines the persistent dilemmas involved in this area of medical practice: justifying involuntary treatment in a democratic society; balancing family, community, and patient interests; and maintaining high-quality medical care for the chronically ill. It is my hope that whatever insights may come from this juxtaposition of past and present will contribute to improving present-day care for the mentally ill and their families.

The first hurdle to understanding the historical origins of American psychiatry lies in comprehending how completely the specialty at its inception was identified with the asylum. Today, psychiatrists do not practice exclusively or even predominantly in mental hospitals. Once they have completed their residencies, only a small minority — a little over 18 percent — care for patients primarily in hospitals. The majority — almost two-thirds of all psychiatrists involved in patient care — regard the private office as the real locus of their work. Although they maintain hospital admitting privileges and hospitalize patients when necessary, their professional identity is not closely bound up with the mental hospital.[1]

In sharp contrast, the mental hospital was the *only* site of practice for psychiatrists in the mid-1800s; indeed, their very claims to be medical specialists depended on this institutional legitimation. The APA's founders did not call themselves psychiatrists — that term was a turn-of-the-century import from Germany — but rather "asylum doctors" and "medical superintendents." The original name of their professional society was the Association of Medical Superintendents of American Institutions for the Insane, and none but asylum superintendents could be members. Only in the late nineteenth century did both the Association's membership and rationale begin to broaden beyond its asylum origins, as reflected in its name changes: In 1892, it became the American Medico-Psychological Association, and in 1921, the American Psychiatric Association.

These fundamental changes in where psychiatrists practice and what they call themselves point to an even deeper divide between past and present. Put simply, the scientific basis of psychiatry today bears virtually no resemblance to nineteenth-century psychiatric theory and practice. Kirkbride and his generation stand on the other side of an intellectual watershed so wide that it would be far easier for them to understand the practice of a seventeenth-century physician than that of a modern-day psychiatrist. This intellectual divide is marked by two rich traditions that have developed since the late nineteenth century: the psychodynamic tradition associated with Sigmund Freud, which emphasizes early childhood experience and family dynamics; and the biological tradition, which focuses on brain physiology and chemistry.

Despite their often antagonistic relationship to each other, the "two psychiatries," psychodynamic and biological, are both critical to the late twentieth-century specialty's scientific legitimacy. This duality is reflected in the complex diagnostic system that psychiatrists of every therapeutic persuasion share, the *Diagnostic and Statistical Manual of Mental Disorders (DSM)*. The latest revised version, *DSM III-R*, classifies mental diseases under sixteen basic categories divided into multiple sub-groupings, each of which can be described along five "axes" marking the biological, psychological, and social dimensions of the disorder.[2]

The complexity of modern psychiatric diagnosis is mirrored in the range of therapeutic strategies and professional co-workers modern practitioners may call upon in caring for patients. Depending on their symptoms and prognoses, patients may be treated with a combination of drugs, psychotherapy, and social supports. More than one hundred drugs are now available to relieve the symptoms of mental illness. The varieties of psychotherapy are almost equally diverse, with duration ranging from short to long term, formats ranging from individual to group, and orientations ranging from psychoanalytic, to cognitive, to behavioral. To help ameliorate the disruptive social impact of mental disease, psychiatric practitioners may refer patients to a variety of social services available (if often too sparingly) to assist them. Recognizing that mental disease has complex biological, psychological, and social ramifications, psychiatrists often treat patients in conjunction with other professionals who possess complementary areas of expertise, such as psychiatric nurses, psychiatric social workers, and clinical psychologists.

Compared to this formidable array of treatment options, the nineteenth-century specialty's etiological theory, diagnostic terminology, and therapeutic strategies seem unbelievably crude. Their etiological theory, which had its roots in classical Greek medicine, might best be described as a simple stress model of mental illness. The early asylum doctors believed that any shock to or disturbance of the body's functions could derange the mind, and vice versa. In their view, the cause of mental illness could usually be found in the patient's immediate past, in a physical illness, period of prolonged stress, emotional trauma, or overindulgence in debilitating vices such as alcohol abuse or masturbation. The nineteenth-century diagnostic system was correspondingly simple. In contrast to the Byzantine complexities of *DSM III-R*, Kirkbride and his colleagues made do with only four basic categories of mental disease: mania, the "high form" of the disease characterized by excitement and delusions; melancholia, the "low form" distinguished by lethargy and depression; dementia, a form marked by mental stupor and evidence of organic brain damage; and monomania, or partial insanity, a form evidenced by delusional thinking about a single subject.

From our post-Freudian perspective, the absence in nineteenth-century psychiatry of any interest in early childhood experience is particularly striking. To be sure, the founding generation of psychiatrists subscribed, in a very general sense, to the widely held belief that proper discipline in childhood ensured adult mental stability. Yet when it came time to account for an individual patient's mental afflictions, they rarely traced the problem back to childhood, but rather sought its cause in some more recent experience. Although they could be fierce in their condemnation of sexual or alcoholic excess, asylum doctors seemed primarily intent on devising explanations of mental disease that absolved the sufferer as well as family from excessive guilt. They emphasized, as Kirkbride once wrote, that mental disease could be found "among the purest and the best of all dwellers upon earth, as well as those who are far from being models of excellence."[3]

This preference for simple, soothing explanations for patients and their families reflected the difficult task early psychiatrists faced in convincing them that insanity was a curable disease. For all the fear that mental illness still inspires, most people today are likely to know someone who has recovered from such an illness and gone on to live a productive life. In Kirkbride's time, the lay public, and even many physicians, saw little chance for recovery from madness. By emphasizing natural causes within the individual's control and stressing the value of asylum treatment, early psychiatrists attempted to reduce the fear and hopelessness surrounding mental disease. In addition, they had to combat a persistent identification of mental illness with sin and supernatural affliction. Although by the nineteenth century "enlightened" opinion no longer countenanced the belief that the insane were possessed by devils, the sense that they had some special spiritual or moral stigma remained strong. Thus simply asserting the identification of insanity with disease, that is, "medicalizing" the condition, became a means to reduce the moral opprobrium attached to it.

But in making the case for the medical treatment of insanity, the founding generation did not stress the kind of therapeutic modalities we now see as central to the practice of psychiatry, namely drug treatment and psychotherapy. To be sure, Kirkbride and his fellow superintendents regarded drug therapy as an indispensable part of asylum treatment. Although they had far fewer pharmaceutical remedies available than do modern psychiatrists, they could effectively modify some of the most distressing symptoms of mental disease. Bleeding and purging helped to reduce the overstimulated system, while narcotics and sedatives soothed nervous irritation and produced sleep. Yet while they regarded these interventions as invaluable, no physician of Kirkbride's generation would have asserted that drugs alone were likely to effect a cure. Patients usually came to them only after their own doctors had exhausted the standard medical remedies for insanity; had those measures worked, they would not have needed institutional care. Not surprisingly, then, nineteenth-century asylum physicians did not invest drug treatment with the kind of expectations that twentieth-century pharmaceutical breakthroughs have conditioned us to expect.

The early asylum doctors likewise had no concept of psychotherapy as a medical modality. As I show in *The Art of Asylum-Keeping*, Kirkbride did practice a simple form of "talk therapy," but his methods more closely resembled the techniques of religious conversion common in his day than the psychoanalytic techniques later pioneered by Josef Breuer and Sigmund Freud. What Kirkbride referred to as his "conversations" with patients were aimed more at what psychiatrists today call "remoralization," that is, restoring the individual's self-esteem and confidence about returning to the outside world. Although apparently quite successful with some patients, this kind of dialogue was extremely limited in extent and scope. Kirkbride practiced it almost unthinkingly, without any systematic attention to technique, much less reflection on the as-yet-unrecognized dynamics of transference and counter-transference.

Instead, Kirkbride and his contemporaries lavished their attention on what seems from a modern perspective a very frail therapeutic creed indeed: the healing influence of the hospital itself. Perhaps no aspect of nineteenth-century psychiatry is harder to understand than the extraordinary faith the founding generation invested in the institutional regimen known as "moral treatment." The difficulties in understanding their therapeutic philosophy begin with the very term "moral treatment," which conjures up images of doctors as moral police bent solely on indoctrinating patients in middle-class mores. While enforcing prevailing standards of acceptable behavior was certainly one aim of moral treatment, there was more to its rationale than simply that. The word "moral" had another set of meanings in the mid-1800s, which later became subsumed under the modern term "psychological." The category of "moral" was opposed to the material; it encompassed the mind, emotions, and soul, which existed independent of the physical body yet could be influenced by the manipulation of sensory and emotional impressions. Thus moral treatment aimed to alleviate the psychological causes of mental disease by radically changing the individual's environment and daily regimen.

Assuming a reciprocal connection between mind and body, moral treatment premised that *confinement in the asylum itself* could exercise a direct healing influence on the mind. Given that insanity

was characterized by irregularity in mental and physical functioning, its treatment logically should include the imposition of order,
harmony, and balance, in terms of both visual stimuli and behavioral patterns. To counteract the overstimulation and stresses of
modern life thought to cause mental disease, the sufferer should be
removed from the everyday world and immersed in a "new kind
of existence," to use Kirkbride's words.[4]

The power of moral treatment depended upon a perception of
the asylum building that is difficult to recapture. In order to
understand why nineteenth-century psychiatrists invested so
much in what historian David Rothman has called "moral architecture," one must first appreciate the distinctive "built environment" in which they lived. In the early 1800s, when the mental
hospital began to assume its monumental form, large buildings of
any sort were still very rare. The vast majority of Americans lived
in rural areas where even the finest homes had few pretensions to
grandeur. In big cities such as Philadelphia, buildings less than
three stories high, closely packed together with very narrow
frontages on the street, were the norm. The grandest public buildings that cities had to offer were still remarkably modest in scale,
and the potential of landscape architecture to enhance their dramatic impact was little exploited.[5]

Thus Thomas Story Kirkbride came of age in a culture that was
just beginning to appreciate the power that grand buildings and
skillful landscaping schemes could invoke. Put in the context of
the time, the scale of the hospital buildings and landscaping plans
Kirkbride envisioned and executed was remarkably innovative.
The impressive mass of the hospital building, the simplicity and
predictability of its exterior lines, the lofty dimensions of its ceilings and windows, the sweep of its hallways and staircases, and the
impressive vistas offered by the carefully landscaped grounds
made an ambitious architectural statement. One hundred and fifty
years ago, families and prospective patients accustomed to untidy
landscapes and modest buildings must have felt themselves under a
powerful influence when they entered those grounds and walked
those halls. Even today, when our standards of the architecturally
impressive are much higher, the Kirkbride Building at Forty-
ninth and Market Streets has a grandeur that the modern hospital
buildings adjacent to it lack.

Undergirding this grand asylum design was an unabashedly hierarchical conception of medical authority. The founding genera-

tion of psychiatrists sought, and to a considerable measure obtained, absolute authority over their vast institutional dominions. Kirkbride and his asylum brethren believed that the proper execution of moral treatment required the chief physician's total dominance, or "one man rule," as it was called. In an era when physicians in general hospitals had relatively limited administrative authority, they successfully argued that ensuring the moral order of the asylum required total control of every institutional detail. Far from seeing it as a bureaucratic burden, psychiatrists prized their administrative power and jealously guarded it against potential competitors. In contrast to the modern mental health team approach, they were notably reluctant to delegate authority to those beneath them in the asylum hierarchy, or to invite into the asylum other professional groups with an interest in mental illness, whether they be clergymen or neurologists.[6]

For all their ardency in seeking absolute authority, their success in achieving it exacted a high price from Kirkbride and his colleagues. At the pinnacle of the asylum hierarchy, the chief superintendent's position was a stressful and lonely one. Having sought "one man rule," he was now entirely accountable for the institution's success or failure. At the same time, the proper execution of moral treatment depended heavily on the assistant physicians, ward supervisors, and attendants who, by virtue of this hierarchical conception, were excluded from full partnership in the asylum's conduct. While they reigned supreme within their own institutions, asylum doctors still had to answer to hospital board members and state legislators when their administrative affairs, particularly their finances, proved unsatisfactory, as they often did.[7]

Perhaps inevitably, the therapeutic potential Kirkbride ascribed to his grand asylum design ultimately lost its power. As monumental architectural designs and sculpted landscapes became increasingly common features of urban life, the impact of the asylum building diminished. The buildings themselves proved extremely expensive to keep up and quickly became dismal and shabby from the hard wear they received from their inmates. Performing a difficult job with limited resources, the asylum staff found it hard to maintain high standards of care, especially for the chronic cases. Most disillusioning of all, the hospitals built with such hope gradually filled up with patients who simply did not get better, a living reminder of the limitations of moral treatment.

So quickly did this declension of moral treatment occur that the first generation of asylum doctors was also the last to believe wholeheartedly in the redemptive character of the asylum. As I show in the last part of *The Art of Asylum-Keeping*, both changes in the larger political atmosphere and contradictions inherent in moral treatment itself brought about its demise within the span of Kirkbride's own lifetime. The rise of the new "scientific psychiatry" of the late nineteenth century, with its greater attention to accurate diagnosis and emphasis on the somatic origins of mental illness, represented an explicit rejection of moral treatment's claims both to scientific rigor and to therapeutic efficacy.

While modern practitioners will probably find little relevance in Kirkbride's preoccupation with hospital architecture and management, they will nonetheless recognize the persistence of many premises of moral treatment in contemporary institutional psychiatry. Psychiatrists and historians have long noted the kinship between nineteenth-century moral treatment and what today is called "milieu management." Despite the many profound changes in treatment philosophy that have occurred, a well-conducted mental hospital still serves many of the same functions it did in Kirkbride's time: protecting the patient from impulses toward self-injury or violence toward others, providing a sense of safety and containment, reducing stimulation and stress, reestablishing the bounds of socially acceptable behavior, and restoring self-confidence.[8]

Likewise, anyone acquainted with the modern mental hospital, either as a health care provider or as a patron, will find familiar my historical depiction of the complex interaction among physician, asylum staff, family, and patient. If much has changed in our perceptions of mental disease, the discontinuity between medical ideals and ward realities, the conflicts between family needs and patient rights, and the tensions generated by involuntary commitment, have by no means abated.

One of the great strengths of *The Art of Asylum-Keeping*, in my assessment, is its inclusion of both families and patients as actors in the nineteenth-century "discovery" of the asylum. At the time I wrote the book, this perspective on the asylum had been little explored. The historical portrayal of the mental hospital was still dominated by the social control interpretation, which tended to portray psychiatrists as agents of the emergent capitalist state, intent chiefly on confining the dangerous elements of the working classes. Yet in looking at the impetus behind the nineteenth-century asylum, I was far more forcibly struck by its uses as a form of family protection.

The overwhelming majority of patients, poor and rich alike, were committed not by policemen or welfare agents, but by their own relatives. Far from being identified with the poor, the influential early asylums were private institutions that catered to an upper- and middle-class clientele. Long before they would go to hospitals to be treated for other diseases, affluent Americans chose to patronize mental hospitals, despite the stigma and expense they entailed. Explaining that preference led me to understand the kind of burdens mental disease imposed on the family at a time when its stability was seen as particularly crucial to the preservation of the social order.

Then as now, the family's motivations in seeking to commit relatives to mental hospitals are easily oversimplified and criticized. The sociologist Andrew Scull once described the asylum as "a convenient place to get rid of inconvenient people," a choice of wording that suggests families acted chiefly to preserve their own comfort.[9] I do not doubt that some of Kirkbride's patrons had less than noble reasons for their actions. Yet the overwhelming testimony of their letters to him, which number in the thousands, suggests a more desperate quality to their situation. Many seemed reluctant to acknowledge their relatives' mental impairment until it took extreme forms, and most tried every alternative within their personal and financial means to avoid institutionalization.

Today, psychiatrists prefer that whenever possible the family be involved in treatment. My account of the historic asylum shows that, far from being a recent development from family systems theory, the collaboration between doctor and family dates back to the very beginnings of modern psychiatry. Kirkbride's psychiatric philosophy was strongly influenced by the needs and concerns the patient's family brought to treatment. But whatever the confidence created between doctor and family members, their therapeutic alliance rarely included the patient as a willing partner. Unlike other forms of illness in which the sufferer voluntarily chose to go to the hospital, commitment for insanity involved curtailing the patient's rights. Although in the nineteenth century a small minority admitted themselves to the asylum, the vast majority of inmates were confined against their will. Some felt they were quite sane; others believed they were sick but still feared or resented being sent to a mental hospital. Then as now, the highly contested character of mental illness and the fundamentally antidemocratic tendencies of involuntary commitment created a persistent source of conflict.

By modern standards, the absence in nineteenth-century asylums of any consideration of the patients' rights or interests, as opposed to the concerns of the family or doctor, is quite striking. In Kirkbride's day, commitment laws were very informal and heavily weighted in the family's favor. Relatives needed only to obtain certificates of insanity from one or two physicians in order to commit a patient. Once hospitalized, patients had no formal avenue through which to protest their confinement or treatment. Their mail could be censored, and their opportunities to get legal advice were limited. Compared to their English counterparts, American asylums were slow to develop external checks on abusive or neglectful treatment.

The disregard for what we today consider the most elemental patient rights to an impartial review of mental status or protection against abuse should not be seen as unique to the American mental hospital. For all its rhetoric about social and political equality, nineteenth-century America was a deeply paternalistic society in many respects. Free white men of sound mind might be, at least in theory, masters of their own fates, but everyone else lived a far less egalitarian existence. After all, the asylum originated in an era when slavery was still practiced, women could not vote, and parents could beat their children without fear of interference. Those Americans who lost their reason also forfeited their right to independent action, becoming part of the dependent classes whose interests were thought best looked after by others. The concept of patients' rights as we understand them has evolved only in the last few decades.[10]

However circumscribed those rights may have been, my account of nineteenth-century asylum life suggests that patients still found powerful ways to influence and resist treatment. The philosopher Jeremy Bentham's Enlightenment ideal of the all-encompassing "panopticon" notwithstanding, the nineteenth-century mental hospital never attained the authoritarian atmosphere of a total institution. Its boundaries proved too porous, both literally, as evidenced by the constant stream of patients escaping through its carefully landscaped grounds, and figuratively, as even a psychiatrist of Kirkbride's standing found himself dragged into court by disgruntled patients.

Perhaps more importantly, *The Art of Asylum-Keeping* suggests how dangerous it is to generalize about "the" patient experience of the asylum. Individuals confined within its walls responded to the hospital experience with emotions ranging from fury to indifference to gratitude. Readers accustomed to negative images of mental hospitals may be most surprised at the evidence I found that patients often felt they benefited from their asylum stay. In juxtapositioning the stories of three ex-patients — Wiley Williams, the young man from Georgia who shot Kirkbride in the head; Ebenezer Haskell, the litigious carriage maker who repeatedly took him to court; and Eliza Butler, the young evangelical woman who became his second wife — I attempt to show the futility of making one story out of the patient experience of the nineteenth-century asylum.

Rereading *The Art of Asylum-Keeping* a decade later, in light of the post-structuralist revolution in critical theory, I am struck by how, inadvertently, I anticipated the much-heralded decline of the historical "master-narrative," that is, a unified, linear version of the past. In deciding to make both family members and patients significant actors in my history of the asylum, I was forced to abandon the quest for a tidy story line. Instead, the book proceeds as a series of contesting views of the hospital written from the standpoint of the family members, doctor, staff, and patients. In attempting to convey their multiple points of view, I found it impossible to derive any single historical "truth" from their asylum experiences.[11]

Were I writing the book today, I would add and clarify certain perspectives. For example, recent work on Southern medicine in general and Southern asylums in particular has made me realize how deeply Kirkbride's vision of the asylum as a microcosm of American society depended on its all-white character. Nowhere in the book do I note the important fact that the Pennsylvania Hospital for the Insane did not accept African-American patients. Thus the emphasis I place in *The Art of Asylum-Keeping* on Kirkbride's "democratic" vision of the asylum has to be severely qualified by noting its limitation to whites only.[12]

I would also want to clarify and deepen my analysis of the ways gender relations shaped the nineteenth-century asylum. Stimulated largely by Elaine Showalter's provocative 1985 book, *The Female Malady*, I have thought much more deeply about whether the asylum played a peculiarly oppressive role in women's lives. As I have argued at length elsewhere, I disagree with the oft-repeated assertion that nineteenth-century psychiatrists believed women to be more liable to insanity than men. Kirkbride's generation believed that men and women were liable to insanity for different reasons, but that they fell prey to its ravages in roughly equal numbers. My reading of nineteenth-century case records suggests that Victorian gender roles were pathogenic for *both* men and women. At the same time, I find it far more difficult than do many feminist literary critics to read women asylum patients' symptoms and behaviors as a form of nascent feminist protest.[13]

The Art of Asylum-Keeping raises another gender-related issue that requires further commentary in light of recent developments. In the last few years, sexual relations between psychiatrists and patients have become the focus of increased concern both within the psychiatric community and among the general public. Feminists have been particularly critical (rightly so, in my opinion) of the specialty's past reluctance to confront the ethical problem of therapists who have sex with patients.[14] Given this ongoing controversy, the fact that Thomas Story Kirkbride's second wife had once been his patient at the Pennsylvania Hospital for the Insane may surprise and even shock some readers. Critics of psychiatry's record on sex and ethics might see in this behavior on the part of one of the APA's founders yet one more proof of its long-standing insensitivity to the issue. Indeed, by the ethical standards being taught to young psychiatrists today, Kirkbride's marriage to Eliza Butler would represent a transgression of the doctor-patient relationship. But without denying the legitimacy of the contemporary ethical code, I would argue that such an interpretation of Kirkbride's conduct would be profoundly ahistorical.

In the first place, the ethical code that governed medical practice in his day was based on an entirely different conception of the doctor-patient relationship. To be sure, *sexual* relations between doctors and patients had been clearly proscribed as early as the Hippocratic oath, which was codified sometime before the first century A.D. But by nineteenth-century standards, what Kirkbride did was not considered "having sex with a patient." He married

Eliza Butler some seven years after she had left the Pennsylvania Hospital. In contrast to perceptions today, when psychiatrists are taught the dictum "once a patient, always a patient," their formal therapeutic relationship was considered long over. Moreover, their sexual union was legitimated by the institution of marriage.

In a more general sense, contemporary concerns about emotional parity between doctor and patient were absent from nineteenth-century debates about ethical behavior. The prevailing standards of that time required that physicians prescribe appropriate treatments and treat their patients with respect; but the usual definitions of "appropriate" and "respectful" did not privilege patient autonomy, emotional or otherwise. As I stressed before, however democratic American political rhetoric may have been in the mid-nineteenth century, medicine was a deeply paternalistic enterprise. Patients, particularly women, were expected to defer to and depend on their physicians. The fear that physicians might unfairly exploit their *emotional* authority over the patient, to the detriment of the latter's autonomy or well-being, was rarely voiced.[15]

For their part, psychiatrists had yet to realize that the treatment of mental disease required a particular sensitivity to these issues. As mentioned earlier, psychiatrists in this pre-Freudian era seem remarkably innocent of any understanding of the potentially treacherous processes of transference and cross-transference. This is not to deny that those processes were at work, but rather to stress how little aware physicians were of their ramifications.

Most likely, therapeutic relationships between male doctors and female patients did on occasion evoke romantic or erotic feelings in one or both parties. Yet given the pervasive denial of female sexuality, particularly among women of Butler's class, it seems likely that such feelings were systematically repressed by most physicians and patients. In her specific case, the extant evidence concerning Butler's hospital stay does not suggest that her treatment had any sexualized overtones of the sort that can be discerned in some case histories of the period.[16] As further testimony to the paternalism that governed both medical and marital relations, Butler's progression from patient to wife seemed to strike all concerned as quite natural. Husband and wife saw no need to conceal their past relationship; on the contrary, Eliza Butler Kirkbride regarded herself as living proof of her husband's powers as a healer. So far as I can detect, neither suffered any professional or social ostracism as a result of their marriage. Far from regarding him as a vulgar seducer, Kirkbride's professional brethren seem to have approved the match and hoped for its success. At least one acquaintance regarded the Kirkbrides as a model for the kind of prophylactic marriages that might benefit people with a history of mental illness. Rather than being seen as a reproach to professional standards in psychiatry, their story was regarded as a vindication of moral treatment.[17]

That the Butler-Kirkbride romance jars modern sensibilities is evidence of the profound transformations in doctor/patient and male/female roles that have occurred since World War II. In the context of their own times, the relationship between Thomas Story Kirkbride and Eliza Butler did not transgress the accepted bounds of the doctor-patient relationship. However much we may applaud the changes in ethical thinking that have taken place in recent years, it is by the standards of the nineteenth century, not the late twentieth, that their behavior should be judged.

I would like to thank Patricia Smith and her colleagues at the University of Pennsylvania Press for helping me to realize a long-time ambition to see this book available in paperback. I am also pleased to have *The Art of Asylum-Keeping* appear in the series, "Studies in Health, Illness, and Caregiving," edited by Joan Lynaugh. In addition, I want to acknowledge the colleagues who have sustained my interest in the history of American psychiatry over the last ten years. I thank Caroline Morris of the Pennsylvania Hospital for her many good services, as archivist and friend; and James Hoyme, Jane Century, and Olivia Reinhart of the Institute of the Pennsylvania Hospital for their encouragement of my continued involvement in its history. My collaboration with Lynn Gamwell on a new pictorial history of nineteenth-century American psychiatry has expanded my visual appreciation of the past. Fellow historians of psychiatry, including Joan Jacobs Brumberg, Patricia O'Brien D'Antonio, Ellen Dwyer, Gerald Grob, Kenneth Hawkins, Constance McGovern, Mark Micale, and Jack Pressman, continue to instruct me. My "family psychiatrist," Randy Sellers, has helped me to put the historical practice of psychiatry in better contemporary perspective. Last but not least, my work as well as my life have been greatly enriched over the last few years by the company of my husband, Christopher Sellers. To all these steadfast colleagues and friends, I would like to dedicate this new incarnation of *The Art of Asylum-Keeping.*

Notes

1. These percentages are calculated from data from the American Medical Association, *Physician Characteristics and Distribution in the U.S., 1993,* comp. by Gene Roback, Lillian Randolph, and Bradley Seidman (Chicago, 1993), p. 55. The data are derived from questionnaires completed by the practitioners themselves. The percentages reflect only those psychiatrists who list patient care, as opposed to administration, research, and teaching, as their primary professional activity; they account for 32,118 of the nation's 35,496 psychiatrists.

2. American Psychiatric Association, *Diagnostic and Statistical Manual of Mental Disorders,* 3d ed., revised (Washington, D.C., 1987). *DSM-IV* is in preparation. For a useful account of the intellectual politics behind *DSM-III,* see Mitchell Wilson, "*DSM-III* and the Transformation of American Psychiatry: A History," *American Journal of Psychiatry* 150:3 (March 1993):399–410.

3. This quote appears in the *Report of the Pennsylvania Hospital for the Insane, 1858,* p. 37.

4. *Report of the Pennsylvania Hospital for the Insane, 1863,* p. 24.

5. David J. Rothman, *The Discovery of the Asylum* (Boston, 1971), p. 84. My appreciation of these historical issues has been further enhanced by reading Kenneth Hawkins, "The Therapeutic Landscape: Nature, Architecture, and Mind in Nineteenth-Century America," Ph.D. dissertation, University of Rochester, 1991.

6. On the position of physicians in general hospitals, see Charles E. Rosenberg, *The Care of Strangers: The Rise of America's Hospital System* (New York, 1987), especially pp. 47–68.

7. Patricia O'Brien D'Antonio's recent work on the Friends Asylum provides a particularly insightful perspective on the asylum from the staff's point of view. See Patricia D'Antonio, "The Need for Care: Families, Patients, and Staff at a Nineteenth-Century Insane Asylum," *Transactions and Studies of the College of Physicians of Philadelphia,* 5th ser., 12:3 (1990):347–66; and "Staff Needs and Patient Care: Seclusion and Restraint in a Nineteenth-Century Insane Asylum," *Transactions and Studies of the College of Physicians of Philadelphia,* 5th ser., 13:4 (1991):411–23.

8. J. Sanbourne Bockoven, Eric T. Carlson, and Norman Dain were among the first to point out the similarities between nineteenth-century moral treatment and modern milieu management. See note 8 to my original Introduction (p. 332). For a sense of how milieu management figures in contemporary practice, see Lloyd I. Sederer, ed., *Inpatient Psychiatry: Diagnosis and Treatment,* 3d ed. (Philadelphia, 1991).

9. Andrew Scull, *Social Order/Mental Disorder* (Berkeley, Calif., 1989), p. 231.

10. For a historical account of changing concepts of patient rights and medical ethics in general, see David J. Rothman, *Strangers at the Bedside: How Law and Bioethics Transformed Medical Decision Making* (New York, 1991).

11. Post-structuralist theorists such as Jacques Derrida, Jacques Lacan, Jean-François Lyotard, and Michel Foucault have championed a critical perspective that stresses the indeterminacy of language and questions the validity of a single critical viewpoint. For an influential discussion of the decline of the master narrative, see Jean-François Lyotard, *The Post-Modern Condition: A Report on Knowledge*, tr. by Geoff Bennington and Brian Massumi, Theory and History of Literature, vol. 10 (Minneapolis, Minn., 1984).

12. On the issues of race and asylums, see Todd L. Savitt, *Medicine and Slavery: The Diseases and Health Care of Blacks in Antebellum Virginia* (Urbana, Ill., 1978), pp. 247–79; and Samuel B. Thielman, "Southern Madness: The Shape of Mental Health Care in the Old South," in *Science and Medicine in the Old South*, edited by Ronald L. Numbers and Todd L. Savitt (Baton Rouge, La., 1989), pp. 256–75.

13. Elaine Showalter, *The Female Malady* (New York, 1985). For my own more recent attempts to grapple with similar issues, see Nancy Tomes, "Historical Perspectives on Women and Mental Illness," in *Women, Health, and Medicine in America: A Historical Handbook*, edited by Rima Apple (New York, 1990), pp. 143–71; and "Feminist Histories of Psychiatry," in *Discovering the History of Psychiatry*, edited by Mark Micale and Roy Porter (New York, 1994), pp. 348–83.

14. For a useful overview of this debate, see Armand M. Nicholi, "The Therapist-Patient Relationship," in *The New Harvard Guide to Psychiatry*, edited by A. M. Nicholi (Cambridge, Mass., 1988), pp. 22–28.

15. For an excellent discussion of nineteenth-century medical ethics, see Martin Pernick, "The Patient's Role in Medical Decisionmaking: A Social History of Informed Consent" (the President's Commission for the Study of Ethical Problems in Medicine), *Making Health Care Decisions*, 3 vols. (Washington, D.C., 1982), vol. 3, pp. 1–34.

16. Several years after *A Generous Confidence* was published, I discovered two large collections of Eliza Butler Kirkbride's personal papers. My perusal of them only confirmed the impressions I had formed of their relationship based on the original materials I consulted. For a more detailed account of Butler's illness, based on the additional papers, see my article, "Devils in the Heart: Historical Perspectives on Women and Depression in Nineteenth Century America," *Transactions and Studies of the College of Physicians of Philadelphia*, 5th ser., 13:4 (1991):363–86.

No doubt Kirkbride's general reputation as a "Christian and a gentleman" protected him from suspicions concerning his behavior toward Butler. His demeanor as a physician might be contrasted with that of his slightly younger medical colleague, the neurologist S. Weir Mitchell. In his famous "rest cure," Mitchell seems to have openly employed his maleness as a therapeutic tool with women patients. He supposedly started to undress and get in bed with one patient who refused to get up when he told her to do so. See Ann Douglas Wood, "'The Fashionable Diseases': Women's Complaints and Their Treatment in Nineteenth Century America," in *Clio's Consciousness Raised*, edited by Mary Hartman and Lois W. Banner (New York, 1974), pp. 9–10.

For an excellent exposition of mid-nineteenth-century views of female sexuality, see Nancy Cott, "Passionlessness: An Interpretation of Victorian Sexual Ideology, 1790–1850," *Signs* 4 (1978):219–36.

17. My impression that Eliza Butler Kirkbride seemed not to suffer socially for her past illness was recently confirmed by an interesting and I think quite impartial source: a credit reference prepared on her by an agent of the R.G. Dun Company, forerunner of the Dun and Bradstreet Corporation. Agents hired by the company were usually lawyers or other respectable men of the community. A report on Eliza Kirkbride was filed in June 1885, which noted: "Is the 2nd wife and a former patient of Dr. Kirkbride, who died some time ago . . . stands well socially, is well spoken of, pays her debts, and is worthy of cr[edit]." See Philadelphia, vol. 163, p. 156, R.G. Dun Collection, Baker Library, Harvard University Graduate School of Business Administration.

PREFACE

No matter how easily the facts concerning its existence can be established, writing the history of a mental hospital is necessarily a difficult enterprise. From the day I first began this book, I have been constantly reminded of the subject matter's inherent volatility. Not only has the historical literature on the nineteenth-century asylum movement been marked by rhetorical extremes, but the current state of the mental health care system also evokes strong opinions. Both the historical and contemporary discourses have been dominated by polar images of the mental hospital: one image of a medical institution infused with humanitarian values, the other of a prisonlike structure dedicated solely to confinement. Did the asylum arise to provide a new and valuable medical service to an unfairly stigmatized class of the physically ill, or did it function only to imprison more effectively various groups, such as the poor, the immigrant, and the eccentric, who simply threatened the middle classes? These have been the sorts of crudely framed questions forced on me, whether I liked them or not, throughout the course of my research.

Yet, for all the heated debate, I soon realized that remarkably little had been written about how asylums actually worked, either as social or medical institutions. Although historians had thoroughly investigated the scientific and professional aspirations of early psychiatrists and charted the evolution of public policy toward the mentally ill, certain key participants in the asylum's historical development, notably the patients and their families, remained virtually invisible in historical accounts. At the time I began my study, we knew very little about families' motivations for seeking commitment or their expectations of hospital care. Similarly, the patients themselves were shadowy figures, appearing only as passive recipients (or victims, depending on the scholar's prejudices) of medical treatment.

So, despite all the previous work on the subject, it seemed to me that a crucial aspect of the asylum's rationale and function, that is, the social needs it served for the patients' families and the institutional experience it afforded the patients, still needed historical explication. Mindful of the well-known figures who had preceded me in the field – Gerald Grob, David Rothman, and most intimidating of all, Michel Foucault – I undertook yet another history of the mental hospital with this goal in mind: to reconstruct daily life in the asylum from the patients' and patrons' viewpoints.

This does not mean that I ignored the asylum's medical rationale or personnel, however. The scientific beliefs and professional goals of the chief physician of the Pennsylvania Hospital for the Insane, Thomas Story Kirkbride, have been a central focus throughout my analysis for two reasons. First, he, more than any other figure in the institution, determined its form and function; in most respects, the Pennsylvania Hospital was a concrete embodiment of his asylum philosophy. Second, Kirkbride's conception of the asylum had an influence far beyond the walls of his own institution: Between 1850 and 1880, mental hospitals throughout the United States were built and organized according to the "Kirkbride plan" he had devised. Because Kirkbride was a very important but little understood figure in both the insane asylum and the early American specialty of asylum medicine, I felt it imperative to explore his medical philosophy in detail.

Still, despite my focus on Kirkbride's conception of asylum medicine, *A Generous Confidence* is not primarily a history of medical ideas, the professionalization of psychiatry, or the evolution of mental health policy, although those developments inevitably figure in my historical analysis. Rather, I think of it as a social history of medical practice, concerned primarily with the interaction between scientific concepts and social needs. I assume that because of his professional status, Kirkbride had the dominant role in determining the medical and social rationale of the asylum. But his medical practice could not help but be affected by the expectations and behaviors of those he treated, so that his scientific beliefs were inevitably molded by his desire to secure the "generous confidence" of his patrons and patients. Thus, I analyze asylum treatment in this book as a collaborative, although not necessarily harmonious, enterprise involving doctor, family, and patient.

My study attempts to delineate the social context of asylum treatment by focusing on two questions: Whom did the asylum serve and how did it function simultaneously as a medical and a social institution? It assumes that concepts of disease and preferred methods of treatment had both a medical and a social rationale. The asylum regimen incorporated the prevailing scientific concepts of insanity, which had an independent existence and authority of their own, at the same time that it embodied the dominant social values and structures of the larger culture. The institution's medical and social rationales were mutually compatible and reinforcing; as such, they can hardly be examined independently of one another without losing sense of how the asylum actually functioned. In other words, I present the mental hospital here as both a therapeutic setting and an institution of social control, on the assumption that the two functions were not as mutually exclusive as the "treatment–incarceration dichotomy" predominant in the historical literature would lead us to believe.[1]

For various reasons, I chose a private rather than a state mental hospital for this line of analysis. In the first place, Gerald Grob had already done an in-depth study of the Worcester State Hospital, and there existed no comparable history of a private institution.[2] Given that corporate, that is, charitable as opposed to profit-making, private mental institutions were the first to be founded in this country and served as models for the state hospitals, this struck me as a serious omission in the historical literature.[3] To remedy the lack, the Pennsylvania Hospital for the Insane seemed a particularly apt choice, because of Kirkbride's standing in the specialty and his work on asylum design. Also, the patron–physician–patient interaction, which I thought the likeliest way to approach the social context of medical practice, would be easier to observe in a hospital dependent on private rather than on state funds. As I will argue, the problems of clientele and public image concerned the state hospital superintendents as well, but in a much more indirect fashion. Finally, I was especially interested in the asylum's appeal to the upper echelons of society. The reasons middle-class reformers might have had for confining poor or immigrant lunatics seemed obvious, if the social control theory had any validity at all; but why would members of the elite wish to put their own relatives in a mental hospital? The answer, I was sure, lay in the links between the asylum and the *family*, rather than in any particular social class. Without the involvement of the state as an intermediary, the private hospital allowed me a clear focus on the family dynamics involved in its utilization.

No scholar can claim to be without personal opinions on the subject she treats, and I am no exception. Therefore, I think it best to make my biases clear at the outset, and state my position on the medical model of mental illness. Personally, I accept the argument advanced by John Wing and other moderates that the definition of mental disorders, as well as the definition of any disease, involves both physiological and social processes. At the same time, I have tried to maintain an objective, or agnostic, stance toward my historical subject matter, describing beliefs and practices as they were rather than as I might wish them to be.[4] For historians, I believe this to be the only appropriate position to take; due to the imperfect nature of the historical records we must rely on, we can add very little to the debate over the true nature of mental illness or the validity of the medical model. What historians can do is illuminate the circumstances that made a particular medical innovation, in this case hospital treatment of insanity, increasingly popular at a certain point in time; the latter question has been my primary concern in this book.

With these assumptions in mind, I have tried to write a balanced account of the nineteenth-century asylum. To my way of thinking, the physicians and lay people involved in its development were neither completely altruistic nor unrelievedly self-interested in their goals; and as a result, the institution they created represented an all-too-human blend of medicine, morality, and expediency. Readers convinced that nineteenth-century doctors were totally scientific and benevolent in their goals will no doubt find me too critical of Kirkbride and his asylum, whereas those who believe psychiatry to be devoid of any scientific legitimacy whatsoever will find me too charitable. I can only hope that both kinds of critics will find the book useful and interesting, in spite of their disagreement with my personal viewpoints.

My historical interpretation of Kirkbride and his asylum philosophy does not easily lend itself to any recommendations for contemporary policy toward the mentally ill. But as I suggest in the Conclusion, I have come to believe that the mid-nineteenth century may well have represented a highpoint in hospital care of the chronic insane. The early asylum doctors such as Kirkbride may have lacked sufficient commitment to modern scientific in-quiry, as their critics have so often noted, but a devotion to moral duty made at least some of them excellent custodians of the hope-lessly ill. The objectification of patients as clinical material and the abandonment of concern for cases lacking scientific interest came only in subsequent generations. So, in this one regard, it might be argued that our modern mental health-care system has hardly improved on Kirkbride's vision of moral treatment.

A final note on terminology: To avoid anachronism, I have eschewed modern terms such as "mental illness" and "psychiatry" in my discussion of nineteenth-century medical practice, relying instead on the language Kirkbride and his generation used, that is, "insanity" and "asylum medicine." I have departed from Kirk-bride's personal preference, however, in that I use the term "asy-lum," a word he disliked because, as he put it, it implied that the insane needed "a place of refuge or security, as though they had committed some crime, or been banished from the sympathies as well as the presence of society."[5] But since his contemporaries commonly employed the term, I have used it for the sake of convenience.

In writing *A Generous Confidence*, I have contracted a number of intellectual debts, which I would like to acknowledge here. The greatest of these is to my dissertation director, Charles E. Rosen-berg, who guided me through every stage of its preparation. Most importantly, in his own exacting standards of scholarship, he has shown me what it means to be a truly fine historian. I hope that in some small way this book will repay the "generous confidence" he has always had in me. I have been doubly fortunate in having worked with another excellent scholar during the laborious busi-ness of turning a dissertation into a book. Over the past few years, Gerald Grob has been a generous and insightful critic of my work. His understanding of the history of mental hospitals and mental health policy has given me a much needed perspective on Kirkbride and his accomplishments.

Two other, younger colleagues have made a special contribution to the book. With a sociologist's critical eye and a historian's familiarity with the sources, Andrew Abbott read through my narrative and made a number of excellent suggestions for clarifying its analytical judgments. Although I have not been able to answer all of his critical queries, his exhortations to be more rigorous have forced me to write a better book. Finally, Janet Tighe has been an unfailing source of intellectual companionship during my forays into nineteenth-century medical history. Her familiarity with psychiatry and the law has made her a well-informed audience, and her patience and good humor have made her an invaluable friend.

Behind every good book, I am convinced, there must be a good archivist. Certainly, without the cooperation of Caroline Morris, the Archivist of the Pennsylvania Hospital, my work on Kirkbride would have suffered. She has assisted me in too many ways to be recounted. No historian could ask for a more competent or cooperative librarian with whom to work, and I never cease to be thankful that the archives of the "nation's oldest hospital" are in her safekeeping.

Numerous other colleagues and friends contributed their insights on various chapters of the manuscript: Ellen Dwyer, Barbara Rosenkrantz, Andrew Scull, and Maris Vinovskis all deserve special mention. Joan Brumberg not only supplied scholarly wisdom but also helped me survive the "finishing-your-book blues." Ronald Angel and Henry Williams gave me much needed technical assistance. My colleagues in the History Department at Stony Brook gave me their moral support as well as allowed me, at some cost to themselves, a two-year leave of absence to complete the manuscript, a generosity for which I am very grateful. The Rutgers–Princeton Program in Mental Health Research, headed by David Mechanic, paid for my leave and, perhaps more importantly, furnished me with a congenial set of colleagues and a pleasant place to work. Of the various librarians I consulted, Christine Ruggiere and her staff at the College of Physicians deserve special thanks for their assistance in tracking down references. June Strickland of the Institute of the Pennsylvania Hospital Library has also been very helpful. Barbara Beresford, Patricia Charity, Teresa Fetzer, Marie Merz, and Gerda Schmidt assisted me by typing innumerable drafts of the manuscript; Donna Rothbart and Thea McGann Capone produced the final copy cheerfully and in record time. Dr. George Layne of the Institute of the Pennsylvania Hospital deserves special thanks for the many hours he devoted to selecting and reproducing the book's illustrations. The staff of Cambridge University Press and the copy editor, Helen Greenberg, did an excellent job of shepherding me through the process of editing and producing the book. Last but not least, I received financial support for my project from the American Council of Learned Societies, which awarded me a Grant-in-Aid for Recent Recipients of the Ph.D. in 1979; and the National Institute of Mental Health, PH Grant No. PHS MH 16242.

Two friends, Suzanne Phillips and Susan Tomasky, have made their chief contributions to this book by keeping me sane while writing it. I hope that they will now think their efforts worthwhile. My husband, Lawrence W. Burnett, has supplied the daily infusions of love and patience so necessary to sustain the scholar. Although I have not acceded to his frequent requests to include a disguised reference to himself in my discussions of the nineteenth-century patients, and have no intention of trying to sell the movie rights to the "Kirkbride Story" (a scheme he is sure would make us rich), I do want to thank him for his loving companionship.

The book is dedicated to all my family; I hope they will be proud of it.

Nancy Tomes

INTRODUCTION: THE HISTORIAN AND THE ASYLUM

If a band of tourists bound for a visit to the nation's oldest medical institution, the Pennsylvania Hospital, were to get lost on the wrong side of the Schuylkill River, they might very well stumble across another Pennsylvania Hospital at Forth-ninth between Haverford and Market streets. The visitors would no doubt be confused, for as any guidebook would note, the original Pennsylvania Hospital is at Eighth and Spruce streets, in the heart of downtown Philadelphia. That institution's West Philadelphia branch, the Institute of the Pennsylvania Hospital, or, as it was called in the nineteenth century, the Pennsylvania Hospital for the Insane, rarely appears on any sightseer's itinerary. Whereas thousands of visitors come each year to admire the colonial general hospital, whose cornerstone Benjamin Franklin laid in 1755, few visit the historic asylum, which opened almost a century later, in 1841. To be sure, the eighteenth-century "Pine Building" is far more elegant and impressive in appearance than the nineteenth-century "Kirkbride Building," the only part of the old mental hospital still standing. (The original hospital building at Forty-fourth and Haverford streets was closed in 1959, and eventually torn down to make way for a public housing project.) Even in the asylum's prime, it was considered "architecturally unpretentious." Now, surrounded on all sides by the ghetto, the Kirkbride Building seems overwhelmed by its urban setting.[1]

Despite its unprepossessing appearance, the Pennsylvania Hospital for the Insane has as secure a place in medical history as its more famous progenitor. During the long and distinguished career of Thomas Story Kirkbride, the asylum's chief physician from 1841 to his death in 1883, it was considered one of the best mental hospitals in America. A founder of the American Psychiatric Association and a national authority on asylum construction and design, Kirkbride played a crucial role in establishing the psychiatric specialty in this country. In his day, visitors came from far and wide to observe the model asylum in operation. Kirkbride's example did much to make "moral treatment," a hospital regimen employing both medical and psychological measures, an acceptable alternative to home care of the insane in the nineteenth century.

Although still a very important component of the modern mental health care system, the traditional mental hospital developed by Kirkbride and his peers today has a more tenuous hold on public esteem than did its historic predecessor. Many private institutions such as the Institute of the Pennsylvania Hospital have maintained good reputations, but mental hospitals as a whole have come to be viewed with considerable distrust and skepticism by both the public and health care policymakers. Of course, since they first began to proliferate in the early 1800s, mental institutions have never been universally popular; critics have been denouncing them as ineffective, personally oppressive, and uneconomical for more than a century. But only recently has the actual utilization of mental institutions begun to decline. Due to new administrative policies and innovations in drug therapy, the resident patient population of American mental hospitals in the mid-1970s was slightly less than one-half the 1955 total. In the last decade, a widely publicized de-institutionalization movement has accelerated the relocation of chronically disabled patients from the mental hospital to residential-care facilities. This shift has been accompanied by a wide-ranging attack on the mental hospital's therapeutic and moral efficacy by scholars as well as journalists. Now, more than at any time since Kirkbride's era, the very right of the mental hospital to exist appears to be widely disputed.[2]

In reality, the term "de-institutionalization" is somewhat misleading. Recent treatment statistics suggest that the new mental health care system has not abandoned the mental hospital, but rather relies less heavily upon its services. Responsibility for certain classes of patients has been transferred from the traditional mental hospital to the community mental health center and the general hospital's psychiatric wards. As a result, some mental institutions have closed down or curtailed services. But the majority seem in little danger of disappearing; in fact, their admission rates have increased even as their patient census has declined because more patients are being admitted for shorter periods of time (the so-called revolving door syndrome). Thus, it appears that the mental hospital has survived the de-institutionalization movement, at least for now, to become part of a new, more specialized set of psychiatric institutions. At the Pennsylvania Hospital, for example, there now exist three types of treatment facilities for mental disorders: the Hall-Mercer Community Mental Health Center; the psychiatric wards of the Eighth Street hospital; and the Institute, which provides a variety of inpatient and outpatient services.[3]

The fact remains that the traditional mental hospital championed by Kirkbride and his contemporaries no longer occupies the dominant position in the mental health care system that it once held. Moreover, unlike Kirkbride's time, its aims are often thought of in custodial rather than therapeutic terms. At best, many observers regard confinement in a modern mental institution as an unavoidable evil, necessary to ensure that patients receive drug therapy, or do no harm to themselves or others. Critics also dispute the notion that the experience of institutional life itself has any inherent therapeutic benefit, other than strengthening the patient's resolve to get well and get out of the hospital. Nowadays, the central tenet of Kirkbride's medical philosophy, that all the insane were best treated in a mental hospital, would find few adherents.

The contemporary critique of the mental hospital makes it all the more difficult to comprehend the enthusiasm that Kirkbride and his generation felt for the institution. If the mental hospital's premises are so inherently flawed, we must wonder why it was established in the first place. The answer to that question lies in the historical circumstances surrounding the asylum's emergence as an innovation in medical care. I hope that this study, by illuminating the complex social origins of the nineteenth-century mental hospital, will contribute to a better understanding of this troubled and troubling fixture of modern society.

The outlines of the Pennsylvania Hospital's history have long been included in the standard histories of American psychiatry. As any survey notes, Benjamin Franklin's hospital was the first medical institution in the colonies to treat insanity. By including lunatics among the charity hospital's proper objects of care, the founders joined with other enlightened reformers of the day to break with a long tradition of regarding insanity as a problem beyond human intervention. For centuries, most Western Europeans had regarded mental disorder as a spiritual affliction that only divine intercession could cure. Even physicians who thought insanity had a physical basis considered it almost impossible to cure. Therefore, to assume that lunatics should receive the "benefit of regular advice, attendance, lodging, diet and medicines," much less that they might be cured by such measures, was a revolutionary view in the mid-eighteenth century. The hospital founders' characterization of insanity as a disease that institutional care might cure marked an important advance in the medicalization of madness.[4]

Although enlightened for its time, the medical regimen provided at the eighteenth-century general hospital reflected the prevailing view of the mad as subhuman creatures. "Rational humanitarianism," as Albert Deutsch termed this form of hospital treatment, consisted of no more than imprisonment partially tempered by scientific and humanitarian concerns. Due to its limited number of accommodations, only the most dangerous and disruptive lunatics were ever taken to the Pennsylvania Hospital. Although not all its patients had violent histories, the hospital's provisions for the insane took their character from the most "furious, fierce and dangerous" inhabitants. The lunatics lived in basement "cells" built "as strong as a prison." Even the most progressive managers and physicians tended to regard the insane as an exotic species of wild animal. That epitome of the Enlightenment scientist, Benjamin Rush, who served as attending physician to the Pennsylvania Hospital from 1783 to 1813, advocated techniques to subdue lunatics that effectively cast the physician as an animal tamer. The practice of allowing visitors to pay a small fee in order to visit the lunatics' quarters further contributed to the zoo-like atmosphere of the early hospital.[5]

As the humanitarian and scientific values associated with the Enlightenment gained ground in the late eighteenth century, this standard of institutional care slowly began to change. Despite his occasional lapses in sensitivity, Benjamin Rush's career at the Pennsylvania Hospital is often held up as an example of the new reform spirit. With the managers' cooperation, Rush experimented with more active medical and psychological measures, a varied daily regimen, and better classification of patients in the decades from 1780 to 1810. Seemingly unaware until the 1800s of similar methods being used by Phillipe Pinel at the Bicêtre and Salpêtrière hospitals and by William Tuke at the York Retreat, the physicians and officers of the Pennsylvania Hospital had in fact begun to implement the rudiments of what came to be known as "moral treatment": a medical regimen employing psychological techniques that emphasized the human, rather than beastlike, nature of the insane.

Moral treatment, as European reformers christened the asylum reform program, rejected the notion that those who had lost their reason partook of "the nature of. . .animals."[6] Inspired by a more optimistic view of human nature, which had roots in both the secular humanism of the Enlightenment and the pietistic doctrine of evangelicalism, the new therapy appealed to the lunatics' supposedly innate capacity to live a moral, ordered existence. If treated like rational beings, the reformers reasoned, the insane would act more like rational beings. To further their reawakening, moral treatment prescribed a round of occupations and amusements designed to stimulate the patients' latent reason and capacity for self-control.

The principles of moral treatment eventually inspired the Pennsylvania Hospital's officers to build a new hospital for the insane. By the late 1820s, the patients' accommodations and regimen had been improved as much as the confines of the old building would allow. The hospital's location in the heart of Philadelphia placed fixed constraints on its privacy and spaciousness. At first, the managers hoped to expand simply by erecting a separate asylum near the old Eighth Street hospital. But the hospital's physicians and contributors eventually convinced the board that the advantages of a rural location far outweighed the inconvenience of operating a second hospital some distance from the first, and a large plot of land in West Philadelphia was purchased for the new asylum.

The Pennsylvania Hospital for the Insane, which began receiving patients in 1841, presented a therapeutic profile quite different from that of its predecessor. In place of the old general hospital, with its relatively unspecialized features, desultory regimen, and decidedly working-class ambiance, stood an imposing structure designed exclusively for the treatment of insanity. Surrounded by ornamental lawns and gardens, the impressive asylum building offered more varied accommodations, including large, comfortable apartments for the wealthy. An extensive program of lectures, gymnastic classes, and other amusements formed the basis of the asylum's moral treatment. These attractions drew patrons from all over the country, including the most elite families of Philadelphia, and the Pennsylvania Hospital for the Insane soon acquired an air of opulence (albeit tempered by its Quaker heritage) that was quite foreign to its parent institution.

During Kirkbride's lifetime, the Pennsylvania Hospital for the Insane became closely associated with the new specialty of psychiatry, or "asylum medicine," as it was called until the late nineteenth century. In 1844, Kirkbride joined with twelve other asylum superintendents to form the Association of Medical Superintendents of American Institutions for the Insane, now known as the American Psychiatric Association; significantly, the organization of this medical specialty (the first such association in the United States) predated the formation of the American Medical Association by three years. Throughout his career, Kirkbride remained a leading figure in the profession. His treatise *On the Construction, Organization and General Arrangements of Hospitals for the Insane*, first published in 1854 and revised in 1880, established him as the acknowledged American authority on asylum construction and design. State hospitals across the country were built according to the "linear" or "Kirkbride" plan it outlined. Perhaps more importantly, Kirkbride's skill at professional diplomacy helped to pilot asylum medicine through its critical early years.

Kirkbride's career closely paralleled the rise and fall of moral treatment as a distinct therapeutic philosophy. In the early 1840s, when he first took charge of the Pennsylvania Hospital for the Insane, American superintendents had just begun to develop their own philosophy of asylum medicine that combined eighteenth-century medical systems with the innovations of Tuke and Pinel. This philosophy, as codified in the association's "propositions" on asylum design and administration written by Kirkbride, dominated the profession for the next three decades. Yet increasingly in the 1860s and 1870s, the weaknesses inherent in both the intellectual and administrative positions advocated by the association created dissension within the field. Physicians committed to new medical theories and lay critics concerned with welfare policy challenged the specialty's consensus on matters such as asylum design, the care of the chronic insane, and the role of the state hospital as a public charity. At the same time, the institutional base of moral treatment, the mental hospitals themselves, began to deteriorate rapidly; as chronic and indigent cases accumulated, therapeutic ideals gave way to custodial measures, particularly in public facilities. Observing their institutions becoming ever more crowded, many asylum superintendents grew pessimistic about the curability of mental disease. In the last decade of his life, Kirkbride tried to mediate the disagreements among his colleagues and restore confidence in the asylum, but with little success. Before his death in 1883, he saw the advent of an era of bad feeling among the various medical and governmental factions involved in caring for the insane, as well as increasing public distrust of the mental hospital.

Thus, the history of the Pennsylvania Hospital between 1751 and 1883 spans a critical period in the evolution of American psychiatry. In its first century and a half, the institution underwent a significant sequence of developments: the emergence of the asylum as a structure distinct from the general hospital, the establishment of asylum medicine as a separate medical specialty, and the dominance of moral treatment as a therapeutic philosophy. The Pennsylvania Hospital's evolution not only reflected these major trends but to a significant degree shaped them, particularly through the careers of Benjamin Rush and Thomas Story Kirkbride.

Few historians would dispute the preceding sketch of the Pennsylvania Hospital's development or its significance for the history of American psychiatry. But the nature of the social changes involved in the asylum's emergence as a specialized medical institution has been the subject of considerable debate. As might be expected with such a controversial topic, the history of the nineteenth-century mental hospital has been marked by strong partisanship. Depending on the scholars' personal allegiance to a particular medical or social philosophy, their interpretations of moral treatment and Kirkbride's role in promoting it have varied considerably. Some historians have seen the asylum's past as a tribute to the scientific and humanitarian vision of psychiatry, whereas others have pointed to the same developments as concrete proof of the specialty's intellectual and moral failings. Consequently, no scholar can venture into the field without becoming aware of the very different ways in which historians have viewed the asylum movement.

In many respects, Albert Deutsch's survey, the *Mentally Ill in America*, first published in 1937 and revised in 1949, still remains the dominant historical interpretation of American moral treatment. Writing within the "Whig" or Progressive tradition, which presents history as the upward climb of civilization, Deutsch chronicled the mental hospital's rise as the triumph of enlightened values over the brutal, ignorant traditions of the past. In the evolution of what he called "scientific psychiatry," Deutsch regarded the mid-nineteenth-century asylum as a radical improvement over previous conditions and praised Kirkbride as the "most prominent American psychiatrist of his time"; yet, he faulted Kirkbride's generation of asylum doctors for their obsessive concern with hospital administration, characterizing their institutions as no more than "well-conducted boarding houses." Moral treatment, Deutsch concluded, was hampered by insufficient scientific knowledge of insanity and its proper treatment. Thus, its decline in the 1870s and 1880s represented the inevitable march of medical progress. Although Deutsch's faith in the psychiatric wisdom of his own time now seems unwarranted, his evaluation of the early superintendents as mere managers and his chronology of moral treatment's rise and fall remain widely accepted.[7]

To be sure, in the 1950s and 1960s, a few scholars took issue with Deutsch's opinion of moral treatment as a psychiatric therapy. The popularity in the 1950s of "milieu treatment," an institutional regimen quite similar to moral treatment, stimulated a more respectful appraisal of the nineteenth-century asylum's therapeutic rationale. Although not denying its failures, J. Sanbourne Bockoven, Eric Carlson, and Norman Dain stressed the soundness of moral treatment's basic principles, that is, the value of a small hospital with a highly structured daily regimen. Dain's *Concepts of Insanity in the United States, 1789–1865*, the most influential work to emerge from this reevaluation of moral treatment, presented a detailed and sympathetic account of its intellectual rationale and practice. Yet in the end, Dain's argument still adhered to Deutsch's schema in that he implied that the evolution of scientific knowledge inevitably led to moral treatment's demise.[8]

Subsequent studies, rejecting the Whig approach to medical history altogether, adopted a far more critical perspective on the nineteenth-century asylum movement. The popularity in American history of the "social control" thesis, which views all reform as an effort by the wealthy and powerful to preserve their dominance over the rest of society, made cynicism concerning psychiatry's professed aims acceptable, indeed expected. Christopher Lasch, a leading exponent of the social control argument, summed up the iconoclastic dissent from the old-style institutional history in these words: "I have never found very convincing those explanations of history in which our present enlightenment is contrasted with the benighted conditions of the past; in which history is regarded as 'marching,' with occasional setbacks, and minor reverses, toward a better world." Instead, he found it personally and intellectually more exciting to explore the "underlying ambiguity" of reform. In the same spirit, scholars in the 1960s and 1970s began to look at the repressive qualities of nineteenth-century asylum treatment.[9]

The work of the French structuralist Michel Foucault was instrumental in fostering a more critical view of the asylum's past. His *Madness and Civilization*, first published in the United States in 1965, essentially reversed the old Whig formula by arguing that moral treatment represented a retrogression, a "gigantic moral imprisonment" necessitated by the exigencies of capitalist development. Contrasting the "easy, wandering existence" of the medieval madman to the oppressive plight of the nineteenth-century asylum patient, Foucault left little doubt as to which era practiced the more humane philosophy. In his account of the asylum's origins, Tuke and Pinel (and, by implication, Kirkbride as well) appeared not as liberating heroes but as the agents of bourgeois repression and conformity. Foucault used the asylum's history to expose what he saw as the central folly of Western society, the myth that scientific positivism brought enlightenment to the world.[10]

In a much more subdued fashion, David Rothman's *Discovery of the Asylum* also challenged the reality of nineteenth-century improvements in the care of the insane. Rothman's work subtly suggested that the informal, household-centered welfare policy of the colonial period was less oppressive than the rigid institutional disciplines adopted later. In place of the humanitarian and scientific values that older histories invoked as the impulse behind moral treatment, Rothman used a different dynamic to explain the asylum's development; its "discovery," as well as the rigid structure it assumed, was a response to the fluid, rapidly changing state of American society. By controlling dependent and deviant groups more closely, nineteenth-century reformers such as Kirkbride were attempting to maintain the dominance of their rural, native-born values. The asylum doctors' therapeutic goals hardly mattered, Rothman implies, since the "highly rigid and repressive system" they invented quickly degenerated into a "harsh and mechanical discipline." For all his iconoclasm, Rothman's conclusions about moral treatment bore a curious resemblance to Deutsch's curative-to-custodial theme.[11]

Since, as other scholars quickly pointed out, European asylums of a very similar type developed during the same time period, Rothman's central argument, that the asylum represented a unique response to American social conditions, did not bear up well. Subsequent versions of the social control argument focused instead on capitalism or modernization to explain the discovery of the asylum in both Europe and the United States. Lasch and Michael Katz, two Marxian advocates of the social control thesis, emphasized how the mental hospital and other nineteenth-century institutions, such as the public school and the penitentiary, fostered the same "single standard of citizenship," a rigorous self-discipline well suited to a rapidly industrializing society. To their way of thinking, the medical concepts and practices involved in asylum treatment were nothing more than scientific rationalizations of middle-class morality. Generally, the social control approach divested the mental hospital of its scientific legitimation and analyzed it entirely as an instrument of class domination.[12]

Richard W. Fox's *So Far Disordered in Mind*, which appeared in 1978, illustrates this revised version of the social control argument. Criticizing Rothman for conceiving of social control as an "abstract conflict" between vaguely defined groups of "controllers and their victims," Fox attempted to delineate the social processes involved in commitment more precisely. To this end, he did a quantitative analysis of early-twentieth-century court records for San Francisco. From his data, Fox concluded that the insane were usually hospitalized for "odd" or "peculiar" ideas and behavior rather than what he considered to be severe disabilities. Thus, he argued that the mental hospital existed less to provide the mentally ill with care than to remove their disturbing presence from society. The hospital functioned to "mark" or isolate individuals "who implicitly rendered their negative witnesses to the power of cultural norms." So, like Foucault, whom he greatly admired, Fox presented the asylum's development as one aspect of a larger historical process by which "bourgeois cultural attitudes took hold of burgeoning urban centers."[13]

In comparison to the works previously discussed, Gerald Grob's studies of the nineteenth-century mental hospital do not fit comfortably in either the Whig or social control schools. *The State and the Mentally Ill* (1966), a history of the Worcester State Hospital, and *Mental Institutions in America* (1973), a survey of mental health policy to 1875, presented the development of the mental hospital as a complex interaction involving psychiatry's professional aims, changes in the social welfare system, and conditions within the institutions themselves. In his interpretation, Grob disavowed the formulas of progressive history, instead presenting the demise of moral treatment as a tragic failure of social policy rather than the inevitable triumph of scientific psychiatry. At the same time, he avoided the conventions of the social control school, insofar as he depicted those involved in asylum reform as having genuine scientific and humanitarian concerns along with professional and class interests. As might be expected of a medical historian, Grob assumed that the mental hospital had a medical legitimation independent of its social function. Although his more conservative line of analysis earned less attention than Rothman's bold synthesis, Grob's work has largely superseded Deutsch's survey as the most reliable and comprehensive overview of the nineteenth-century mental hospital.[14]

The recent historical controversy over the mental hospital's purpose has been paralleled, and to some extent inspired, by sociological debate over the nature of mental illness. The skepticism regarding the asylum's scientific legitimation evident even in Grob's work is but one aspect of a larger scholarly questioning of psychiatry's foundations. As historians cannot help but be aware, over the last twenty years the "societal reaction" or "labeling" school of sociology has disputed the definition of insanity as an illness. What our society calls mental disease, psychiatrist Thomas Szasz and sociologist Thomas Scheff, among others, have argued, is in fact a socially constructed form of deviance whose "symptoms" represent the transgression of basic social norms rather than signs of a pathological process. The whole notion of "mental disease," the argument follows, is nothing more than a convenient fiction that allows physicians, with society's acquiescence and approval, to control a particularly troublesome group of social misfits. Erving Goffman's analysis of the mental hospital as a "total institution" took this logic a step further by classing the asylum with the prison and concentration camp. Generally, those in the labeling school have assumed, as did Goffman, that the mental hospital has a punitive, not a therapeutic, purpose and is devoid of any real benefit for its inmates.[15]

Without a doubt, the questioning of assumptions that has arisen out of both the historical and sociological debate over the mental hospital's purpose has envigorated the history of American psychiatry. The revisionist historians' break with the stultifying traditions of the old Whig school has certainly produced more broadly conceived, provocative studies of the nineteenth-century asylum. But whereas the "treatment–incarceration dichotomy," as Gerald Grob has termed it, once forced a healthy reexamination of historical preconceptions, it now threatens to become stultifying in its own right, insofar as scholars feel forced to choose between two equally overdrawn stereotypes: the asylum as "gigantic moral imprisonment" or the triumph of scientific and humanitarian zeal.[16] To cast further research in either of these molds promises to add little to our understanding of the mental hospital's history.

One way to move beyond the treatment–incarceration dichotomy is to focus attention on certain neglected actors in the asylum drama, the patients and their families. Although previous studies have made the motivations and activities of lay reformers, asylum doctors, and state legislators increasingly clear, the identities and attitudes of these important parties to commitment remain obscure. Contemporary historical conceptions of reform no longer allow the convenient Whig assumptions that the progress of moral treatment was inevitable, or that physicians and humanitarians commanded an immediate audience for their ideas. Yet historians still know remarkably little about the profound changes in popular attitudes toward institutionalization that must have accompanied the asylum's rapid expansion; similarly, they have not explored the methods medical men used to enhance the social, as well as medical, legitimacy of their new specialty. Thus, it has become imperative to establish the asylum's social context and identify its sources of support within the larger culture.[17] Without more detailed knowledge of both asylum practice and popular attitudes toward insanity, the central trend of this period, that is, the growing acceptance of hospital treatment, can be only imperfectly understood. For the asylum was not the sole creation of doctors or lay reformers, as previous histories have implicitly assumed, but an institution sanctioned by the whole society to meet certain commonly perceived needs.

The format of *A Generous Confidence* reflects my basic assumptions concerning the social definition of disease. Chapter 1, which examines the treatment of the insane at the Pennsylvania Hospital from 1751 to 1840, investigates the asylum's relationship to the general hospital and suggests some internal, institutional factors involved in the evolution of moral treatment. Using Kirkbride's biography as a focus, Chapter 2 sketches the professional and intellectual background of early asylum medicine; it ends with a summary of American medical theory concerning insanity at the time Kirkbride first became an asylum superintendent. With this groundwork laid, Chapters 3 to 5 present the asylum from the viewpoint of patron, doctor, and patient in turn. Their interaction serves as the matrix for my discussion of the medical and social dimensions of asylum practice.

The most direct link between the nineteenth-century asylum and the larger society was forged by the institution's lay clientele, that is, the families of the insane. Chapter 3 describes their attitudes toward insanity and the mental hospital, as revealed in their letters to the asylum superintendent. In recounting the events leading to a relative's commitment, Kirkbride's patrons often specified the symptoms they considered evidence of insanity and the types of deviant behavior they could not or would not tolerate in the home. Not only do their accounts suggest the boundaries between sane and insane behavior, they also reveal the many ways in which the patrons' motivations for seeking commitment and their expectations of asylum care influenced Kirkbride's medical practice.

My profile of the mid-nineteenth-century asylum's clientele also suggests a strong association between institutional growth and changing notions of the family's responsibility for health care. The asylum's rapid development can perhaps be best understood as the resolution of an increasingly painful domestic situation. Moral treatment proved to be a popular medical innovation among all classes precisely because it furnished families with a justifiable alternative to the care of difficult, disruptive relatives in the home. As we shall see, rising expectations of domestic life, as well as greater faith in the asylum's efficacy, predisposed nineteenth-century families to commit insane relatives more readily, and for a broader range of reasons, than did their eighteenth-century ancestors.

When the patients' families are considered as a primary influence on asylum practice, the early profession's preoccupation with asylum construction and design becomes more understandable. As Kirkbride well understood, the superintendent's success ultimately depended on his ability to match his patrons' needs with appealing institutional measures. Chapter 4 examines both the theory and practice of asylum medicine as a response to the family's concerns discussed in the previous chapter. The first section outlines the psychiatric "persuasion," the set of beliefs about mental disease and its treatment that Kirkbride promoted to assuage the family's guilt and anxiety concerning commitment of a relative. The remainder of the chapter shows how, in his professional writings and his own asylum practice, Kirkbride sought to manipulate every aspect of the hospital environment so as to have it coincide as closely as possible to the therapeutic ideal he projected for it. His treatise on design specified the building and staff arrangements he deemed essential to the successful practice of moral treatment. And, as the record of his own administration shows, Kirkbride's prescriptive advice was based on his own experience of the serious problems seemingly insignificant details of management could engender.

Kirkbride's asylum philosophy and practice both reveal the internal contradictions inherent in his conception of moral treatment: how to restrain the patients without giving the hospital a prisonlike appearance; how to create an institutional environment that was simultaneously awe-inspiring and comfortable; how to accommodate a variety of social and mental classes in one hospital while providing roughly equal treatment for all. Much of Kirkbride's professional energy went into the resolution of these "design dilemmas," to use Dolores Hayden's term. But far from reflecting a bureaucratic or managerial turn of mind, Kirkbride's preoccupation with asylum design was intimately related to his therapeutic goals. In his asylum practice, he strove to create a special "moral architecture," a set of spatial and social arrangements that would promote a "generous confidence" in his healing powers.[18]

As might be expected, the patients did not always develop this generous confidence in Kirkbride's ability. Chapter 5 looks at their response to involuntary hospital treatment as another element in the evolution of nineteenth-century asylum practice. Unlike the victims of other serious disorders, who might be expected to accept or even demand treatment, the mentally ill were usually unwilling patients. The unspoken alliance that united the superintendent and the patron rarely included them as equal or cooperative partners. Yet, they did not remain passive or powerless actors in the asylum drama, as their letters, case records, and diaries show.

Chapter 5 begins by examining the various measures the superintendent employed to cure or control his patients, including drug therapy, occupations and amusements, rewards and punishments, and individual conversations with the doctor. By these means, some patients accepted the doctor's characterization of their ideas or behavior as symptoms of disease, followed the regimen he outlined, and became well again. The diaries and letters of one young female patient, whom Kirkbride later married, illustrate the process of a cure and the qualities that led many patients to trust and respect their doctor. Conversely, other patients continued to resist, and by their rebellious behavior posed a constant threat to the superintendent's psychiatric persuasion. For all his authority, Kirkbride's security as an asylum superintendent was sometimes deeply threatened by noncompliant patients; one former inmate shot him in the head and another bested him in court, to cite two extreme examples. By destruction, escape, suicide, and legal action, patients continually showed that they could evade the physician's control, thereby detracting from the asylum image he wished to project. As my discussion of patient-related controversies will show, troublesome inmates played a significant role in the demise of moral treatment.

Of course, the influence of Kirkbride's patrons and patients on his medical thought and practice was exceedingly complex. Although viewing asylum medicine as an interactive process, this study does not adhere to a simplistic "marketplace model" of the causal link between social expedients and medical ideas. Certainly Kirkbride's asylum philosophy was not dictated solely by his concern to attract well-paying patrons; the linkages that shaped the therapeutic consensus, or persuasion, shared by doctor and patron (and so often resisted by the patient) were far more complicated than that. But the social context of psychiatric practice did encourage physicians to select or emphasize certain ideas and therapeutics over others on the basis of their relative utility in medical care.

This measure of utility encompassed far more than the need to make asylums financially secure, although that was surely a consideration. But in the case of insanity, the family's need to have some comprehensible explanation of the disorder's etiology and prognosis was a far more pressing concern. The asylum doctor's desire to assuage their fears and guilts must have been a factor influencing his conception of mental disease. Even more subtly, the nature of the clinical setting itself shaped asylum medicine in an era when it had no separate academic center for study. The circumstances under which physicians observed the disorder had to affect their theorizing about its etiology. For example, the complexities of the nineteenth-century "pathway to the mental hospital" ensured that asylum doctors became involved with commitment proceedings at a very late stage, and could rely only on the family's account of the disorder and its causes. Surely this circumstance must have hindered the specialty's development of etiological and diagnostic concepts.

Chapter 6 places the composite portrait of the nineteenth-century mental hospital drawn in Chapters 3, 4, and 5 within a larger context by examining the influence of Kirkbride's asylum philosophy on the evolution of American psychiatry. At first glance, one might well wonder how representative of general conditions Kirkbride's practice in an affluent private institution could have been; certainly, the superintendents of state hospitals did not possess the same advantages he enjoyed. But for various reasons, which I detail at the beginning of Chapter 6, the dynamics of his asylum practice were representative of the specialty as a whole. The need to build a therapeutic consensus that would legitimate the asylum as a new form of treatment concerned all asylum superintendents, whether in state or private practice. The histories of other doctors and hospitals, including Kirkbride's own circle of friends – David Tilden Brown at Bloomingdale, John Curwen at Harrisburg, Charles Nichols at the Government Asylum, and Isaac Ray at Butler – reveal that they all shared the same pressures and challenges in asylum practice. Running a mental hospital was like "living over a volcano," as Nichols once put it; such a perception could not fail to influence the profession's collective mentality.[19] Only by comprehending the common "perils of asylum practice," as I have called them, can we make sense of the apparent rigidity, indeed shrillness, with which the older asylum doctors defended their professional stance in the 1870s and 1880s. Their stubborn refusal to abandon the principles of Kirkbride's asylum philosophy, as codified in their propositions on construction and management, stemmed directly from their experience of asylum practice. Only by maintaining the superintendent's one-man rule and keeping the asylum to a manageable size did the brethren feel they could derive a degree of professional satisfaction commensurate with the rigors of their work. Thus, the internal history of the asylum implies a fuller understanding of the specialty's development.

In a deeper sense, I will argue, Kirkbride's linear plan came to stand for a certain vision of the state mental hospital and its place in American society. As Kirkbride envisioned public facilities of the insane, they were not to differ dramatically from his own institution. Although offering less luxurious accommodations, they were to be exactly like their private counterparts in design and organization. Mixed state institutions, which served the professional and artisan classes along with the indigent, and treated chronic as well as curable cases, were the only type of public hospital Kirkbride felt appropriate for American society. In a way, his linear plan embodied the system of class relations his generation believed to exist in the mid-nineteenth-century city: Equality of opportunity mediated class distinctions; rich and poor lived in separate neighborhoods, but within a neighborly distance of one another. Conversely, the hospital plans proposed by his younger critics, which called for large public hospitals to be built exclusively for the chronic, indigent insane, struck Kirkbride and his brethren as inherently un-American. As they saw it, the "cottage" hospital and its derivatives tacitly accepted the permanent existence of a large pauper class and rigid social distinctions. So, the highly charged debates of the 1860s and 1870s concerning hospital architecture involved far more than administrative issues. The rival hospital plans represented different conceptions not only of the state hospital's purpose but also of the very nature of American society.

The ultimate rejection of Kirkbride's asylum philosophy, a rejection he lived to see, heralded the larger direction of late nineteenth-century medical thought. The postbellum debate over asylum design involved two different and competing medical world views: the older, characteristically mid-century view of Kirkbride's generation, with its fusion of moral and medical imperatives into a commonsense approach to scientific truth; and the aggressive new gospel of laboratory medicine, whose youthful practitioners strove (at least in theory) to divorce moral values from scientific investigation. In asylum work, as in all other areas of medicine, the vision of youth won out, and the conception of the asylum as a moral universe gradually gave way to the more modern vision of the hospital as a vast laboratory.[20]

In a broader sense, the declining appeal of Kirkbride's asylum philosophy reflected the new social realities of late nineteenth-century America. Civil war, industrial expansion, and rapid geographic and population growth all combined to transform the rural society of Kirkbride's youth into an industrial nation. The new facets of institutional life he lived to see (and regret) – the differentiation of public and private services, the growth of state regulation, and the acceptance of a more rigid, impersonal system of class relations – merely reflected this larger transformation. Kirkbride's linear plan, along with the antebellum notion of social relations it embodied, simply proved unequal to the scale of late nineteenth-century social problems and class distinctions.

So, the history of the Pennsylvania Hospital for the Insane, as presented in the following pages, can be read on two levels. First, it is the history of a medical innovation and, as such, chronicles the rise and fall of moral treatment as a therapeutic paradigm. Second, it follows the evolution of American society, writ small within the walls of one institution, throughout the nineteenth century. Through the medium of institutional and individual biography, these two levels of history come together in an immediate and compelling way.

1

From hospital to asylum

In the winter of 1841, a strange traffic began between the Pennsylvania Hospital in the center of downtown Philadelphia and the countryside some two miles west of the city limits. A carriage load at a time, first the men, then the women, almost one hundred lunatics, were removed from the nearly ninety-year-old hospital at Eighth and Pine streets to a new institution set in the isolated, rolling farmland near the small village of Blockley (see Figure 1). Most of the patients who made the journey had not been outside the hospital for many years. Some traveled in the wristbands they had become used to wearing at all times; others had long been in seclusion. All had been categorized as hopelessly insane patients for whom active medical or psychological treatment no longer was necessary.

As each carriage load of patients settled into their new quarters, they found life in the asylum to be quite unlike their experience of the old general hospital. Instead of infrequent visits from a succession of different physicians, who also had charge of the sick wards, they were constantly under the eye of one doctor, the hospital superintendent, and his assistant, who had responsibility for no patients but themselves. Moreover, the chief physician, a slight, soft-spoken young Quaker named Thomas Story Kirkbride, seemed bent upon disarranging their long-accustomed institutional routine. First he removed the restraints from the "dangerous" patients and let them move freely in the wards, which were barren of the "tranquilizer chairs," leather cuffs, and straitjackets they had been used to seeing at the old hospital. Then, after receiving baths and clean clothes, the inmates sat down together to take their meals in a regular dining room, equipped with ordinary utensils and crockery, amenities unknown in the old institution. During the day the doctors did not allow them to sit

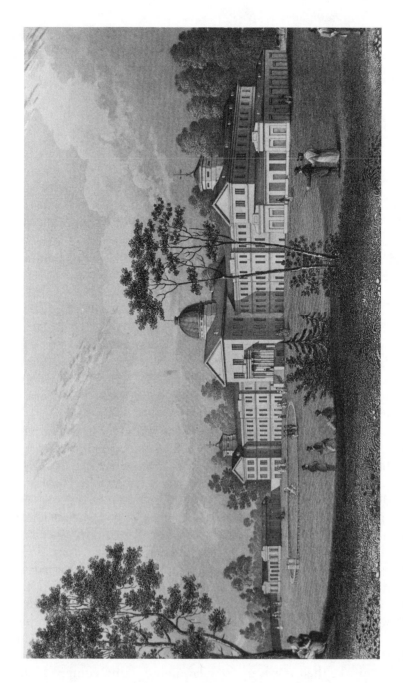

Figure 1. Engraving of the original Pennsylvania Hospital for the Insane as it appeared in the *Report of the Pennsylvania Hospital for the Insane for 1845*.

about unoccupied, but kept after them to read, play checkers, or work around the grounds. Once a week the patients were expected to sit quietly through a Bible reading, and were given gingerbread if they behaved nicely. When individuals became violent, they were not placed in restraint but given a stern warning to stop, and if the misconduct continued, were confined to their own rooms until calmer. Upon making a pledge to cease misbehaving, they could immediately regain their freedom.[1]

In his journal, the young superintendent recorded the effect of this new regimen on what he himself characterized as a set of "most unpromising cases." Kirkbride found that given relative freedom from restraint and expected to conform to a sane standard of behavior, his new charges did not become more violent or disorderly; quite the contrary: They took greater care of their personal appearance and seemed more alert and sociable. It was impressive, Kirkbride wrote, to see almost all the chronic patients sit with "perfect order and decorum" during his lengthy Bible reading (no doubt eagerly awaiting their gingerbread). Individuals long thought incapable of any rational activity read, played games, and did algebra. Their occasional outbursts of violence, when met with nonviolent but firm resistance, almost always yielded quickly and without mishap. Referring to the new hospital regimen in his first *Report*, Kirkbride stated that "from this freedom of action, and from these indulgences we have found nothing but advantage." Long-established cases of insanity might not be completely cured by the new methods, he concluded, but their "habits" could be radically improved. Kirkbride felt sure that the same techniques applied to recent cases would produce even more dramatic results.[2]

Thomas Story Kirkbride's handling of the chronic patients during his first months at the new Pennsylvania Hospital for the Insane reflected the influence of moral treatment, a philosophy of hospital care for insanity that dominated American asylum medicine in the nineteenth century. The basic tenets of moral treatment grew out of late eighteenth-century asylum reform movements in England and France. By freeing chronic patients from physical restraint and treating them as capable of rational behavior, the young superintendent quite consciously modeled himself on the European movement's most famous advocates, William Tuke in York, England, and Philippe Pinel of the Bicêtre and Salpêtrière hospitals in Paris, France. Independently of one another, Tuke and Pinel had implemented a hospital regimen for insanity based upon minimal physical correction, incentives to self-control, and firm paternal direction. By the early nineteenth century, educated physicians throughout Western Europe and the United States had espoused their principles of moral treatment as representing the first truly humane and scientifically correct mode of treating insanity.[3]

Although Kirkbride's practice of moral treatment followed well-known European precedents, it also reflected indigenous American developments. The new asylum was as much an outgrowth of the old Pennsylvania Hospital as a copy of the York Retreat or Bicêtre. From its earliest years, the insane had comprised as much as half of the resident patient population of the general hospital. In the late 1700s and early 1800s, recurring problems of housing and amusing a socially and mentally heterogeneous set of lunatics predisposed its managers and physicians to try their own experiments with new methods of treatment. Long before they could have heard of Tuke or Pinel, the Pennsylvania Hospital's officers had adopted many of the same attitudes and techniques that the European reformers later espoused. So, the managers' decision to build a separate asylum reflected the internal history of the Pennsylvania Hospital as well as the influence of European innovations. In its building design, regimen, and unified medical direction, the new Pennsylvania Hospital for the Insane embodied almost a century of institutional experience with the insane.

TREATMENT OF INSANITY AT THE PENNSYLVANIA HOSPITAL, 1752–1840

In 1748, a Philadelphia physician named Thomas Bond returned from a trip to England much impressed with the new voluntary hospitals he had seen in London and the larger provincial towns. Determined to see such an institution built in Philadelphia, Bond approached some influential friends, among them Benjamin Franklin, and together they began to canvass support for the plan. In 1751, thirty-three prominent citizens petitioned the colonial assembly for a charter and a grant of money to found a provincial hospital. A year later, the Pennsylvania Hospital received its first patients in a small rented house on Market Street, and the work of building the new hospital began. In 1756, the institution moved to the three-story brick building at Eighth and Pine streets, which still stands on the grounds of the modern Pennsylvania Hospital.[4]

The voluntary hospital plan advanced by Bond and Franklin appealed to the philanthropic tastes of colonial Philadelphians because it served a variety of needs. A man paid ten pounds to become a contributor, which allowed him the privilege of attending a yearly meeting to discuss the hospital's general policies and elect its Board of Managers. The twelve managers actually governed the institution, setting its fiscal and administrative policies, appointing a medical staff, and supervising the steward and matron. In this fashion, the hospital's financing and governance provided a wide base for public participation and identification through an open contributorship while maintaining actual control of its management by a small elite. Both managers and contributors had the privilege of recommending servants and poor neighbors for treatment. By exercising this right selectively, they favored the "worthy" over the "idle and vicious" poor; whereas the former were always welcome at the Pennsylvania Hospital, the latter had to rely on the far less pleasant accommodations at the almshouse. Thus, the hospital not only reduced the burden of caring for sick dependents but also reinforced and symbolized a properly deferential relationship between rich and poor. For the managers, association with the hospital had additional benefits. By the mid-eighteenth century, philanthropic activities had become one asset in the competition between political factions in the city. The Quakers in particular tried to use charitable enterprises such as the Pennsylvania Hospital to shore up their declining political power in the colony. Although the Board of Managers included non-Quakers as members, Friends dominated the early hospital's management in both numbers and influence.[5]

The Pennsylvania Hospital also played an important role in the rise of Philadelphia's medical elite. During their medical training in the leading European centers of Edinburgh, Paris, and London, the city's leading physicians, among them Thomas Bond, John Morgan, and the Shippen brothers, had become thoroughly convinced of the hospital's value in the clinical study of medicine. To put the American profession on the same sound foundation, they were determined to build their own hospital, which would provide the clinical practice and teaching facilities necessary for a proper course of medical education. Since clinical experience enhanced a doctor's professional skill and prestige, ambitious young men eagerly competed for posts as attending or resident physicians at the new hospital. The Pennsylvania Hospital soon became an integral part of the system of medical education and professional organization that made Philadelphia the premier medical center of the colonies.[6]

From its inception, the care of the insane was a central goal of the voluntary hospital plan. In explaining the need for a provincial hospital, the founders' petition to the colonial assembly explicitly mentioned the growing number of lunatics in the colony and the disruptions they caused. Some "going at large are a Terror to their Neighbours, who are daily apprehensive of the Violences they may commit," the petition stated; "others are continually wasting their Substance, to the great Injury of themselves and their Families." Invoking the success of London's Bethlehem Hospital, the founders expressed their faith that the insane might be cured if "subjected to proper management for their recovery." The hospital, by providing lunatics with proper accommodations (i.e., ones from which they could not escape) and forcing them to accept medical regulation, would provide two essential services: confinement and cure.[7]

This provision for the "reception and Relief of Lunatics" in the new hospital reflected a long-standing medical jurisdiction over insanity.[8] The conception of madness as disease dated back to classical medicine and the Hippocratic texts. Throughout the medieval period, a tradition of medical rationalism continued to dispute the widespread popular belief that mental disorder had a supernatural or demonic origin. By the eighteenth century, this tradition had gained considerable ground outside the medical profession. The notion that madness was a disease appears to have been commonplace among the educated classes of eighteenth-century Anglo-American society. This does not mean that lay people no longer recognized a spiritual dimension of insanity; on the contrary, they continued to think of it as a disturbance of the soul as well as the body. In traditional conceptions of disease, mind and body were inextricably linked, so that lay person and doctor alike naturally saw a troubled spirit as particularly vulnerable to mental and physical disease. The important shift in thinking evident by the eighteenth century was this: The origins of mental disorder were now securely located within the individual, in the internal imbalance of psychic and physical energies; supernatural agencies no longer had a legitimate place in eighteenth-century conceptions of insanity.[9]

Although eighteenth-century society did not necessarily assume that insanity was a curable disorder – even many doctors were convinced that it rarely yielded to medical remedies – still, some optimism centered on the development of hospital treatment. For example, in the late 1600s and early 1700s, Edward Tyson, the physician in charge of the Bethlehem Hospital, claimed to have cured two-thirds of the lunatic patients by active medical treatment combined with simple kindness. It was undoubtedly to Tyson's work that the Pennsylvania Hospital founders referred in their petition when they invoked the "long experience" of the Bethlehem Hospital, which proved that two-thirds of the insane might be cured with proper medical care. A more optimistic view of insanity's curability also permeated the voluntary hospital movement, and many of the new institutions founded in the mid-eighteenth century included wards for the insane.[10]

It was the hospital's association with medicine, and the implicit assumption that doctors might somehow successfully intervene in the course of mental disease, that led eighteenth-century colonial philanthropists to view the hospital as superior to other available forms of institutional care for the insane. The Philadelphia city almshouse, for example, had been sheltering homeless and unruly lunatics since the 1730s.[11] To accommodate the growing number of insane persons, the charitably inclined might simply have expanded this nonmedical facility or founded a private almshouse administered on similar lines. They chose instead to build a hospital, because it could *treat* as well as *confine* the insane. Thus, although almshouse and hospital both reflected a general concern with poverty and disorder, they had quite different social profiles: one defined by the provision of poor relief, the other by the practice of medicine.[12]

Despite the overriding importance that eighteenth-century benefactors of the insane attached to its therapeutic rationale, the early Pennsylvania Hospital provided a rather stark institutional existence for the insane. In its earliest years, the hospital furnished its inmates with little more than regular food, relatively clean accommodations, and occasional medical attention. The lunatics lived in barred basement cells subject to extreme temperatures and poor ventilation. Leg chains, manacles, and straitjackets were frequently used to confine them. The sole attendant assigned to their care was a "cell keeper," a low-status male employee paid even less than the nurses and groundskeeper. In good weather, he turned the residents out of the cells into the "crazy yard," a fenced-in enclosure on the hospital grounds, so that they might get fresh air and exercise, but otherwise made no effort to amuse or employ them. The attending or senior physicians, who visited all the hospital wards twice weekly, usually confined their attention to recently admitted or violent cases of insanity.[13]

In part, the prisonlike character of the Pennsylvania Hospital's early accommodations for the insane merely reflected the violent character of its inhabitants. The limited space available for confinement virtually ensured that only the most dangerous and disruptive lunatics were placed in the hospital. As accounts of the patients' behavior before commitment make clear, derangement itself did not prompt institutionalization. The family and community apparently tolerated, or rather had to endure, bizarre behavior as long as the mad person remained relatively peaceful. In order to be considered fit candidates for commitment, lunatics had to disrupt the familial or communal order in some very serious fashion. Many of the hospital's inmates had committed violence against themselves, their relatives, or their property before admission. A farmer who burned down his barn to rid it of rats, a woman who murdered her infant, a vagrant who broke the tombstones in the Jewish cemetery – these were among the hospital's early patients.[14]

Other lunatics had not actually harmed anyone but were so disruptive or menacing that their family and neighbors wanted them removed from the community. For example, the justice of the peace sent to the hospital a chair maker who "hath frequently behaved in a very disorderly manner to ye great Terror of his Family, and Annoyance of his Neighbors." In another case, a merchant repeatedly "disturbed [and] insulted diverse individuals, as well as a whole society [i.e., the Friends] in the places of their religious worship" before his commitment. Occasionally, a charitable person would support an incapacitated, homeless lunatic in the hospital, but more often, the quieter pauper cases were kept at the almshouse. So, in most cases, the hospital officers had good reason to regard the lunatic patients as dangerous characters in need of strong restraint.[15]

But the institutional milieu of the early hospital did not simply reflect the "fierce, furious and dangerous" nature of its inhabitants. Nineteenth-century asylum patients, as we shall see in later chapters, were also a relatively violent lot, yet their treatment was significantly different. Clearly, traditional perceptions of madness, as well as the lunatics' actual behavior, shaped their institutional treatment in the eighteenth century. The early hospital officers, like the rest of their contemporaries, tended to assume that the insane were less than human. Edward Cutbush, a former resident physician, wrote in 1794, "madmen, if suffered to have their liberty, resemble beasts rather than men." Even the most enlightened of the early managers and physicians believed that the insane, by virtue of losing their reason, had reverted to a brutish state. Thus, what was considered humane treatment for the time still reflected traditional notions that the insane, like animals, were impervious to extreme temperatures or needed to be shackled in heavy chains.[16]

The institutional origins of moral treatment

Gradually in the late eighteenth century, this grim conception of insanity and its treatment began to change. In asylum care, as in childrearing, prison discipline, and other dimensions of social life, there developed a tendency to replace physical punishment and restraint with gentler, more psychologically oriented forms of discipline.[17] The roots of this important change were many and complex: The evolution of Enlightenment concepts of human nature, the maturation of commercial capitalism, and the changing nature of social relationships in a more egalitarian, open society all played a part in the "domestication" of asylum treatment. The exact relationship between such broad social developments and the hospital's evolution is difficult to determine, but we can isolate some of the institutional dynamics precipitating changes at the Pennsylvania Hospital in the decades from 1780 to 1830.

Although usually less than one-fourth of the hospital's total admissions, the insane made up one-half of its resident institutional population by the 1780s because of their longer periods of hospitalization and lower rates of cure, compared to the physically ill patients.[18] Many of the chronic insane were paupers who had to be supported entirely at the hospital's expense. Generally, lunatics tended to be more expensive to keep than other patients. As a committee appointed in 1790 to examine the hospital's financial condition reported, the lunatics' individual rooms required more fuel to heat them than did the sick wards; attendants compelled to subdue "strong and turbulent" patients demanded high wages; hot and cold baths had to be provided for the lunatics' use; and their clothing, bedding, and crockery had to be replaced frequently due to their excessive destructiveness and dirtiness.[19] So, the managers, finding more than one-half of their scarce institutional resources devoted to the care of the insane, naturally saw improving the cure rate as a financial as well as a humanitarian goal.

The insane also placed constant pressure on the Pennsylvania Hospital's institutional resources because of their social heterogeneity. In sex, age, marital status, and class, the hospital population of lunatics was extraordinarily diverse. Although skewed in admission rates, 70 to 30 percent, the ratio of men to women residents in the institution was roughly 60 to 40 percent, since female patients tended to remain longer.[20] All age groups except the very young were represented in the hospital. Surveys in 1794 and 1812 found that 85 percent of the lunatics were between twenty and fifty. A more thorough census done in 1828 found 6 percent between fifteen and twenty, 81 percent between twenty and fifty, and 13 percent over fifty.[21] Among the women patients, 50 percent were married, 31 percent single, and 19 percent widowed at the time of admission. Among the men, 58 percent were single, 35 percent married, and 7 percent widowed.[22]

Although the Pennsylvania Hospital was originally intended to serve only the poor, its facilities for the insane quickly attracted a much broader clientele. A high percentage of the lunatic patients, 50 percent as opposed to 15 percent for the sick, paid for treatment. Some of the hospital's patrons came from the wealthiest ranks of Philadelphia society. Millionaire Stephen Girard, for example, kept his wife, Mary, in a private room at the institution for almost twenty-five years. More modestly situated farmers and artisans also found the cost of maintaining relatives in the hospital preferable to caring for them at home. Occupational data on the male patients collected in the late 1820s and 1830s show that the hospital's facilities for the insane had become quite skewed toward the wealthy: 18 percent were seamen and unskilled laborers, 48 percent were skilled laborers or shop clerks, and 34 percent were proprietors and professionals.[23]

In all these respects – class, marital status, age, and sex – the social variability of the lunatic patients made their disposition within the hospital exceedingly complex. Eighteenth-century notions of propriety and deference made it seem desirable to separate the various ranks of patients, that is, rich from poor, male from female, old from young; yet the original building plan, which provided only the basement cells and a few large upstairs rooms for the insane, made such separation difficult. Probably the single most important factor precipitating improvements in the hospital accommodations was the wealthier patrons' requests for more spacious private rooms. Families who were willing to pay for better accommodations to ensure a relative's "ease and comfort," as one man expressed it, provided an important incentive for growth.[24]

The steadily increasing demand for institutional care, coupled with the accumulation of chronic cases, prompted the first major expansion of the Pennsylvania Hospital's facilities for the Insane in the 1790s. During the preceding decade, overcrowding had become a critical problem within the institution. Two, sometimes three, lunatics had to be housed in every cell and quiet cases placed on the sick wards, measures the managers felt to be so "improper and unsafe" that they could not be continued for long. In addition, the noise emanating from the crowded lower-story cells continually disturbed the sick patients living above them.[25] To rectify these problems of institutional discipline, the managers decided to raise money for an entirely new wing, to be used solely by the lunatics. The "new house" or "West Wing," begun in 1792 and completed in 1796, on the hospital lot due west of the original building, could house eighty patients in varied accommodations. Although the two hospital wings or "departments," as they began to be called, were eventually linked by a connecting building, sick and insane were effectively separated under the new plan. In effect, the West Wing constituted the Pennsylvania Hospital's first asylum and became the prototype of the nineteenth-century Philadelphia Hospital for the Insane.[26]

The opening of the new house was but one aspect of a broader program of change carried out by the hospital's personnel. Hoping to increase cure rates and thereby lessen the chronic patients' steady drain on the hospital's treasury, the managers proved receptive to new forms of medical treatment for the lunatics. Benjamin Rush was certainly the most influential if not the only physician to introduce innovations in the institution's medical regimen.[27] Attempting to regulate the disordered blood circulation that he felt caused derangement, Rush experimented with alternating hot and cold shower baths; a "gyrator," which spun the patient around on a board to increase the pulse; and a tranquilizer chair, which bound the lunatic at the head and limbs to reduce the blood flow to the brain. For recent or violent cases, Rush devised a regimen of bleeding, purging, and blistering that quickly reduced the patient to a weakened, and therefore more manageable, state. "Heroic treatment," as his therapeutic combination came to be known, remained standard practice at the hospital well into the 1830s.[28]

The hospital physicians and officers also practiced a psychological counterpart to heroic treatment: an effort to frighten, shame, reason, or divert the lunatics into more rational behavior. Accounts of the hospital from this time period describe many dramatic confrontations between the patients and their keepers. To give one example, Benjamin Rush recorded Steward Francis Higgins's methods used with a woman named Sarah, whose "profane and indecent conversation and loud vociferations" had offended and disturbed the whole institution. At first, Higgins attempted to silence Sarah by "light punishments and threats," but having no success, he placed her in a tub and told her to prepare for death, saying, "I will give you time enough to say your prayers, after which I intend to drown you, by plunging your head under this water." Sarah immediately said a prayer "such as became a dying person" and promised to reform. "From that time on," Rush reported, "no profane or indecent language, no noises of any kind, were heard in her cell."[29]

In less dramatic ways, the hospital officers worked to expand the occupations and amusements available for the patients in the West Wing. The new building had dayrooms for the various classes of inmates and a larger, more pleasant crazy yard for their use. Rush and his colleagues tried to implement several schemes to employ the lower-class patients in manual labor, but eventually abandoned them "for want of a system and some additional help and superintendence." The wealthier patients fared better, having a steady supply of books, games, and writing materials with which to amuse themselves. Some patients had flutes, and the women's dayroom had a pianoforte and a "grand harmonium." A velocipede and carriage provided occasional rides for the inmates.[30]

In addition, the managers tried to improve the hospital regimen by providing more and better attendance. Additional male cell keepers and female nurses were hired for the West Wing, and a few "companions" or educated attendants of a "higher grade" occasionally were employed to "superintend the Lunaticks, to walk with them, converse with them, *etc.* in order to awaken their minds." Sensing the need for more uniform, orderly direction of the West Wing, the managers experimented with having one lay officer to oversee its operation. In 1813, they hired a "Director of the Insane Department" and his wife "to manage the said Department in all its branches when it does not interfere with the general superintendence of the Steward." Evidently the couple did not suit, for they left after a year's service. A "Matron of the Insane," Alice Harlan, who served from 1821 to 1829, had more success in unifying the administration of the West Wing. But when Harlan retired, the managers abolished her position, noting that "experience had shown that the powers and responsibilities of Steward and Matron should devolve upon those officers exclusively as heads of this institution." Thereafter, the hospital matron, who was usually the steward's wife, supervised the insane division under his direction.[31]

As a result of these varied improvements, the institutional milieu of the West Wing was considerably more genteel than the atmosphere of the old hospital. Removed from the old basement cells to more hotel-like accommodations, the insane, not surprisingly, seemed less fearsome. Playing on the harpsicord or working at their crafts, they hardly recalled the wild beasts of Rush's generation. Perhaps in response to their more civilized surroundings, the patients did indeed become less outrageous in behavior. Whether the reality or simply the perception of the patients changed, the image of the furious, fierce, and dangerous madman so prominent in early hospital folklore gradually gave way to a more romantic vision of the insane as victims of human passion and frailty.

Nowhere is the romantic character insanity began to assume in the early nineteenth century better illustrated than in a little notebook kept by Manager Samuel Coates, recording the life histories and interesting traits of some forty inmates he had known in his long service at the Pennsylvania Hospital. Although Coates's account contained elements of the older, more ferocious view of madmen, he gave much more pronounced emphasis to their human qualities. In the process of recording the lunatics' tragic life stories, literary accomplishments, and shrewd sayings, the manager made them appear sympathetic and intriguing characters. Moreover, his anecdotes attest to the lively institutional culture nurtured in the West Wing. Not all the patients simply sat in their rooms; some gave sermons, others wrote poems, and many developed strong attachments to those around them. Although deprived of their reason, Coates's lunatics still possessed thoroughly human talents and emotions.[32]

Thus, a domestication of asylum treatment at the Pennsylvania Hospital was well underway by the 1820s. Pressures on the institution's resources encouraged the managers and physicians to introduce new measures designed to improve the cure rate and more effectively control the patients. In the process, the concept of therapeutic confinement that shaped the hospital's original provisions for the insane took on a different meaning. Active medical therapeutics, psychological treatment, and manipulation of the hospital milieu all became integral parts of the medical rationale for institutional care. In adopting these measures, the hospital's officers had been convinced not only of the greater humanity but also the therapeutic superiority of this course of treatment.

Their confidence was not necessarily based on statistical evidence of success. From 1790 to 1830, the hospital's cure rate remained at around 17 percent and its rate of improvement 12 percent.[33] Thus, slightly less than one-third of the patients responded favorably to hospital care. Yet, although hardly overwhelming, at the time these statistics were cause for optimism rather than disillusionment, in light of the still common feeling that insanity could not be cured at all. The hospital officers reasoned that only recent cases could be cured quickly; because most of the inmates had long-standing mental disorders, they could hardly be expected to respond to the new treatments. Perhaps the most dramatic support for the belief in the hospital regimen came from the demonstrable effect of heroic measures on maniacal patients. The power of certain therapies, particularly bleeding and purging, to bring an uncontrollably violent individual into a weakened and therefore manageable state confirmed the officers' belief in the value of medical treatment. Although the resultant change might only be temporary, it still offered proof that medical therapeutics could alter behavior in significant ways.

In a more subtle sense, the lively patient society of the West

Wing must daily have reinforced the officers' conviction that hospital treatment represented a superior mode of managing the insane. Despite the suffering that was an unavoidable aspect of madness, patients still could be made to conform to certain expectations of sane behavior. When given the opportunity by indulgent managers and physicians, the lunatics created a remarkably vigorous community of their own, as Coates's accounts of his poetry-writing, sermon-giving inmates demonstrated. To maintain an institution in which even incurable lunatics could make the most of their human qualities provided justification enough for the hospital officers' labor.

The officers' commitment to the new therapeutic regimen that had gradually evolved at the Pennsylvania Hospital eventually led to their decision to build a separate asylum. As in the 1780s, an internal crisis prompted expansion of the institution's facilities for the insane. Despite repeated efforts to improve the hospital's accommodations, recurrent problems of overcrowding and lack of privacy once again threatened to jeopardize its efficacy. Increasingly, it appeared that only a new location and building could preserve the ideals of treatment to which the officers had become devoted.

By the late 1820s, overcrowding again strained the Pennsylvania Hospital's resources. Even with a new "lodge" for the wealthier female patients built in 1825, and reappropriation of the twelve cells in the basement of the East Wing, the hospital still had insufficient housing for the insane. More than one hundred patients and their attendants were crammed into a building designed to hold at most eighty. The small site occupied by the West Wing intensified problems caused by overcrowding. The building and exercise grounds covered less than three-quarters of an acre. In this confined space, the noise made by the violently insane disturbed not only the West Wing but the homes adjacent to the hospital as well. Overcrowding also diminished the advances made in the patients' regimen. "Is classification desirable?" asked William Malin, the hospital clerk and an outspoken advocate of asylum reform. "How can it be effected while more than one hundred persons of both sexes and every grade of insanity are crowded into the West Wing?"[34]

The hospital's accessibility to the public further exacerbated the difficulties caused by overcrowding. Despite the officers' repeated efforts to discourage visitors, the West Wing remained a "convenient lounge for idlers" who regarded its inmates as a form of public entertainment. Even members of the city's best families routinely included visits to the Pennsylvania Hospital (which one lady described as "chiefly inhabited by lunatics") on the agenda of fashionable amusements. Ignoring signs asking them to stay out of the West Wing and prying open the "venetian" doors installed to provide privacy for its hallways, visitors plagued the patients constantly. Nothing deterred the curious, an indignant Malin complained to the managers. "The morbid curiosity displayed by a majority of the visitors to the Hospital is astonishing, and their pertinacity in attempting, and fertility in pretexts and expedients, to gain admission to the 'mad people' is not less so," he wrote. "Even females who have tears to bestow on tales of imaginary distress, are importunate to see a raving madman, and do not hesitate to wound the diseased mind by the gaze of idle curiosity, by impertinent questions, and thoughtless remarks," Malin concluded.[35]

Under such conditions, medical supervision of a large and diverse group of lunatic patients was exceedingly difficult. To make their medical regimen more systematic, the resident physicians suggested in 1828 that one doctor be appointed to attend the insane. A unified system of medical attendance would be "of great benefit to the patients," they felt: A resident having exclusive care of the lunatics would be "better qualified to give that information to the attending physician that would enable him to direct the best medical and moral treatment." The resident physicians' letter concluded, "if these duties are properly performed, they will consume so much time, that none will be spared for other business." The residents may also have realized that a medical officer might avoid the conflict with the steward that had undermined the manager's previous experiments with lay directors of the insane department. Although their advice was not immediately heeded, it contributed to the growing dissatisfaction with the existing arrangements for the insane.[36]

In a letter to the managers written in 1828 and later published as a pamphlet, William Malin summed up the arguments for a new asylum. None of the recurring difficulties caused by overcrowding, public location, and insufficient supervision could be solved in the hospital's present location, he wrote; the "disadvantages... connected with the public situation and contracted space" of the hospital were ones "which no system of management may hope to obviate, and which preclude the possibility of keeping up a salutary discipline." In contrast, a new asylum located a few miles out of the city would automatically provide adequate isolation, ample room for new buildings and recreation areas, and the disciplinary benefits of a unified management. Such a separate mental hospital, "situated in a large open space, united the advantages of a country atmosphere with the peculiar conveniences of the city," wrote Malin. In summing up, he invoked his most persuasive argument: that the new location would improve the cure rate. "The founders of existing asylums for those afflicted with mental maladies do not appear to have been sufficiently impressed with the importance of providing for their *cure*," he wrote; their aim was rather "to *secure*" the patients. Yet "a review of the errors of their predecessors and contemporaries" would soon convince the managers that "an asylum for the *cure* of insanity" could be built, "an asylum which shall prove a lasting monument of their wisdom, benevolence, and public spirit."[37]

Malin's appeal to the managers' wisdom did not immediately succeed, for the financing and organizing of a whole new hospital less than forty years after construction of the West Wing seemed a prohibitive task. But eventually, in 1831, the managers resolved to build a separate asylum for the insane, "with ample space for their proper seclusion, classification and employment." At first, they wanted to construct the new building on a nearby lot that the hospital already owned, fearing that an asylum located any distance from the parent institution could not be properly supervised. But the contributors and physicians objected to such a plan, agitating instead for a location outside the city. In 1835, the managers abandoned the idea of a city asylum and appointed a subcommittee to find a rural site for the new institution. The next year, the managers purchased an 111-acre farm in West Philadelphia, four miles west of the old hospital and about two miles outside the city limits, near the village of Blockley.[38]

Significantly, although Malin and other supporters of the new asylum plan must have read about William Tuke's Retreat and Philippe Pinel's work at the Paris hospitals, their appeals for change never mentioned them. They looked no further than "a review of the errors of their predecessors," as Malin put it, to convince the managers of the need for change. Their interest in asylum reform apparently stemmed from concern over internal institutional problems, not admiration of foreign precedents. Thus, the adoption of moral treatment at the Pennsylvania Hospital must be viewed more as a response to institutional experience than as an emulation of European innovation.

In light of this orientation, the similarities between the regimen that evolved at the Pennsylvania Hospital and the reforms associated with Pinel and Tuke are indeed striking. As early as the 1790s, well before the managers and physicians of this provincial hospital could have been familiar with European developments, they had begun to experiment with the basic features of moral treatment: psychological manipulation, separation and classification, amusements and employments. To be sure, American developments differed from the European movement in important respects. The Americans remained more reliant on active medical therapeutics, such as bleeding and purging, and countenanced more physical restraint of the insane, differences in approach that persisted in Kirkbride's generation of asylum doctors. But in all other respects, the transatlantic development of moral treatment was remarkably parallel.[39]

These similarities no doubt reflect the basic cultural heritage shared by the Western European societies. The Enlightenment, the development of Quaker humanitarianism, and the rise of bourgeois society have all been invoked as explanations for the simultaneous appearance of these reforms. But their growth might as well – and more concretely – be explained in terms of the common institutional forms shared by Americans and Europeans. The Pennsylvania Hospital's founders modeled their establishments on the eighteenth-century English hospitals with which they were familiar. In succeeding years, their treatment of the insane followed parallel, if not identical, lines. In England, as well as in France and Italy, conditions of overcrowding and neglect of the insane in general hospitals and private madhouses produced asylum reform movements. At the Pennsylvania Hospital, Americans experiencing similar difficulties evolved similar solutions. The common pattern of problems and solutions was rooted in the shared institutional structure of European and American hospitals.[40]

At another level, the Pennsylvania Hospital's history suggests the importance of institutional factors in the evolution of a new medical rationale for treating insanity. In the founders' estimation, the Pennsylvania Hospital provided a superior form of confinement to the almshouse. Initially, this confinement consisted primarily of cells and chains, only slightly tempered by Quaker humanitarianism. But the necessity of controlling an ever-increasing, more diverse patient population forced the hospital's managers and physicians to expand and elaborate their concept of therapeutic confinement. Experimenting with new medical and moral means to control and improve the inmates' behavior, they found ample evidence to confirm the conviction that hospital treatment was indeed effective. The power of heroic treatment to modify, if only temporarily, the violence of a maniac; the usefulness of psychological techniques when employed by authoritative individuals such as the doctors, managers, and stewards; the richness of the patient culture sustained by a sympathetic milieu; and even the value of a good building design – all these developments seemed to justify hospital care. The hospital's original concept of therapeutic confinement had broadened into a larger vision of the physician and hospital as uniquely equipped to control disruptive behavior and effect personality change through medical intervention. The history of the old Pennsylvania Hospital illustrates, in microcosm, the forces that converged to create the distinctive form and spirit of the nineteenth-century insane asylum.

THE ASYLUM AND ANTEBELLUM SOCIETY

In appearance and organization, the Pennsylvania Hospital for the Insane that opened early in 1841 was markedly different from the eighteenth-century general hospital. In place of a loosely structured, casually regulated institution treating all forms of illness stood a hospital specially designed to provide intense, regimented treatment for one disease, insanity. Situated about two miles outside of the city limits, the new hospital possessed a degree of seclusion impossible to obtain in the old building, while being a convenient distance from the city. The 100 acres of land surrounding the asylum's site ensured ample grounds for the exercise and employment of its inmates. The building designed by architect Isaac Holden, which provided a central section with two wings, could accommodate 160 patients, all properly separated and classified. Most important, the new hospital's administrative plan called for one medical officer to be its head, rather than relying on a rotating staff of visiting physicians; the asylum superintendent was expected to live on the hospital grounds and devote himself entirely to asylum practice. Under the exclusive control of one doctor, the asylum promised to offer a more consistent, ordered regimen than had been possible in the old hospital.

But for all its newness and grandeur, the Pennsylvania Hospital for the Insane represented no sharp break with the past, but only an elaboration and amplification of the eighteenth-century hospital's Enlightenment rationale. William Malin might accuse his predecessors of seeking to secure rather than cure the insane in order to dramatize his cause, but in fact, his aims and theirs were almost identical. Eighteenth- and nineteenth-century reformers had the same basic goals: to protect the family and the community by confining the insane, while at the same time attempting to cure them. Both generations of hospital advocates believed in the therapeutic power of institutional design and milieu to modify insanity's symptoms, and stressed improved classification and amusements as a means to that end. In sum, the innovations associated with the nineteenth-century asylum movement represented changes in *degree* rather than *kind;* the distinctive features of the new asylum were but the working out, on a larger and grander scale, of the founder's Enlightenment conceptions of insanity and its proper treatment.

While recognizing the underlying continuity between the new asylum and its eighteenth-century predecessor, we must not lose sight of their differences. In spite of the organizational and ideological elements they shared, the two institutions operated in very dissimilar social contexts, which could not help but influence their operation in manifold ways. Basic aims and structures persisted, but their expression changed to suit the time. These changing institutional fashions reflect the large forces transforming American society during the early national period.

The primary agency of change was the massive economic and demographic transformation that took place between 1790 and 1840.[41] During these decades, population growth and improved transportation fostered an increasingly specialized national economy in which western grain and lumber and southern cotton were traded for Northern manufactured products. Steadily growing demand for foodstuffs and household goods encouraged technological innovations such as the cast iron plow, the automatic flour mill, the cotton gin, and the power loom, which made production more efficient, thereby lowering prices and creating more demand for products. The rapidly expanding urban centers that provided the financial and marketing services needed to transact transcontinental commerce grew at a phenomenal rate; in 1840, Philadelphia had a population of 220,000, ten times its size at the time of the American Revolution. Through the cities flowed a population constantly on the move: settlers heading west to claim cheap homesteads, immigrants hoping to find new opportunities in a foreign land, and farmers' sons and daughters attempting to make a living as clerks and teachers. Although migration had always been an integral aspect of American life, the volume of the population movement reached unprecedented levels in the early nineteenth century.

The expansiveness of American economic and social life during the early national period brought to fruition the leveling tendencies inherent in the American Revolution. With the extension of white male suffrage, eighteenth-century politics of deference gradually gave way to the boisterous new politics of the common man. Amid huge election parades, rallies, and riots, increasing numbers of voters cast their ballots in the state and national elections. In analogous fashion, the post-Revolutionary disestablishment of state churches ushered in a new era of denominational competition, and the Second Great Awakening extended a new spiritual franchise to all Americans. Rejecting the old Calvinist doctrines of limited salvation and innate human depravity, revivalists such as Charles Grandison Finney preached about the availability of God's grace to all who sought it. Reformers embued with the belief that individual transformation could produce a heaven on earth formed voluntary associations to attack such long-established social evils as slavery, prostitution, and drunkenness. In its own distinctive fashion, Jacksonian perfectionism carried Enlightenment faith in human progress to its logical, if extreme, conclusion.

Although egalitarianism and perfectionism became its touchstones, Jacksonian social philosophy seemingly overlooked certain increasingly salient consequences of economic and social change. The advance of commercial capitalism may have created more economic opportunity, but it hardly obliterated class distinctions or inequalities of wealth. In fact, the social distance between the rich and poor steadily widened, as graphically illustrated by new patterns of residential segregation in large cities such as Philadelphia. Yet for most citizens, the seeming fluidity of American society, the greater ease with which one might go up and down the social ladder, at least as compared with the eighteenth century, justified the inequalities that resulted. As Stephen Thernstrom has argued convincingly, nineteenth-century Americans believed that equality of *opportunity*, that is, access to economic, political, or religious institutions, rather than equality of *condition*, ensured the fairness of their social institutions.[42]

The scope and intensity of early nineteenth-century economic and social change could not help but leave its mark on institutional forms. Like the economy and society in which they functioned, nineteenth-century institutions became much more highly specialized and strictly organized than their predecessors. The pressures created by expanding numbers of the poor and disorderly elicited similar responses from officials in charge of almshouses, jails, and hospitals. As their institutions grew larger, they simply had to become more concerned with regimentation. Separation and classification of inmates, development of more rigid, all-encompassing regimens, specialization and expansion of staff, and isolation from the disruptive intrusion of visitors were all useful strategies in controlling large inmate populations. Thus, the mental hospital resembled other institutions that were forced in the early nineteenth century to develop new strategies for managing their diverse and disorderly inmates.[43]

But the similarities among nineteenth-century institutions such as the penitentiary, public school, and asylum reflected more than shared internal dynamics. Their institutional economics also reflected the broader cultural trends of their time. Could we but set the colonial Pennsylvania Hospital alongside its asylum progeny, the changes wrought by a century of economic and social development would be strikingly apparent.

In the first place, the Pennsylvania Hospital for the Insane existed in a far wealthier society than had its eighteenth-century predecessor. By the late 1830s, the growth of commercial capitalism had produced an unprecedented level of material ease and abundance. As the mill, forge, and loom were transforming the interior of the American household, so too did economic development leave its mark on the new asylum. Although still far from sumptuous in its appointments, it could approximate a homelike comfort unimaginable in the old colonial institution. The quality and abundance of furnishings, the convenience of indoor plumbing and forced-air ventilation, and even the ornamental use of cast-iron fixtures were made possible by nineteenth-century technological innovation and mass production. For all its bucolic setting, the new hospital's physical properties were very much the product of the nascent industrial revolution.

Prosperity also underwrote a broadening of the asylum's clientele. The original general hospital had been financed by the city's mercantile elite to serve only the deserving poor. But soon after it opened, the hospital managers discovered that its specialized facilities for the insane, unlike its wards for the sick, could attract a steady paying clientele. As mentioned earlier in the chapter, the increasing demand for asylum treatment among those classes able to pay for it proved a significant factor in the managers' decision to expand the institution. Rather than serve any one class, the new hospital was explicitly organized to serve the needs of a broad-based clientele. The assumption that asylum treatment for insanity was no longer a charity the rich provided the poor, but rather a medical service any member of society might purchase, reflected a larger reorientation of nineteenth-century social relationships. Like the society that supported it, the asylum was classless, not because it ignored class distinctions but because its wards were open, at least theoretically, to all who could afford them.

The role in the asylum movement played by individuals such as William Malin and, later, Thomas Story Kirkbride, who both moved from modest rural backgrounds into the rapidly expanding urban professional classes, points to another significant dimension of institutional change. In the mid-eighteenth century, philanthropy had largely been the province of wealthy merchants, who founded charities such as the Pennsylvania Hospital to preserve a properly deferential relationship between themselves and the worthy poor and otherwise to advance their position in society. In contrast, the nineteenth-century asylum movement was dominated by the new urban middle classes who found in reform a satisfying way to order not only the new social environment they lived in but also their own lives. Although concerned in a general sense with uplifting the poor, the new reformers expressed an equally if not more compelling concern with individual improvement and the moral order of the family. They believed that in a rapidly changing society, the reformation of the individual, rather than the preservation of hierarchical class relationships, was the most direct way to ensure social improvement and social order.[44]

The broadening of the asylum's appeal to both reformers and patrons was paralleled by a new intensity in its aims and methods. Jacksonian reform recognized no social problem as insoluble, no matter how well entrenched it might appear, and insanity was no exception. As befit the optimism of the era, the asylum's advocates created a "cult of curability," a conviction that insanity would quickly yield to proper treatment.[45] Naturally, this ambitious outlook engendered a far more intensive regimen than had prevailed in the colonial general hospital. Physicians and lay reformers alike believed the transformation of individual patients could be achieved only by an all-encompassing, intrusive program of treatment. And although those involved in asylum reform as a rule had little sympathy with "enthusiastic" or revival religion, which they believed often caused madness, their notions of a cure bore a marked resemblance to the process of conversion, as we shall see in a later chapter. In both the religious and medical processes, guilt, emulation, and incentives to self-control were used to reshape individual behavior. By such measures, reformers expected the asylum virtually to eliminate insanity, a claim far beyond the modest expectations of Rush's generation.

It was within this context of attitudes and expectations that Thomas Story Kirkbride took charge of the Pennsylvania Hospital for the Insane in 1841. Over the next forty years, his mental hospital continued to reflect larger social concerns with class and social order, particularly the need to reconcile class distinctions with an egalitarian social philosophy, and the reliance on individual uplift and emulation to eliminate deviant behavior. The specific connections between asylum and society developing in the decades between 1840 and 1880, particularly the role of the family in the commitment procedure, will be explored in more detail in subsequent chapters.

But before we can understand the asylum's social function, we must first delineate its medical rationale. Throughout these decades of change, the asylum was perceived and operated first and foremost as a *medical* institution. Alone among the specialized facilities that developed in the early nineteenth century, it was an exclusively medical jurisdiction. Thus, in the asylum's operation, broader cultural concerns with individual reformation and social uplift were expressed and legitimated within a framework of medical concepts and authority; hospital design, administration, and therapeutics united both medical and social imperatives. To explore more fully the social functions Kirkbride's new hospital would assume, then, we must first understand its medical foundation. For it was in the familiar language of health and disease that the doctor and patron determined the hospital's proper role in their society. Using Kirkbride's professional biography as a focus, the next chapter explores the general nature of nineteenth-century medical authority and examines the specific medical concepts that early asylum doctors developed to explain insanity and its treatment to their lay clientele.

2

Christian and physician

Upon completion of their new asylum building in the fall of 1840, the Pennsylvania Hospital managers had to make their final and most important decision concerning its future: the choice of the asylum superintendent, the physician who would have complete control over every aspect of its operation. As the managers well knew, the superintendent's competence would determine both the financial and therapeutic success of the institution. Naturally wanting the best man they could obtain, the managers tried first to hire Samuel Woodward, the distinguished head of the Worcester State Hospital. When the eminent Woodward declined, they began to consider younger, less well-established candidates. In October 1840, they decided upon Thomas Story Kirkbride, a former resident at the Eighth Street hospital, who possessed a modest local reputation and some prior institutional experience in treating the insane.[1]

For the thirty-one-year-old Kirkbride, the decision to accept the managers' offer was also a weighty one. Describing it later as "a post for which I had felt little anxiety, and to attain which I had taken little pains," the young Quaker physician was reluctant to abandon his plans to specialize in surgery, a field in which he had already displayed considerable talent. For years Kirkbride had worked toward the goal of becoming an attending surgeon at the Eighth Street hospital, an ambition he soon seemed likely to realize, only to have another, quite different institutional opportunity come his way. Finally, after long deliberation, the young physician decided to accept the asylum position. For both himself and the managers, it turned out to be a fortunate choice. Thomas Story Kirkbride went on to serve for forty-three years as the hospital's chief physician and achieved national eminence within the specialty of asylum medicine. His personality left such an indelible imprint upon the institution he headed that for years after his death it was still known to many as "Kirkbride's" rather than as the Pennsylvania Hospital for the Insane.[2]

This fusion of institutional and individual identities reflected not only Kirkbride's force of personality but also the larger role the medical profession played in legitimating the early mental hospital. Despite the fierce medical competition and strong antiauthoritarian sentiment of the day, doctors acquired sole jurisdiction over this large and costly new medical establishment. They used their institutional supremacy as chief physicians to mold the asylum in their own image so that it embodied their particular scientific and moral principles. From their institutional stronghold, the asylum superintendents set about building public support for their new specialty and the innovative medical services it offered.

The superintendents' success as "moral entrepreneurs" depended partly upon the unusual strains insanity placed upon the tradition of home medical care, a situation that will be examined in the following chapter, and partly upon the personal and professional attributes that they brought to their work, the subject of this chapter.[3] To understand how physicians such as Kirkbride came to wield an uncommon degree of power both within the asylum and the larger society, we must consider several factors: their personal backgrounds, the general respect physicians commanded in the mid-nineteenth century, and the specific concepts of insanity that asylum doctors devised to justify its treatment to their lay clientele. Kirkbride's biography nicely illustrates the personal and professional qualities that combined to give the asylum superintendents their unusual position of authority. By examining his family background and medical training, we will better understand not only the persona of a major actor in this particular asylum drama (to unfold in later chapters) but also the formation of a new medical specialty.

THE MAKING OF AN ASYLUM SUPERINTENDENT

Like the overwhelming majority of early-nineteenth-century Americans, Thomas Story Kirkbride came from a rural background. He was born on July 31, 1809, in a stone house built by his father on a 150-acre farm in eastern Bucks County, Pennsylvania, just above the town of Morrisville. Thomas was the first of seven children, two sons and five daughters (only five of whom lived to adulthood), born to John and Elizabeth Story Kirkbride. The elder Kirkbride was a prosperous farmer who cultivated fruit trees and raised livestock for the local market. He also operated a small plaster mill on the farm and ran a ferry from a landing on his property, which fronted on the Delaware River, across to Trenton and Bordentown, New Jersey.[4]

Although at an early age Kirkbride decided (with his father's blessing) not to take over the family farm, he still acquired a knowledge of agriculture and love of improvements from his father that would prove immensely useful in asylum management. More importantly, the demeanor of a country boy – an observer once described him as a good-natured "farm product" – undoubtedly gave Kirkbride a rapport with the many asylum patrons and patients who also came from rural families. The traditional agrarian virtues of hard work, pragmatism, and moderation in living that they all shared became an integral part of his conception of asylum treatment.[5]

Another significant element in Kirkbride's personal history was his religious upbringing. He was descended from a very old and distinguished Bucks County Quaker family. His first American ancestor, Joseph Kirkbride, came to the colony in 1682 as a member of William Penn's original plantation. Arriving as a runaway apprentice with only a bundle of clothes and a flail, Kirkbride's great-great-grandfather Joseph went on to become a prominent merchant, assemblyman, and leader in the Bucks County Society of Friends. Kirkbride's paternal grandparents carried on the family's Quaker tradition in a more modest fashion. As a youth, Jonathan Kirkbride distinguished himself by a "gift of ministry" that his coreligionists felt bore unmistakable "evidences of divine origin." Although too "delicate" to do heavy farm labor, he possessed strength enough to travel about the countryside preaching at Friends' meetings. His wife Elizabeth, a "meek-spirited" woman as befitted such a husband, also served the Society throughout her long life as an elder, overseer, and clerk of the Women's Monthly Meeting.[6]

Although Jonathan and Elizabeth's son John, Kirkbride's father, did not show any special talent for the ministry, he did maintain the family religious tradition in his own household. As the Society's discipline required, young Thomas received his early education in "guarded" or religious schools run by Friends in Morrisville and Fallsington. Besides attending the Falls Monthly Meeting in Fallsington, the Kirkbrides worshipped with other families in their neighborhood during the intervening weeks.[7]

Shortly before Kirkbride left home to pursue his medical education, the closely knit religious community he had known as a child was rent by controversy. Between 1819 and 1827, the Philadelphia Yearly Meeting had become increasingly divided over the teachings of Elias Hicks, a minister from Long Island. Hicks believed in equality among all believers to the point of questioning the divinity of Christ, the authority of the Bible, and the concept of the Trinity. The revelations of his own conscience prompted Hicks to call on all Friends to withdraw from worldly affairs, including scientific and intellectual pursuits, participation in organizations that had non-Friends as members, and any activity that even remotely benefited southern slavery. Since a great many Friends participated in just such worldly matters, Hicks's denunciations created bitter controversies within the Society. The Philadelphia Yearly Meeting became so badly divided over his testimony that in 1827 it split into two factions, Orthodox and Hicksite.

Although many rural Friends became Hicksites, the Kirkbride family, including Thomas, joined the Orthodox Meeting, a preference that suggests the conservative nature of their religious views. The Orthodox faction, which was heavily influenced by Anglicanism and Methodism, developed the churchlike as opposed to the sectlike tendencies of Quakerism. Rejecting the Hicksite doctrine as tantamount to Unitarian heresy, they stressed right belief, especially the doctrine of Christ's redemptive power and the divine inspiration of the Bible, as the basis for church membership. Orthodox Friends tended to leave doctrinal disputes for the church elders to decide, and accepted the premise that worldly success was closely correlated with a capacity for spiritual leadership. On the whole a wealthier and more urbanized group than the Hicksites, the Orthodox Friends contemplated modern society and secular affairs with less trepidation than did the more Antinomian members of the society.[8]

Kirkbride's youthful affiliation with the Orthodox Meeting anticipated the restrained bent his religious faith would take in later years. Throughout his life, he adhered to certain distinctive features of the Society's discipline, eschewing public display, wearing simple clothing, and maintaining a "detachment from the world."[9] Yet, his religious observances remained very unobtrusive. Kirkbride had no sympathy with the radical, separatist tendencies that had always been inherent in the Society's doctrine. By joining the Orthodox Meeting, Kirkbride reconciled his religious principles with full participation in the secular world, including a career in medicine.

In retrospect, it was a wise choice for a future asylum superintendent. At the time Kirkbride entered the specialty of asylum medicine, the interdenominational rivalry generated by antebellum revivalism had made churchgoers and nonbelievers alike wary of sectarianism in public office; they feared any use of public power to advance the cause of a particular denomination. In addition, some observers believed that revivalism had contributed to a rise in insanity, and the fact that the insane often had religious delusions lent credence to this supposition. Thus, for various reasons, an evangelical Christian would have been considered a highly unsuitable choice for asylum work. On the other hand, the majority of citizens respected piety and probably would not have accepted an avowed atheist for a physician; they preferred him to be both a devout and learned man.[10]

Kirkbride's image as both a "Christian and Physician," to use one patron's phrase, allowed him to satisfy his clientele on both counts.[11] His conservative Quakerism marked him as a devoted Christian, yet one who eschewed the potentially divisive and destabilizing forces of enthusiasm and had no religious designs on his charges. Such a steady and emotionally predictable faith made an Orthodox Friend a particularly appealing counselor in an age of religious unrest. At the same time, as we shall see later, Kirkbride's religious background equipped him with some basic techniques of personality transformation, that is, reflection, repentance, and submission to a higher authority, that he would use to "convert" his patients to sanity.

The Society of Friends had always regarded medicine as a suitable profession for its members, so a youth such as Thomas Story Kirkbride, who by his own account had a "naturally delicate constitution" unsuitable for farming, would naturally consider it as an occupation. Kirkbride's father particularly wanted his eldest son to become a doctor after a serious and painful illness left him with a new appreciation of medicine's value. According to Kirkbride, upon his recovery, his father decided that "if his son ever manifested any taste for the profession he should study medicine and from that time he left nothing undone that he thought likely to advance that object." So as a boy, Kirkbride "began to regard medicine as his path in life."[12]

In preparation for a medical career, John Kirkbride provided his son with what was for that time a very thorough and expensive secondary education. First, Thomas attended a Trenton school run by the Reverend Jared Fyler, a Presbyterian minister, where he spent four years in classical studies; then he took an additional year at John Gummere's boarding school in Burlington, to complete a course in higher mathematics, primarily algebra. Both schools had excellent local reputations and attracted many affluent students. In particular, Gummere's school had a number of West Indian planters' sons, with whom Kirkbride formed several boyhood friendships; this early social experience probably contributed to his later success with southern planters, who patronized his asylum in large numbers.[13]

Upon finishing his secondary education, Kirkbride was ready to begin his medical training. In his time, it should be noted, entry into the medical profession required no formal schooling at all, much less an academy education of the quality Kirkbride had received. Most doctors possessed only a common school education. So, although he did not attend college, Kirkbride was among the best-educated doctors of his day. In the 1820s, only a tiny minority of his male peers went on to obtain a college degree.[14]

Kirkbride began his medical career at a particularly turbulent period in the profession's development. The same economic and social forces that made politics and religion so competitive and faction-ridden in the 1820s and 1830s also affected medicine. Increasing cultural and ethnic diversity, rising expectations of health, and a general antiauthoritarian spirit combined to make medical careers in the Jacksonian era somewhat more precarious than they had been in previous decades. Yet, regular physicians with a certain kind of education and social background continued to maintain their credibility among large segments of American society. To plumb this reservoir of respect for the medical profession, which Kirkbride would draw upon, first as a general practitioner and later as an asylum doctor, we must pause briefly in recounting his professional biography to survey the popular attitudes toward health, disease, and doctors that would shape his career as an antebellum medical man.

Popular health and medicine in the antebellum period

In most respects, nineteenth-century Americans had reason to consider themselves a particularly healthy people. Theirs was, on the whole, a benign climate and an abundant land. Although enjoying the affluence generated by an increasingly diversified economy, most Americans (nearly 90 percent in 1820) still lived on farms, safe from the health hazards of city living. A vastly improved transportation system made it possible to distribute the material benefits of economic growth to even the most isolated frontier communities. Improved housing, new forms of consumer goods, and a more varied diet gave the average citizen of the early nineteenth century an unprecedentedly high standard of living.[15]

Yet, the new prosperity had its costs, especially for the health of the nation's city dwellers. Population concentration and improved transportation increased the circulation not only of trade goods but also of epidemic diseases such as cholera. Crowded, unsanitary urban living conditions bred endemic contagious diseases, including typhoid fever and tuberculosis. Changing social mores, particularly the growing sexual commerce of prostitution, facilitated the spread of venereal infections. In addition, the sedentary habits, rich diet, and availability of stimulants accompanying the new affluence increased a number of minor but still uncomfortable ailments such as dyspepsia, constipation, and "nervousness." The frequent uproars occasioned by economic speculation, popular politics, and religious revivalism further strained the mental and physical well-being of the citizenry. Although by no means absent from rural areas, these unsalubrious aspects of change worked with particular force on town and city residents, and large urban centers such as Philadelphia were regarded as particularly unhealthy.[16]

In response to the dangerous aspects of their changing physical and social environment, Americans took a fervent interest in their health. Of course, the desire to stay well, or, failing that, to relieve injury and disease as quickly and painlessly as possible, was hardly a novel aspiration. Nineteenth-century Americans were the heirs of a long tradition of popular concern with personal hygiene and domestic medicine; the Jacksonian interest in popular health was but a variation on an ancient preoccupation with individual health and morality. Still, if one compares late eighteenth and early nineteenth century popular health manuals with older texts, it is evident that the quest for health in the new republic gradually attained a distinctive flavor of its own.[17]

In an era of heightened individualism and social opportunity, personal responsibility for one's health took on added rhetorical urgency. Observers noted that the competitive pace of modern life was more than enough to make one sick, thus necessitating ever more exacting precautions concerning one's health. Authors of health manuals frequently pointed out that physical vitality was a crucial prerequisite for getting ahead; as a man's position in life increasingly came to depend (at least theoretically) upon his own talents, it was all the more important that he be vigorous in order to succeed. Women, although disqualified by their sex from the same competition, had to be careful of their health in order to be the good wives and mothers the upwardly mobile men of the republic needed. For both sexes, personal responsibility for health became bound up with other contemporary efforts to maintain order and cohesion in a fluid society. Regulating the bodily functions served as an immediate and satisfying way to respond to a rapidly changing social environment. Thus, Jacksonian reformers made personal hygiene and morality a major focus of the individual reformation that they sought not only for the disorderly elements of society but also for themselves.[18]

Perhaps the most distinctive aspect of the Jacksonian personal health movement was the breadth and depth of its appeal. The democratization or popularization of health concerns affected all but the poorest classes of society. Americans used their unprecedented degree of affluence and leisure time to pursue physical well-being with a vengeance. Public education, which by the 1820s had made most Americans literate, at least in the North, enabled them to read extensively at the same time that the so-called print revolution began to make books and magazines more affordable; advice books and medical manuals became a bookseller's staple, and health-related articles abounded in the newly popular magazines. With their characteristic fervor for self-improvement, Americans in towns and cities flocked to educational lectures on physiology, anatomy, and the like. Visits to mineral springs and spas became a standard form of vacation for many middle-class families. Again, although more common among affluent city dwellers, these forms of health-seeking behavior appeared among prosperous farmers and artisans as well. Good health, it would seem, had become the aspiration of every American citizen.[19]

Patronage of doctors was an integral aspect of the growing nineteenth-century health consciousness. To advise them on healthful regimens and to treat their illnesses, Americans employed a wide range of healers. But ironically, their increased demand for and expectations of medical care did not necessarily strengthen the regular doctors' professional position. On the contrary, growing dissatisfaction with heroic treatment, that is, bleeding, purging, and the use of mercury, led to the proliferation of medical sects hostile to the medical establishment. Thomsonianism, with its herbal-based system of therapeutics, flourished in the 1820s and 1830s, followed by homeopathy, a German-imported school of medicine employing highly diluted drug mixtures, in the 1840s and 1850s. The sectarians' popularity, combined with the antebellum aversion to centralized authority, led to the repeal of medical licensing laws in many states. Not only did the regular physicians lose what little power they once possessed to restrict their competitors' practice, they also could not control the expansion of their own ranks. The spread of proprietary or commercial medical schools led to the rapid overproduction of undereducated doctors. To a surfeit of regular and sectarian medical men was added a variety of lay healers, including patent medicine salesmen, diet reformers, and hydropaths. So, by the mid-1840s, the medical consumer could choose from a broad range of competing medical outlooks and treatments.[20]

The regular medical establishment loudly bemoaned this state of affairs, claiming that the quacks and crackpots made it impossible for an honest physician to earn a decent living. Yet, their complaints of professional impotence, which continued throughout the century, should not be taken too literally, for the regulars possessed considerable advantages in the competition for patients. They maintained control of most medical schools and hospitals, including the oldest and most prestigious institutions, such as the Pennsylvania Hospital, and within these institutional strongholds gained clinical experience that bolstered their claims to scientific superiority over the "irregulars." More importantly, regular physicians retained much of their traditional clientele in both urban and rural areas and remained important leaders within their communities.[21]

Thus, by pursuing a prescribed course of medical training, Thomas Story Kirkbride acquired a professional identity that still commanded considerable respect in his society. Although somewhat weakened and circumscribed by deregulation and competition, the authority of the regular medical establishment provided Kirkbride's career with a firm foundation. It was a foundation built not so much on the doctor's social class (although that was certainly a factor) as on his ability to conceptualize and treat disease in certain predictable ways. Modern observers often assume that because nineteenth-century therapeutics appear woefully unscientific and ineffective by present-day standards, nineteenth-century patients could have had no real faith in them. Such a historical perspective obscures the way in which traditional medical systems of explanation functioned for doctor and patient. As a young physician, Kirkbride acquired a set of theories and skills that allowed him to treat disease in a manner both reassuring and comprehensible to his lay clientele. To understand the faith patrons came to have in Kirkbride, we must examine these medical concepts and procedures in a nonjudgmental fashion, seeing how they operated in a nineteenth-century, rather than a twentieth-century, context of belief.

*Regular medical education and theory in the
Jacksonian period*

Thomas Story Kirkbride began his medical education, as did most doctors in the early nineteenth century, with an apprenticeship to a physician in private practice. In his generation, such preceptorial tutelage often comprised the whole of a less ambitious doctor's training; he might receive a license to practice after serving an apprenticeship of several years. For a more aspiring young man such as Kirkbride, the preceptorial relationship served only as preparation for a formal medical education. It was customary before entering medical school for a student to spend one or two years reading medicine in the preceptor's office and observing his practice. The apprentice assisted his mentor by compounding pre-scriptions, helping with the office trade, and treating simple cases of injury and illness.[22]

Nicholas Belleville, the man Kirkbride chose as his preceptor, was a French-born Trenton physician with an excellent local reputation. After receiving his medical training in Parisian medical schools and hospitals, Belleville came to America in 1777 to serve as a doctor in the Revolutionary army. He soon found the prospects for an American medical practice more enticing than either army service or a return to France. (According to Kirkbride, Belleville was also such a martyr to sea sickness that he dreaded the voyage back home.) He married a Trenton woman and set up a practice in the city and surrounding countryside. The young Frenchman developed professional and personal ties with Philadelphia's late eighteenth-century medical elite, including Thomas Bond, Benjamin Rush, and Phillip Syng Physick. (It was in a letter to Belleville that Rush first announced his concoction of the famous "ten and ten," a powerful purge of ten grains each of calomel and jalap, for which Rush gained great notoriety.) He played an active role in the Medical Society of New Jersey as well as the district and county medical societies centered in Trenton, and in 1811 and 1812 served as a district and county medical examiner. But the prime of Belleville's career had passed by the time he accepted Kirkbride as his last student. Although, as Kirkbride recalled, "he devoted a large amount of time to my private instruction," the medical approach he offered had become relatively old-fashioned by the late 1820s. Kirkbride's choice of preceptor provides the first clue to the position he would achieve within the Philadelphia medical profession as a conservatively trained, respectable practitioner who was nonetheless not a member of the city's innermost circle of elite physicians.[23]

Despite his age, Belleville gave Kirkbride a thorough grounding in the basics of bedside medicine, which formed the mainstay of nineteenth-century medical practice. To explain disease and its treatment to his pupil, Belleville used the same traditional concepts that physicians had employed for centuries. Disease, according to the prevailing view, was produced by an imbalance of substances within the body, variously conceived of as humors, fluids, or electrical impulses. An individual's pattern of interaction with the environment determined the internal balance; thus, overeating, exposure to cold air, or a grave mental shock could disturb the body's equilibrium and lead to disease. Within this conceptual framework, disease was conceived of as a condition or state of the body, that is, a fever, dropsy, or diarrhea, rather than as a specific entity such as malaria or dysentery. Clinical pictures of discrete ailments, each with an identifiable pathological mechanism and a developmental course, had only begun to be developed. Although physicians recognized that certain diseases had distinct character-istics, such as smallpox, or a localized manifestation in one organ, such as a tumor, they thought of most diseases (including insanity) as having a nonspecific origin and effect on the body.[24]

To treat a disease state, physicians had to discover the cause of the imbalance that produced it. To this end, Belleville taught his student to scrutinize the physical clues to the body's internal con-dition: pulse, perspiration, temperature, urine, blood, feces, res-piration, and skin color. Kirkbride had to learn the import of the different states of these indicators, such as the color of the blood, amount of sediment in the urine, strength of the pulse, and sound of the lungs. In a medical era before the clinical thermometer, stethoscope, and X-ray provided new forms of physical diagnosis, such measures constituted the physician's only diagnostic tools. Despite the seemingly primitive nature of their methods, doctors often developed considerable acuity in reading the patient's phys-ical signs. Nicholas Belleville evidently was such an acute clinician. Although he left France before the rise of the Paris School, with its emphasis on careful clinical observation, he had already de-veloped some of its characteristic traits. A former student described Belleville's methods as "curious and minute in investigation – keen in observing – careful and deliberate in deciding."[25]

Once the doctor had read the physical signs, he formed a di-agnosis specifying the nature of the disease state, that is, whether it was a fever, diarrhea, or the like, and the probable site of its origin, that is, a disordered stomach, inflamed brain, or abscessed lung. Once this determination had been made, the physician could decide upon the proper combination of therapeutic measures needed to restore the body's internal balance and return the patient to health. If he could not discover the source of the patient's disease, Belleville advised his students to avoid treatment, saying, "If you do not know, nature can do a great deal better than you can guess." But when Belleville recognized a disease state, he prescribed an active therapeutic regimen. Like his contemporary, Benjamin Rush, he recommended the liberal use of the lancet, in conjunction with purges and emetics, for the treatment of high fevers or respiratory difficulties, symptoms that indicated a bodily state of excessive "excitement" in need of a "depleting" regimen. Belleville ordinarily took 10 to 12 ounces of blood at the first bleeding and increased amounts at regular intervals if the patient's pulse continued to be high. In one case, Kirkbride recorded in his student notebook that his mentor had bled and purged a patient with violent headache and fever three times within twenty-four hours. The patient recovered, but was not grateful for his treatment. Kirkbride noted, "as an example of the unjust reproaches often cast on physicians for their best directed efforts," that the patient's family remarked to Belleville, "Doctor, Mr. H. has recovered, but if he had died, we should have been sure you bled him to death." The young student also recorded his preceptor's opinions on the value of emetics: "I have . . . during a practice of more than forty years, given emetics as much perhaps as any other practitioner . . . and have never in a single instance witnessed any but good effects from their use." For good measure, Belleville bequeathed to his student a favorite recipe for an "emeto-purgative," to be used "whenever he wishes to 'empty the stomach and bowel right well.'"[26]

In addition to the indications and techniques for using venesection, purges, and emetics, Belleville gave Kirkbride recipes containing a wide variety of vegetable and mineral drugs. Among them were a mercurial preparation for syphilis, a decoction of black oak bark and alum for a throat tumor, a hemlock solution to be used as an injection in uterine cancer, and a mixture of nutmeg, sugar, rhubarb, and magnesia for children with diarrhea. As a necessary adjunct to these prescriptions, Belleville impressed upon his student the importance of sound diet and regimen. A man known for "his leanness [and] his abstemious and careful habits," the Frenchman criticized his American patients for their overindulgent life-styles, supposedly telling one group of hard-drinking, gluttonous lawyers, "I will live to stamp on the graves of every single one of your damned set."[27]

Thus, during his year's study with Belleville, Kirkbride learned the basics of traditional medical practice: diagnosis, therapeutics, and regimen. These same skills formed the foundation of practice for all doctors, whether country practitioners or elite urban consultants. The route to prestige, however, necessitated acquisition of a more sophisticated knowledge that was to be obtained only in medical school. So, as the next step in his medical education, Kirkbride entered the University of Pennsylvania Medical School in the fall of 1828.[28]

Although one of the best medical schools in the United States, the University of Pennsylvania's standards did not match those of the best European institutions of its time. Unlike Edinburgh, the university had no entrance requirements and no graded course of lectures; the students attended the same set of lectures for three years before they applied for graduation. Unlike Paris, which offered extensive opportunities for clinical work and dissection, Philadelphia had very limited clinical facilities. Students could attend a course of lectures at the Pennsylvania Hospital, as Kirkbride did, but that opportunity for clinical observation was not integrated with the medical school curriculum. Nathaniel Chapman, Kirkbride's professor of medicine and the dominant figure on the faculty, seems in retrospect to have been a man of mediocre intellect. A "leader among followers," as one historian has characterized him, he taught his students a medical orthodoxy only slightly modified from that of his preceptor, Benjamin Rush.[29]

Although Kirkbride's medical education did not expose him to the most recent advances in medical science, it did introduce him to a more sophisticated intellectual framework for understanding disease and its treatment. In scientific circles revitalized by the Enlightenment, debate over the nature of disease had reached a new intensity in the late eighteenth century. Although physicians remained in general agreement that disease had a nonspecific origin and effect on the body, they by no means agreed upon the physiological mechanisms that produced the disease state. Elite physicians devoted much effort to advancing the claims of their own etiological schemes over those of their rivals and building elaborate nosologies that classified all forms of illness according to their favored concept of causality.[30]

The medical systems developed by William Cullen and John Brown at the Edinburgh School of Medicine had the strongest impact on early nineteenth-century American medicine. Both Cullen and Brown drew heavily upon the seventeenth-century anatomical work of Thomas Willis and Albrecht von Haller, which exposed the body's extensive network of nerves and illustrated some of their basic functions. The determination of the nervous system's role in "sensibility," that is, the transmission of information taken in by the senses to the brain, soon made the nervous system rival the circulation as the mechanism physicians used to explain physiological changes. Cullen based his medical system on the theory that nervous tension and laxity, or "excitement" and "debility," as he termed them, served as the proximate or immediate cause of all diseases. In essentially mechanistic terms, Cullen portrayed disease as the product of "irregular motions of the system" induced by nervous excitement or debility. In health, the vital energy generated by the various organs was balanced and thus produced a regular motion. But let one organ produce too much or too little nervous action, and an imbalanced, irregular motion would inevitably result and eventually cause disease. John Brown modified Cullen's system by characterizing debility not as the immediate cause but rather as the disease state itself. He postulated two types of disease: the "asthenic," or direct debility, which resulted when external stimuli could not balance the body's innate motions or excitability; and the "sthenic," or indirect debility, which existed when external stimuli were so strong that they could not be balanced by the body's own nervous force. Benjamin Rush produced yet a third hybrid medical system based on the premise that nervous excitement and debility caused illness by producing a "morbid excitement" of the circulation. A sthenic or asthenic state of the nervous system induced excitement, but the nerves functioned only by communicating those states to the circulation. Thus, according to Rush, disease always involved an overactive, irregular state of the vascular system.[31]

When confronted with the complexities of these medical systems, the average medical student such as Kirkbride absorbed few of their fine points; unless inclined to scientific disputation, he contented himself with learning the tenets of the system preferred by his professors. Kirkbride mastered the modified version of Rush's system that Nathaniel Chapman favored. His most important acquisition in medical school was not a specific medical system but a set of more general terms and concepts with which to explain disease. Despite their disagreements, the competing eighteenth-century medical theories all conceived of disease as an imbalance produced by irregular actions of the nervous or circulatory system. For all the argument over their precise relationship, American physicians relied heavily on the nervous and circulatory systems to explain the mechanism of sympathy. Thus, as a student, Kirkbride learned to think of disease in terms of irritation, inflammation, debility, and excitement. Superimposed on rather than supplanting the simpler language that Belleville had taught him, this new layer of medical explanation gave Kirkbride a more elaborate intellectual framework within which to comprehend disease.

Using this framework, Kirkbride continued to practice the basic principles of therapeutics that his preceptor had taught him, but learned to apply them in a different fashion. Between the generations of Rush and Belleville and their students, Chapman and Kirkbride, physicians began to consider Americans as less prone to diseases caused by excess energy or excitement, and more susceptible to diseases caused by too little energy, or debility. According to early nineteenth-century doctors, the influence of a civilized, sedentary life had made Americans less robust. Consequently, they did not need a heroic treatment to restore health, but rather a gentle, strengthening regimen to build up their depleted systems. Thus, in medical school, Kirkbride learned a much milder course of therapeutics than that advocated by his preceptor, Belleville. He was instructed to avoid harsh drugs such as mercury, to use sparingly emetics or purges that acted violently on the body, to trust more in the body's own healing powers, and to interfere only cautiously in its internal processes. Local bleeding by cups or leeches replaced venesection as the recommended method for reducing inflammation. The emphasis on gentler techniques did not condone therapeutic nihilism, however. Kirkbride's professors placed great store on medical therapeutics and extended his knowledge of drug actions. In a student notebook, Kirkbride made a chart of the classes of drugs grouped by their physiological effect – emetics, cathartics, diuretics, diaphoretics, narcotics, and emmenagogues – and listed under them more than 110 drugs, each with its proper dosage and modes of application.[32]

Besides the theory of medicine and therapeutics, Kirkbride's medical education included practical instruction in surgery and midwifery. Lack of anesthetics and the risk of infection limited the types of surgery that could be undertaken in his day, but procedures such as bone and joint surgery, setting of fractures, and lithotomies (removal of bladder stones) could be successfully and reliably performed. Kirkbride learned surgical methods with great enthusiasm and, even in his student days, appears to have been tending toward a surgical specialty. His study of midwifery, although less extensive, introduced him to the means of easing a difficult birth.[33]

In contrast, Kirkbride learned very little about the nature of mental diseases and their treatment as a medical student. Anatomy classes included lectures on the nervous system, but the regular coursework rarely mentioned diseases of the mind. In Kirkbride's student papers are references to several books on the subject that he must have read on his own. While Belleville's student, he perused Benjamin Rush's famous 1812 treatise, *Medical Inquiries and Observations Upon the Diseases of the Mind*, but the passages he copied – headed, for example, "Rush's advice on mingling with ladies" and the "dangers of close application to study" – suggest that he read it more as a book of advice than a medical text. In medical school, Kirkbride devoted more serious attention to George Man Burrows's ponderous treatise, *Commentaries on the Causes, Forms, Symptoms and Treatment, Moral and Medical, of Insanity*, published in 1828. This work, hailed as "the most elaborate and complete treatise" on insanity in the English language, summarized both French and English developments in the treatment of mental disease, and most likely provided Kirkbride with his first formal introduction to the principles and methods of moral treatment.[34]

In spite of his early leanings toward a surgical specialty, Kirkbride did have enough interest in nervous diseases to devote some independent research to the topic. Before graduating from the University of Pennsylvania Medical School, every student had to write an original thesis on some aspect of medicine that interested him. Perhaps under the influence of Nathaniel Chapman, who himself was working on the topic in the early 1830s, Kirkbride chose to write his thesis on neuralgia, a class of disorders characterized primarily by "lancinating pain" along the course of a nerve but also including "a large number of highly interesting and important cases – arising from irritation of nervous centres...not characterized by pain, but by some disordered or perverted state of their functions." In his description of neuralgia, Kirkbride mentioned symptoms such as "an extreme disinclination to exertion," a disposition to be agitated by "trifling causes," gloomy spirits, dyspepsia, heart palpitations, and feelings of suffocation. Kirkbride recommended treatments based on the principles of counterirritation, such as the application of leeches and cups, blisters, and tartar emetic ointment. He also advised the use of tonics, liniments, and other soothing remedies. Kirkbride did not neglect moral treatment, although he did not term it such; he recommended employment and exercise on the grounds that a morbid self-absorption often accompanied neuralgia. "The patient's mind should therefore be relieved from apprehension, and active pursuits and cheerful society be recommended." Kirkbride concluded his discussion by stating, "The irritation of nervous masses are at the present day attracting much attention, from many of the most enlightened of the profession, and to this source we shall probably in a few years be able to ascribe many obscure diseases – with practical results of the highest importance."[35]

Kirkbride's early writings on neuralgia are interesting not only because they reveal his conception of nervous irritation as the basis of mental disorder but also because they reflect a general trend toward the expansion of accepted boundaries of mental disease. Clearly, Kirkbride viewed neuralgia as a disease of "infinite variety and...a great diversity of symptoms" whose kinship with more serious mental diseases was obvious. In the 1830s, medical conceptions of the nervous system and its disorders were becoming increasingly flexible, expanding to include not only insanity but also a host of milder ailments. Such milder ills were widespread, especially among the upper classes, and their willingness to seek relief from annoying and often debilitating nervous symptoms created a promising field for medical practice. But, at this stage of his career, Kirkbride's interest in nervous and mental disorders developed no further. He finished his thesis, which he never published, and left medical school in 1832 with no apparent intention of doing further work in the field.[36]

Hospital residencies

After graduating from medical school in 1832, Kirkbride applied for a residency at the Pennsylvania Hospital, which since its foundation had been an important asset to a Philadelphia doctor's career. Not only did a hospital position enhance a physician's knowledge and reputation, it also introduced him to prospective private patients. Naturally, competition for residencies was keen, and acquiring one necessitated personal influence as well as professional ability. Kirkbride had both, yet found himself in a quandary, for the year he applied, another young doctor, "whose friends were my particular ones," also wanted the post; "as both of us could not be elected, I was led to withdraw in his favor, being convinced that my own chance for next year was rendered much stronger by the course," he recalled.[37]

Upon returning to his father's farm to wait until he could apply again for the residency, another opportunity for hospital service soon came Kirkbride's way. His uncle and future father-in-law, Joseph R. Jenks, who was a manager at the Friends Asylum for the Insane, wrote to ask him to apply for the resident's post there. Kirkbride accepted, not apparently from any special interest in the insane but because he hoped that the experience there would help his candidacy at the Pennsylvania Hospital, which had a separate wing for insane patients. "A little reflection satisfied me that holding that position might be of service to me in regard to my election to the Pennsylvania Hospital," he wrote in his autobiography, so in the spring of 1832, Kirkbride took up his residence at the asylum, located a few miles outside Philadelphia in the village of Frankford.[38]

Kirkbride's service at the Friends Asylum gave him his first practical experience with the system of moral treatment developed by Philippe Pinel at the Bicêtre and Salpêtrière hospitals in Paris and by William Tuke at the York Retreat in England. This system, whose intellectual rationale will be discussed in more detail later in the chapter, gave new emphasis to the psychological, or "moral," causes of insanity and developed moral methods to treat them. Tuke and Pinel advised the asylum's officers to create an intimate family atmosphere in which the patient's natural emotions of affection, emulation, guilt, and desire to please could be manipulated to induce sane behavior. The patients' minds were to be constantly stimulated and diverted by amusements such as games, lectures, and parties. Regular physical exercise would tone their bodies and calm their minds. Tuke and Pinel both expressed little faith in the ability of traditional medical therapeutics to modify insanity, so that the only medicines they recommended were directed at curing its physical side effects: gentle purgatives for constipation, mild stimulants for debility, and the like. If moral measures were carefully and diligently implemented, Tuke and Pinel concluded, no restraint or harsh treatment would be needed to control the insane.[39]

Although, as we shall see, Pinel's work had the greater impact on medical theories of insanity, Tuke's institutional practice served as the more immediate model for early American asylums. Samuel Tuke's account of his grandfather William's asylum, *The Description of the Retreat Near York*, published in a Philadelphia edition in 1813, introduced moral treatment to the United States. The York Retreat had a particular impact on American practice because of the personal ties between the Tuke family and the American Friends, notably Thomas Eddy at the New York Hospital and Thomas Scattergood of Philadelphia.[40] The Friends Asylum at Frankford, Pennsylvania, was founded in 1817 by Scattergood and others as an American counterpart to the York Retreat. By establishing a small institution restricted to members of the Society, its founders hoped to create the intimate, familylike milieu Tuke had found so effective in treating the insane. Like its English model, the Frankford asylum originally placed little value on medical treatment. The managers appointed a visiting physician who confined his attention to the patients' physical ailments. The lay superintendent had complete charge of the patients' employment, amusement, and exercise, which were considered the most important facets of asylum care.[41]

In the early 1830s, however, the managers of the Friends Asylum departed from this philosophy and instituted a more vigorous medical regimen. As they explained in their annual report for 1833, the managers had been forced to reconsider the asylum's original policies by the realization that "in the cure of recent cases we had fallen short of the success of some other Institutions." The asylum had been founded, they felt, "with very high and perhaps exaggerated expectations of the results to be produced by moral treatment"; medical treatment had been "depreciated in comparison" and "occupied a subordinate place in the system." After conferring with "anxious solicitude," the managers had decided that this approach no longer served the asylum's purpose, and that they must implement "a more systematic medical treatment of the patients." To this end, they hired two Philadelphia doctors, Robert Morton and Charles Evans, to be the asylum's attending physicians, and Thomas Story Kirkbride to be the resident physician under their direction.[42]

Even after this change in policy, the Friends Asylum's system of medical attendance remained at variance with the governance of other corporate American asylums. By the early 1830s, the practice begun in English asylums of having one senior resident medical officer, or superintendent, in charge of both medical and moral treatment had become commonplace in the United States. From their foundation, both the McLean Asylum in Massachusetts (1818) and the Hartford Retreat in Connecticut (1824) had such a medical superintendent. The same year the Friends Asylum adopted the general hospital scheme of having senior attending and junior resident physicians, the Bloomingdale Asylum (founded in 1821) abandoned it in favor of a single chief physician. For a time in the mid-1830s, the Pennsylvania Hospital managers considered the attending–resident physician plan for their new asylum, but eventually rejected it on the grounds that a single medical superintendent was becoming a universal practice. Despite the trend in other private institutions, the Friends Asylum did not appoint a chief medical officer until 1850. So, the plan of medical attendance under which Kirkbride served in his first asylum post was not the system he himself would later practice.[43]

The attending physicians at the Friends Asylum may have held an anomalous position in its governance, but they nonetheless gave Kirkbride a good grounding in the basics of asylum medicine. Doctors Morton and Evans fully believed in the power of active medical treatment to cure many cases of insanity. In their first report to the managers, they criticized the "commonly received opinion" held among the asylum staff that "insanity is not a disease dependent on physical disorder and therefore amenable to medical skill" but rather a "morbid state of the immaterial principle itself, originating from moral causes and demanding only moral treatment." Not only had this erroneous opinion reduced the asylum to a "state of great inefficiency," the doctors observed; it also ran counter to recent medical investigations that had repeatedly shown "the almost inseparable connection existing between mental derangement and a structural or functional disturbance of the brain." Moral causes produced insanity, they insisted, only by "acting as agents" to produce a morbid physical condition of the brain. Thus, moral treatment could be effective only after medical means had removed physical disease. For this reason, Morton and Evans concluded, they intended to "conform the practice of the house to this pathology of the disease, and to employ in the curative treatment all such medical and moral remedies, as we are able to command."[44]

Under the direction of Morton and Evans, Kirkbride carried out the new plan for medical treatment, recording the results in a casebook, portions of which were copied into the managers' minutes.[45] These abstracts are interesting not only because they reveal the methods of treating insanity that Kirkbride learned at the Friends Asylum but also because they show how the results of treatment were interpreted. The first abstract from Kirkbride's notes concerned a patient who had been admitted "restless, noisy, desponding and extremely adverse to being put under treatment." Deciding that he suffered from a "derangement of the functions of the Brain" due to "too large a supply of blood, produced by a morbid state of the stomach," the physician ordered him "freely cupped over the head and vomited" by the resident. An almost immediate change took place, indicating that the underlying source of the disorder had indeed been removed. As Kirkbride recorded, the patient "became at once calm and comfortable, reconciled to his situation, and willing to conform to whatever was prescribed for him." Moral treatment confirmed his recovery, and he left the asylum cured within six weeks. In a similar case, when "copious depletion" was prescribed for a patient supposedly suffering from acute inflammation of the brain, the attending physicians noted that the man was "so sensible...of the relief procured by the application of the cups to the head that he repeatedly requested Dr. Kirkbride to have them put on."

The new plan of active medical treatment was not confined to the recently afflicted. Morton and Evans reported the measures tried with one long-afflicted patient who had always been considered "beyond the reach of medical treatment." A troublesome woman who showed little interest in any activity except destroying her clothes, she had been repeatedly strapped to a chair, with her hands confined in a muff. After Kirkbride's use of emetics and a shower bath, the patient became more alert, stopped tearing her clothes, and participated in asylum activities. The attending physicians admitted that "though the disease was shaken," in her case "it had acquired too strong a hold to be dislodged"; yet they felt that medical treatment had greatly improved her mental condition.

At the same time Kirkbride learned the value of medical treatment for insanity during his year at the asylum, his training did not neglect the importance of moral measures. Despite the new emphasis given to the medical department, the asylum's lay superintendent continued to exercise full control over the patients' moral treatment. As his other duties allowed, Kirkbride participated in this aspect of asylum care and had the opportunity to see its effect on the most discouraging cases. His notes recorded the case of one longtime asylum resident who was frequently confined because she persisted in "rendering her person and room objects of disgust" by the "most filthy habits." The lay superintendent resolved to try the effect of moving her to a "more agreeable apartment, changing the coarse clothes for finer, and allowing her the use of pen, ink and paper." Kirkbride reported that "she immediately showed herself sensible of the change and took an interest in her new employment."

Yet, the dramatic testimony to the efficacy of both medical and moral treatment that Kirkbride observed as an asylum resident must have been balanced to some extent by less cheering aspects of hospital life. During his residency, there occurred deaths, suicides, and escapes, events that must have had a sobering effect on the young doctor. Late one December night, for example, Kirkbride sent for the attending physicians to examine a patient who, after suddenly recovering his reason, "complained of a strange feeling" and died. On another occasion, Kirkbride visited a patient's room, only to find the inmate dismantling the window in order to make an escape. Only a few months later, a woman patient cleverly arranged her bedclothes so as to deceive the night watcher and used her new-found freedom to hang herself on the hospital grounds. Since "her disposition to destroy herself was such that no cure would fully guard against it," the Visiting Committee assigned no blame for her death; yet, her demise must have made a troubling impression on Kirkbride.[46]

Kirkbride's residency at the Friends Asylum undoubtedly shaped his later practice at the Pennsylvania Hospital for the Insane. Besides giving him his first real experience with moral treatment, Morton and Evans taught Kirkbride the all-important principle that became the foundation of his own asylum philosophy: that medical and moral means were "parts of the same system" and gave "full benefit" only when practiced together. Yet, despite a full trial of the work to which he would later devote his life, the young physician left the Friends Asylum with no intention of pursuing asylum medicine. Although the managers, expressing "great satisfaction" with his "faithful and exemplary discharge of his duties," asked him to stay, Kirkbride refused. Although feeling an "active interest in everything related to the care of the patients and the management of the institution," as he stated later, he still thought only of receiving an appointment to the Pennsylvania Hospital. In March 1833, when he was finally awarded the coveted post, Kirkbride immediately left the Frankford asylum for Philadelphia.[47]

In his new residency, Kirkbride plunged into the more varied medical and surgical practice offered by a general hospital over ten times the size of the asylum he had just left. Along with his fellow resident, he lived on the second floor of the hospital's center building so that he could devote his entire attention to the several hundred patients housed in the East and West Wings. Since the senior, or attending, physicians visited the hospital only twice a week, the daily medical attendance devolved upon the residents. Kirkbride carried out the senior physicians' orders for the patients and handled the emergencies that inevitably occurred in their absence. Despite his many duties, he found time to record cases he thought of special interest in the hospital casebook; entries in Kirkbride's hand included the treatment of puerperal fever, tetanus, and various injuries requiring special surgical procedures. He later rewrote some of these case histories and published them in the *American Journal of Medical Science*. None, it should be noted, involved insane patients.[48]

Despite his apparent lack of interest in studying insanity, Kirkbride treated many lunatics during his residency at the Pennsylvania Hospital. At that time, the West Wing housed more than 100 patients suffering from varying forms of mental disease. From his private notebooks, it is evident that in treating them, Kirkbride carried out the principles he had mastered at the Friends Asylum. When a patient was first admitted, Kirkbride administered a purge, followed by a sedative drug such as opium, morphine, or conium. For the most violently excited patients, he ordered cups or leeches applied to the back of the neck. Occasionally, he prescribed restraint, as in the case of one man, who was "so destructive to the furnishing of his room" that his hands were confined. Kirkbride also must have done more reading on insanity, for he recorded in a notebook several prescriptions used by Dr. Eli Todd of the Hartford Retreat, which he probably acquired from a compendium on the treatment of mental diseases.[49]

During Kirkbride's second year at the hospital, a classmate of his from medical school, William W. Gerhard, served as his fellow resident. After obtaining his degree at the University of Pennsylvania, Gerhard had gone to Paris to study medicine, a common career pattern among the most ambitious antebellum doctors. There he had been "an ardent student, principally in the French hospitals," and a "favorite pupil of the celebrated Louis," according to Kirkbride. Gerhard's mentor, Pierre Charles Alexander Louis, developed the American student's interest in correlating disease symptoms during life with pathological appearances after death. Gerhard entered his residency at the Pennsylvania Hospital eager to carry on this work in its medical wards, and gladly left the surgical and insane wards to Kirkbride's care.[50]

Gerhard was Kirkbride's closest contact with the innovations of the Paris School of medicine, which were then reshaping the medical thinking of elite American physicians. Kirkbride recalled that Gerhard's "wonderful habits of industry and his very accurate manner of making observations, were of not a little use to me."[51] The respect for pathology and statistical methods that Kirkbride expressed in later years, despite his limited use of them at his own asylum, stemmed in part from his youthful friendship with Gerhard. But it is important to note that Kirkbride, whether for lack of money or interest, never acquired the European experience that distinguished the leading scientific men of his generation. Again, as in his choice of preceptor, Kirkbride's medical training did not place him at the very forefront of his profession.[52]

General practice

Still, Kirkbride's medical education and postgraduate training were quite sufficient for him to establish a successful private practice in Philadelphia. In 1836, after finishing his residency at the Pennsylvania Hospital, Kirkbride rented a room at Fourth and Arch streets to serve as a combination of office and living quarters. In setting up a practice, he had several advantages that many young doctors of his generation lacked. His residency at the Pennsylvania Hospital had yielded a number of former patients who came to him for treatment. Acquaintances among the Society of Friends and the hospital managers also referred relatives and servants to his care. Most importantly, Kirkbride enjoyed the "friendly recognition" of two elderly doctors, John Otto and Joseph Parrish, who had begun to curtail their practices and gladly referred clients to the young physician. Due to his infirmities, Otto could not always visit his patients at home, so "on these occasions, he frequently asked my assistance, which I need scarcely say, I was most happy to render," Kirkbride recalled. In this fashion, he concluded, "I became intimate with a large class of patients...with whom I was not likely otherwise to have been acquainted."[53]

Like the general practitioners of his time, Kirkbride had both an office and a family practice. His office clientele consisted mostly of laborers, artisans, and shopkeepers from the immediate neighborhood. Sometimes patients merely saw Kirkbride's sign and walked in; others had accidents in nearby shops or streets and sought the closest doctor's office. A few office patients, including some from the professional class, were referred to Kirkbride because he used a nonmercurial regimen for treating syphilis, which consisted of warm baths, a vegetable diet, and applications of copper sulfide to the ulcer. For an office visit, Kirkbride charged a minimum of $1.00, with additional fees for minor surgery or treatments administered on the spot. In total, office trade comprised about one-third of Kirkbride's practice.[54]

The young physician spent the rest of his time and derived the greater part of his income from family practice. Unlike modern family practice, this meant attending at home any member of the household, including parents, children, and servants, who became ill. During a house call, Kirkbride might perform minor medical services such as lancing boils, treating sprains, or dressing burns for patrons who did not wish to come to his office. Women and children, for example, were usually seen in the home, even for minor ailments.[55] In his family practice, Kirkbride also treated patients with a serious illness or injury who today would be sent to the hospital. Nineteenth-century institutional care existed primarily for the poor; moreover, there was little medical assistance a hospital physician could render a patient that Kirkbride could not provide just as well in the home.[56] So, as a private practitioner, he treated a wide range of acute and infectious diseases: respiratory disorders such as pneumonia, bronchitis, and pleurisy; the ever-present intermittent fevers, and even smallpox and cholera. Children's diseases such as croup, whooping cough, and measles were also common. Although not making midwifery a special interest,

Kirkbride attended difficult deliveries in the families he treated. He even cared for a few cases of nervous diseases, primarily dyspepsia and hysteria.

With his social and medical connections, Kirkbride did quite well in private practice, developing a thriving business among the prosperous artisans in his neighborhood, as well as among the wealthier merchants residing in more fashionable areas. For some of the latter households, the bill for Kirkbride's services, which he usually submitted once or twice a year, could amount to more than $100.00. In his first years, Kirkbride netted approximately $500.00 per annum, a respectable income for a young physician. By the late 1830s, his yearly income had increased to almost $1,000.00. This success boded well for Kirkbride's future, for as he grew older, his practice would naturally increase. Clearly, he did not turn to asylum work solely in search of economic security, as some of his contemporaries did. [57]

Choosing a specialty

Once his private practice began to prosper, Kirkbride started to work toward a new goal: to return to the Pennsylvania Hospital as an attending surgeon, a position that would have placed him at the pinnacle of local success. Unless he sought a chair at the medical school, a prospect that interested Kirkbride less than the opportunity to give clinical lectures at the hospital, he could aim no higher. As an attending surgeon, his professional standing would be solidly established and his private practice greatly increased. When a wealthy family needed a surgeon, they almost invariably chose a hospital man and paid liberally for his services. So, to achieve these advantages, Kirkbride continued to visit the Pennsylvania Hospital, maintaining his connection with the surgeons there, and in his spare time studied and practiced surgery, publishing several papers on cases he had observed as a resident. Although he was still relatively young, his surgical skills had attracted the attention of more established doctors. "I had become known to some of my older brethren as devoting myself to surgery," he recalled in his memoirs, "and was not infrequently called in to aid them in the performance of such surgery as came under their care," he recalled. Kirkbride also acted as attending physician at the House of Refuge, Magdalen Hospital and Institute for the Blind, to gain experience and enhance his chances at the Pennsylvania Hospital, as he had by his service at the Friends Asylum.[58]

By 1840, Kirkbride had every reason to hope that he would be elected an attending surgeon at the Pennsylvania Hospital. He had the necessary ties with its surgeons and managers, as well as a successful private practice. Furthermore, Kirkbride knew that his friend and mentor, J. Rhea Barton, would be retiring from the post that year and would use his influence to have his young colleague succeed him. "My intimacy with the Board of Managers, and the friendly feelings they were kind enough to express in my favor" convinced Kirkbride that his ambition would soon be realized. "Just at this time," wrote Kirkbride, in his autobiography, "occurred one of those incidents that seem beyond the control of men, and which changed the whole course of my life." While walking along Race Street, he met his friend John Paul, a manager at the Hospital, who asked "what would induce me to go over the river, to take charge of the new Hospital for the Insane." Kirkbride replied that he had hoped for another post at the hospital, but agreed to consider the offer.[59]

Kirkbride's ruminations over this unexpected job offer, as recorded years later, suggest his motives in becoming an asylum doctor. His was not a forced choice, for he had the reputation and skills to pursue his surgical ambitions. But a surgical specialty, although a more established field than asylum medicine, had several drawbacks as far as Kirkbride was concerned. "The labor attendant upon the successful practitioner of private surgery, and of hospital surgery in addition," he thought, "must necessarily be great and would demand more than ordinary good health." The night calls, the long hours and rigors of operations, the traveling for postoperative visits all required great physical stamina. His being a "weak and delicate frame" (an opinion confirmed by others who described him), Kirkbride doubted his ability to withstand the physical strain of surgery. In contrast, the asylum position offered a comfortable residence, the farm's old mansion house, and what Kirkbride considered a "rather liberal" yearly salary of $3,000.00. Ultimately, he could have made more money as a surgeon, but only by following a strenuous routine. Evidently, Kirkbride's parents, as well as his young wife, the former Ann Jenks, whom he had married in 1839, approved the change from surgery to asylum work. To them it represented "a certainty in place of an uncertainty." His wife seemed particularly pleased, according to Kirkbride, "knowing as she did, that a successful city practice must necessarily keep me the most of my time from home, while the care of the Hospital for the Insane would be sure to keep me somewhere on its premises."[60]

Yet, for a man as ambitious as Kirkbride, the argument that he chose the asylum solely because it offered a more secure existence is not wholly satisfying. Clearly, he did not take the position because he could not survive in the competitive medical world of the late 1830s. Nor did he make the choice out of an overwhelming interest in treating the insane; his rejection of the Friends Asylum's offer suggests otherwise. It seems much more likely that this ambitious young doctor saw in the asylum a new channel for his professional aspirations. Kirkbride recognized, as he stated in his memoirs, that the new situation provided "the opportunity of starting a new institution, and developing new forms of management, in fact, giving a new character to the care of the insane." He also realized the possibility of "securing for myself a reputation as desirable as that which I might obtain by remaining in the city."[61] As a surgeon, Kirkbride at best could have acquired local or regional fame, but his chances for wider renown were limited. He had not studied abroad, and his academic training, although solid, was not outstanding. As head of a model asylum, Kirkbride may have realized that he had a far better opportunity to achieve a national reputation in the less well-established specialty of asylum medicine.

Another important consideration for Kirkbride must have been the organizational arrangement of the new hospital. Instead of the system of senior attending and junior resident physicians found in the general hospitals of the period, the new asylum was to have at its head one senior medical officer. Furthermore, this officer would have charge of both the medical and moral treatment of the patients. Unlike his counterpart at the Friends Asylum, the lay steward would attend only to housekeeping matters and was completely subordinate to the superintendent. The extraordinary degree of institutional power granted one physician under this arrangement, which, as mentioned before, had become standard for American mental hospitals by the 1840s, must have been one of the chief attractions of asylum work.[62] The medical superintendent possessed a unique opportunity to mold an entire hospital to his own tastes. As an attending surgeon at the Pennsylvania

Hospital, Kirkbride would never have had such administrative power. Since he later worked so diligently to justify and expand the asylum's one-man rule, he could not have been unaware of the potential for power in asylum medicine.

Kirkbride must also have considered the class of patients who would patronize the new hospital. In private practice, he had built up a small clientele among Philadelphia's comfortable classes, but the bulk of his business was still among artisans and clerks. The very wealthy patronized established physicians of their own social rank. With a surgical specialty, Kirkbride might have developed a more elite practice, but it would have taken considerable time and effort. The new asylum presented much easier access to the upper classes. Although they shunned institutional care for any other ailment, affluent families were obviously willing or, perhaps more accurately, driven to seek hospital treatment for insanity. Having treated wealthy insane patients at both the Friends Asylum and the old Pennsylvania Hospital, Kirkbride knew this social fact well. As head of the new asylum, he might become the personal guide and confidant of the best families, not only of Philadelphia but of other cities and states as well.

Kirkbride's professional biography suggests that his recruitment into asylum medicine did not grow out of a well-defined scientific or personal interest in the insane. His religious background was certainly a factor predisposing him to the work, for the Friends had long been associated with asylum reform; but when offered the chance to stay on at the Frankford Asylum in 1833, Kirkbride had turned it down with no apparent regret. What made the difference when a second such opportunity came his way in 1840 was the degree of institutional power it offered. For Kirkbride, an ambitious, successful, but conservatively educated physician outside both the scientific and social elites of his profession, asylum practice represented a means by which he might greatly enhance his power and reputation. An asylum career did entail a risk, however: If successful, it offered a shortcut to an eminence Kirkbride might not otherwise have obtained; if unsuccessful, it meant the blight of a promising, if not outstanding, medical talent. For Thomas Story Kirkbride, the gamble would prove successful.

THE MAKING OF AN ASYLUM SPECIALTY

Once Kirkbride decided to specialize in the treatment of insanity, he had quickly to familiarize himself with the latest developments in American asylum medicine.[63] Almost seven years had passed since he left the Friends Asylum, and during that time the specialty had made significant progress. As of 1841, sixteen mental hospitals based on the principles of moral treatment expounded by Pinel and Tuke had opened in the United States. The earliest and most influential of these included the Friends Asylum at Frankford, Pennsylvania (1817); the Massachusetts General Hospital's McLean Asylum at Somerville, Massachusetts (1818); the New York Hospital's Bloomingdale Asylum in New York City (1821); the Hartford Retreat at Hartford, Connecticut (1824); the Worcester State Hospital at Worcester, Massachusetts (1833); and the Maine Insane Asylum at Augusta, Maine (1840). Within a few years of the Pennsylvania Hospital for the Insane's opening, two more important institutions had begun operation: the New York State Lunatic Asylum at Utica, New York (1843), and the Butler Hospital for the Insane at Providence, Rhode Island (1845). By the early 1840s, the superintendents of the older mental hospitals, some of whom had been in practice for over a decade, had acquired enough experience to begin formulating their own ideas about asylum treatment. Drawing upon the disease concepts dominant in American medical thinking, as well as the doctrines of moral treatment advanced by Pinel and Tuke, the generation of asylum superintendents who held posts before 1845 had already established the outlines of a new theory of insanity and its treatment.[64]

The doctors who pioneered the development of American asylum medicine came from social backgrounds similar to Kirkbride's own. Most were the sons of farmers or doctors in comfortable but not affluent circumstances. Only McLean Asylum's Luther Bell, whose father had served as governor and then senator of New Hampshire, came from a family distinguished by a degree of power and wealth. The early superintendents were all Protestants reared in rural or small-town settings. The older men, such as Samuel Woodward of the Worcester State Hospital and Amariah Brigham of the Utica Asylum, had received little formal education and got their licenses to practice medicine by serving an apprenticeship rather than attending medical school. The younger superintendents, such as Bell, Isaac Ray (Maine, later Butler, Hospital), Pliny Earle (Bloomingdale Asylum), and John Butler (Hartford Retreat), had all been privately educated, many of them obtaining college degrees before entering medical school.[65]

Roughly similar in social background and medical training, the early asylum doctors were drawn even more closely together by the institutional experience they shared. Practicing a unique, specialized form of medicine, they quickly came to regard themselves as "brethren," a term they used among themselves, who had much to learn from one another. Personal ties among superintendents in the 1820s and 1830s developed into a more formal association in the early 1840s. Seeking to advance their specialty by professional organization, thirteen asylum superintendents met in Philadelphia in 1844 to form the Association of Medical Superintendents of American Institutions for the Insane (AMSAII). Samuel Woodward became its first president, Thomas Story Kirkbride its first secretary. The association continued to meet yearly for the presentation and discussion of papers on insanity and asylum treatment. Many of these papers, along with transcripts of the AMSAII proceedings, appeared in the new *American Journal of Insanity*, which began publication in 1844 under the editorship of Amariah Brigham. Together, these two professional organs served as the focus of asylum medicine for the rest of the nineteenth century.[66]

The theory and practice of American asylum medicine, which remained virtually unchanged from the 1840s to the 1880s, necessarily reflected the specialty's institutional base. No separate university centers for research on mental disease existed in the United States until the early twentieth century. Except for a few small private asylums, no extramural forms of specialized treatment for mental disorders developed until the 1870s.[67] Early psychiatric theory consisted of the practical truths of asylum medicine that the superintendents regarded as self-evident. The therapeutic approach Kirkbride learned as a young superintendent and continued to practice throughout his career remained quintessentially an asylum medicine.

Early American asylum medicine: theoretical foundations

The rationale for asylum medicine developed by the early American superintendents represented a synthesis of eighteenth-century medical systems, Pinel's reconceptualization of the psychological causes of insanity, and the theory of cerebral localization postulated by phrenologists. This synthesis gave the asylum doctors a relatively sophisticated intellectual foundation that still incorporated traditional notions of disease. The fundamental premise that disease represented an internal state of imbalance, which might be produced by either physical or mental shocks to the body, remained unaltered; the asylum doctors reworked only the mechanisms underlying the mind–body relationship and the therapeutic scheme needed to restore mental balance.

The oldest mechanism for explaining the mind–body relationship was the humoral theory, which, despite its ancient origins, continued to crop up in nineteenth-century medical thinking about insanity. Nathaniel Chapman, Kirkbride's medical school professor, in his lecture on the role of the "passions of the mind" in causing disease, included an exposition of the humors. A little observation, he assured his students, would persuade them that "the passions possess an extensive dominion over the body and can afford no slender assistance in producing its varied derangements." He explained that "the temperaments depend on an irregular state of the solids and fluids" within the body. Each temperament caused a different propensity to disease. The fair, florid, sanguine individual possessed an "ardent temper" and a predisposition to hemorrhages and violent inflammatory diseases. The dark, fleshy, bilious individual, although "bold and daring," had an "irritable temper" and a tendency to liver disorders and intermittent fevers. The phlegmatic individual, who was usually sandy-colored and plump, had a sluggish, bland temperament and suffered from glandular complaints and obstructions. The melancholic individual, known by his thin, sallow countenance, manifested a "temper petulant and fretful" and was predisposed to hypochondria.[68]

In their definitions of insanity, the medical systems of Cullen, Brown, and Rush recast the mind–body relationship posted by humoralism in more modern terms. Cullen believed mania, the "high stage" of insanity, to be a form of delirium resulting from a "spasm," or contraction, of the arteries brought on by overstimulation of the brain. Melancholia represented the opposite in Cullen's system: a disease caused by insufficient brain action, which produced a state of vascular constriction. Brown characterized mania and melancholia as the sthenic and asthenic forms of mental disease, resulting from too much or too little nerve force, respectively. Rush argued that the sthenic and asthenic states of the nerves caused the "morbid excitement" of the circulatory system. He believed that melancholia and mania represented merely different grades of the same diseased action of the brain's blood vessels.[69]

Despite their disagreement on the fundamental causes of insanity, all three physicians advocated the course of therapeutics originally outlined by William Cullen in his *First Lines on the Practice of Physic* in 1781. Mania, whether defined as an inflammation or a sthenic condition, called for a depleting regimen. Logically enough, Cullen prescribed an "antimaniacal" course of bleeding, purges, and emetics. By reducing the body's internal excitement through a depleting regimen, the mind's functions might return to their normal motions. Conversely, melancholia, an asthenic disorder caused by too little external stimulation, necessitated the use of tonics and stimulants, including liquor and opium. Although emphasizing medical therapeutics, Cullen mentioned a few measures he found useful, such as isolation and restraint for maniacs and diversion for melancholics.[70]

Cullen's recommendations for treatment reveal the relative weight of somatic and psychological factors in explaining the cause of insanity. For eighteenth-century physicians, the proximate, or immediate, cause of insanity always consisted of a somatic disorder. Doctors recognized a wide variety of physical ailments as causes of insanity, including fevers, injuries to the head, skin eruptions, suppression of natural secretions, dyspepsia, tuberculosis, and chills. They classified psychological factors such as grief, unrequited love, fear, and envy as predisposing, or remote, causes that acted on the body, not the mind. For example, anger might cause indigestion, which in turn led to insanity. In eighteenth-century medical schemas, emotions or ideas never affected the mind directly, but always worked through the body to influence the mind.[71]

Despite the secondary role assigned psychological factors in the causation of mental disorders, physicians increasingly recognized their importance in both mental and physical illness. The eighteenth-century interest in nervous diseases undoubtedly contributed to this trend. The work of Robert Whytt and George Cheyne defined a new grouping of diseases recognized as psychosomatic in origin. Thereafter, doctors paid more attention to the role of emotional stress and anxiety in causing neuralgia, dyspepsia, hysteria, "vapors," "fits," and many other common yet debilitating ailments. Cullen sanctioned this new category of ills in this medical

nosology by designating them "neuroses," or "affections of movement or sensation occurring without fever, and not depending on
local disease." The gradual recognition and acceptance of this type
of disease may also have increased interest in insanity and contributed to the growing belief that, like dyspepsia or neuralgia, it
too might respond to treatment.[72]

The work of Philippe Pinel carried the reconceptualization of
the mind–body relationship in insanity one step further by re-
versing the relative importance of psychological and somatic factors in mental diseases. Specifically, Pinel departed from traditional
conceptions of insanity by insisting that mental strains and shocks
were proximate causes and physical conditions predisposing causes.
In other words, he stated that psychological stimuli acted on the
mind directly, disordering its functions. The mind's disorder then
caused bodily disturbances. Thus, Pinel made the bodily ailments
accompanying insanity its *effect* rather than its *cause*. Believing only
a small percentage of mental disorders to involve organic brain
disease, Pinel claimed that most cases of insanity were functional
in nature, that is, disorders of the mind's operation produced by
traumatic events and manifested by psychological symptoms such
as delusions, hallucinations, and loss of memory. Physical ailments
followed in the wake of psychological troubles; the maniac's pulse
would race, the melancholic would become constipated, and eventually both patients might suffer more serious physical illness as
a result. But, at least initially, the insanity itself involved no lesion
or other organic source.

Pinel's other significant contribution to the nineteenth-century
medical theory of insanity was a broader conception of the mind's
function. He viewed the faculty psychology prevalent in medical
thinking as inadequate because it did not accord enough importance to the emotional, or moral, causes of mental disease. The
psychological theories derived from Locke concentrated primarily
on disorders of the intellectual faculties. Pinel's choice of the term
"moral" rather than "psychological" to describe his philosophy
of insanity reflects this distinction; he meant to convey the importance he accorded to the emotions, or "passions," as motivators
of human behavior. By elevating the importance of emotional
factors as causes of insanity, Pinel encouraged interest in the nature
of the emotions and their role in human behavior. For his British
and American adherents, this trend in Pinel's work received in-

creased emphasis from the influence of the Scottish commonsense school of philosophy, which also accorded the emotions a prominent place.[73]

Based on these changes in traditional views of insanity and its causes, Pinel advocated a new style of treatment. In line with his theory of insanity's proximate causes, he abandoned the active regimen associated with Cullen's somatic orientation and emphasized moral methods of treatment. Expanding Cullen's notion of isolation, Pinel emphasized the importance of a quiet, orderly regimen for the insane. The abandonment of restraint, the lack of attention to medical therapeutics – in fact, all the measures associated with moral treatment – reflected Pinel's fundamental reordering of the eighteenth-century medical schema.

The rationale for asylum medicine developed by the early American superintendents constituted a cautious reworking of Pinel's theories to justify more active medical intervention. Although generally regarding Pinel's work as the foundation of their specialty, the American superintendents found certain of his doctrines unacceptable. Pinel, after roundly criticizing his fellow physicians for bleeding and purging the insane, had concluded that medical measures had little value in the treatment of insanity. Since the disease rarely had an organic basis, he reasoned, it could not be modified by the usual medical therapeutics. The American asylum doctors thought these arguments came perilously close to the old notion that insanity was a purely spiritual, or "immaterial," problem. As they well knew, insanity's definition as a spiritual disorder had long contributed to its status as an incurable malady and to theological controversies that most physicians sought to avoid. Even if the public could be made to accept Pinel's belief that a psychological disorder might be cured by psychological means, there would be little justification for its treatment by doctors, for a lay superintendent could administer moral measures as well as a physician.

To legitimate medical domination of the asylum, the superintendents had to rework Pinel's original conception of moral treatment on these crucial points. Much as the managers and physicians at the Friends Asylum had explained its reorganization in the 1830s, American asylum doctors generally argued that Pinel (and Tuke as well) had unfairly rejected the value of medical treatment for insanity. In order to be considered curable, insanity had to be defined as a disease process that physicians could affect by medical measures. At the same time, recognizing the necessity to substitute gentler methods for the incursions of heroic treatment, the superintendents had to put forth a new medical regimen that would be more compatible with the psychological aspects of moral treatment. Thus, in their theoretical conceptions of the definition, diagnosis, etiology, and treatment of insanity, early asylum doctors attempted to justify their redefinition of moral treatment as a medical system.[74]

Using the conceptual framework inherited from the eighteenth-century medical systems, American superintendents first redefined the character of insanity as a disease. No longer was it the disease of inflammation that Cullen, Brown, and Rush had observed; instead, insanity had become almost exclusively a disease caused by nervous irritation and debility. In other words, insanity had become an asthenic rather than a sthenic disorder. The asylum doctors believed that social factors had brought about this shift. Modern individuals rarely possessed the too abundant "vital force" that had so frequently caused insanity in their parents' generation. As Pliny Earle of the Bloomingdale Asylum explained, "during the period in which Dr. Rush was in active life, disease, in all its forms, in this country . . . involved the nervous system less than at the present time." Progress had increased the sources of anxiety and excitement by fostering religious, political, and business uncertainty. Therefore, more people suffered from mental diseases caused by nervous exhaustion. As Earle concluded, "Now disease has gradually more and more deeply affected 'the roots of life' until it has finally fixed itself in the nervous system."[75]

The morbid state of the nervous system manifested itself not so much in the physical deterioration of the nerves as in their disordered operations. Adopting Pinel's conception of a functional disorder, the asylum superintendents believed that the proximate causes of insanity generated abnormal trains of nervous motion, or impulses, that were transmitted to the brain. The brain's normal functioning was thereby disturbed, producing distortions or derangements of the intellect and passions. "All insanity, whether of physical or moral semiology, is proximately owing to a derangement of the functional activity of the cerebral organ," as one doctor stated. If sustained over time, functional nervous disorders could cause organic changes such as hardening or softening of the brain. Once that stage of the disease had been reached, chances for recovery were poor. But, asylum doctors agreed, the majority of cases involved no such organic deterioration and thus were potentially curable. In this fashion, they attempted to make the characterization of insanity as a functional disorder work to their advantage by linking it with a more hopeful prognosis.[76]

The definition of insanity as a functional disease caused by nervous irritation allowed asylum superintendents to use a very flexible etiological scheme. Any event that could be correlated with a change in the individual's psychological state could be considered a proximate cause of the disease. Using the categories of physical and moral causes set up by Pinel, the asylum doctors listed all the shocks that they believed might affect the nervous system of the modern individual. Physical causes included serious illness, suppression of natural secretions, blows to the head, or any physical disruption of the body's normal functioning. Psychological stresses such as grief, fear, disappointment, or any strong emotion were also conceived of as having a physical effect on the nerves. The causes of insanity within such an etiological framework were endless. Pliny Earle had no difficulty listing sixty-one types of physical and twenty-three types of moral causes in an 1848 essay on insanity. Without materially altering the traditional etiology of the disease, asylum doctors simply expanded and refined the list of causes to encompass as many explanations of insanity as possible.[77]

To make the connection between these proximate causes, the functional disorders of the brain, and the derangements of the mind, the asylum superintendents employed a modified form of faculty psychology. The theories of mental organization that they used had developed outside the medical field as a branch of philosophy. John Locke's writings in the late seventeenth century had popularized the concept of the mind as a collection of faculties. Locke believed that the mind at birth was a tabula rasa; as it received sensory impressions from the external or "material" world, it gradually developed certain faculties that operated to analyze this input into ideas. Locke's list of faculties consisted of the intellectual processes of memory, judgment, imagination, reason, and attention. The philosophers associated with the Scottish Enlightenment, better known as the "commonsense school," modified Locke's theories on two counts. First, they included, as did Pinel, the passions as faculties. Second, they objected to Locke's assertion that the mind possessed no inborn propensities. Instead, the commonsense philosophers argued that all human beings were born with certain innate faculties, which developed as they grew older.[78]

Phrenological doctrines, which became popular in America and England in the 1820s and 1830s, linked the commonsense version of faculty psychology with the structure of the brain. Phrenology developed from the work of Franz Joseph Gall, an Austrian doctor who produced a complex theory of cerebral localization in the early nineteenth century. Using case histories of brain injuries and unusual skull conformation, Gall purported to prove that the faculties postulated by the "mental philosophers" resided in specific portions of the brain. Elaborating upon this theory, his followers drew up detailed maps of the faculties' location in the brain, and correlated the size and shape of its sections with the predominance of different personality traits. This, in turn, became the basis for a widely popularized (and vulgarized) "science" of reading character from the conformation of the head.[79]

Although a few asylum superintendents became enthusiastic advocates of phrenology, the majority remained skeptical of the skull readings and charts produced by Gall's popularizers. At the same time, the profession as a whole accepted the premise that the various faculties of the mind were located in different portions of the brain, and that the disordered action of the nerves on specific parts of that organ disrupted or perverted different intellectual and emotional functions. The theory of cerebral location made popular by phrenologists gave asylum doctors a convenient tool with which to explain the link between brain malfunction and mental disturbance.[80]

The faculty psychology promoted by phrenology also served asylum doctors as a useful way to explain individual differences in tolerance to stress. As they well knew, an event that might shatter one person would affect another only slightly. Faculty psychology helped to explain this phenomenon. People were born with a certain combination of innate feelings, or propensities, the asylum doctors reasoned; the individual developed these traits through the years simply by exercising them. "The brain is formed by habits," as one doctor wrote in a paper for the AMSAII's annual meeting. Exercise and discipline of the mind would "call into regular and repeated action certain portions of the brain, and enable

them to manifest easily and powerfully certain mental operations."
The asylum doctors argued that proper mental exercise built a
healthy brain, just as physical exercise developed the muscles.[81]

Combining Pinel's reorientation of eighteenth-century medical
systems with new doctrines of phrenology, the American superintendents evolved a comprehensive rationale for asylum treatment. Their theory of insanity and its causes served to rationalize
both the medical and moral regimens they wished to direct. At
the same time, it equipped asylum doctors with a medical philosophy that allowed them to explain not only the nature of insanity but also the larger moral imperatives facing their society.

The redefinition of insanity as a sthenic disease caused by nervous irritation legitimated the new forms of medical treatment
that doctors were finding useful in the asylum. The sthenic forms
of the disease common in the past had "more seriously implicated
the circulation and hence requires a more heroic method of attack
for its subjection," as Earle argued. But asylum doctors felt that
the copious bloodletting and purging practiced in such cases were
far too drastic for contemporary forms of nervous debility. The
depleting regimen had to be replaced by strengthening measures
such as tonics and narcotics that soothed and restored the nerves.
In this fashion, the superintendents linked the new character of
mental disease to a gentler and (they hoped) more effective therapeutic regimen.[82]

This shift in therapeutic rationale no doubt reflected the success
of new narcotic treatments in the asylum. The redefinition of
insanity as an asthenic disorder roughly coincided with the introduction of morphine into American medical practice. Before the
early nineteenth century, crude opium had been used to treat delirium tremens and melancholia, but its serious side effects, especially on the digestion, had made it unsuitable for extended use.
Because it supposedly exercised a stimulant effect, opium was
never used in cases of mania. Nathaniel Chapman, for example,
warned in the 1827 edition of his standard text on materia medica
that the drug would simply increase the patient's excitement. By
the 1840s, however, asylum superintendents were reporting great
benefits in all cases of insanity from the use of morphine, a derivative of opium that possessed its benefits without so many
unpleasant side effects. Samuel Woodward concluded in 1845,
"The manner in which morphine has been used in this and other

hospitals in this country, continuing it till the symptoms have subsided, then omitting it and seeing them return, then again and again removed by the renewal of the medicine, affords unequivocal evidence of its power to subdue maniacal excitements, relieve the delusions of the insane and restore the brain and nervous system to a sound and healthy state." The efficacy of morphine treatment further confirmed the asylum superintendents' belief that insanity had changed from a disease of inflammation to one of irritation.[83]

The redefinition of insanity as a functional disease caused by nervous debility also justified its treatment in the asylum. Since overstimulation of the nervous system usually caused mental disease, its cure required isolation and quiet so that the "disordered organ," as Amariah Brigham put it, could be left in "absolute repose." Furthermore, the insane needed to be removed from surroundings that had become associated with their morbid thoughts. However peaceful their homes, continuance there inevitably "aggravates the disease, as the improper association of ideas cannot be destroyed," stated T. Romeyn Beck. In the asylum, the patient not only could live quietly but also could be subjected to moral measures that would "awaken into activity the dormant faculties of the mind and . . . dispel delusions and melancholy trains of thought," as Amariah Brigham wrote.[84]

The special requirements for both medical and moral measures in the treatment of insanity necessitated the superintendent's absolute authority in the hospital, the asylum doctors concluded. To achieve the best results, the medical officer had to administer all forms of treatment. The superintendents considered the old practice of having a resident lay steward to direct moral measures and a visiting physician to handle medical care completely unacceptable. Professional influence was brought to bear on those asylums that did not give the medical superintendent sole authority, and by the 1840s, almost all American mental hospitals were operating under the direction of one physician. Those institutions such as the Bloomingdale Asylum that continued to place significant limits on the superintendent's control over asylum affairs received heavy criticism from the brethren. Pliny Earle, who served for five years at Bloomingdale, wrote in 1858, "Throughout the whole country, the Bloomingdale Asylum is the only one which still clings to that relic of the past, a collection of executive officers acting nearly independently of each other." He complained, "None but they who have learned from experience can comprehend the amount and the variety of evils which in its practical operation, flow from this system." The most successful institutions in the country, asylum doctors agreed, were those in which the superintendent was "least trammeled by superior authority."[85]

The superintendents' conceptualizations of insanity and its treatment became the basis not only for their position within the asylum but also for a larger advisory role in society. They believed that their inquiries into insanity had given them knowledge that, if properly applied, could improve the mental health of the whole community. As Edward Jarvis, a doctor in private practice who took an active role in the AMSAII, wrote, insanity "depended on some cause or causes within the control of man." Many cases of insanity might be prevented, he concluded, "if people were warned of these, and would take proper pains to guard against them or repel them." The asylum doctors' flexible etiological concepts allowed them to condemn all kinds of physical and social excesses as sources of insanity. Intemperate use of drugs, tobacco, and alcohol, masturbation, venereal indulgence, and improper diet and exercise were all characterized as physical abuses of the body that had a deleterious effect on the mind. Among the psychological dangers to be avoided were excessive study, reckless business activities, and domestic disharmony.[86] The superintendents placed special emphasis on the pernicious effect of misguided religious enthusiasm. Whereas "true religion" always had a beneficial effect on the mind, "fanaticism," as Earle styled it, had the power to overthrow the mental faculties. Amariah Brigham warned in 1835, "If a number of people be kept for a long time in a state of great terror and mental anxiety, no matter whether from vivid descriptions of hell and fears of 'dropping immediately into it,' or from any other cause, the brain and nervous system...[are]...liable to be injured."[87]

Concerned as the asylum superintendents were about the rising rate of insanity, they presented its increase as the inevitable price Americans had to pay for their advanced civilization. There would always be more mental disease, wrote Brigham, in a society "where people enjoy civil and religious freedom, where every person has liberty to engage in the strife for highest honors and stations in society, and where the road to wealth and distinction of every kind, is equally open to all." Edward Jarvis neatly summed up his contemporaries' view of the relationship between insanity and civilization in 1852:

The increase of knowledge, the improvement in the arts, the multiplication of comforts and the amelioration of manners, the growth of refinement, and the elevation of morals, do not of themselves disturb men's cerebral organs and create mental disorder. But with them come more opportunities and rewards for great and excessive mental action, more uncertain and hazardous employments and consequently more disappointments, more means and provocations for sensual indulgence, more dangers of accidents and injuries, more groundless hopes, and more painful struggle to obtain that which is beyond reach, or to effect that which is impossible.[88]

The special opportunities and rewards of American life made it all the more imperative, asylum doctors argued, to ensure that children received the proper moral education. They urged parents and teachers to see that good habits of mind and body were established during the "formative period of life." As John Fonerden, superintendent of the Maryland Insane Hospital, wrote, "The right growth of the brain in childhood is promoted or hindered by the habits which are formed in the nursery." If parents indulged their offspring and neglected this duty, insanity might very well be the price their children would pay.[89]

Although the flexibility of the asylum doctors' medical system allowed them to comment authoritatively on many social issues, it was not without its weaknesses. The imprecision involved in diagnosing the disease inevitably undercut their authority. Without reliable physical indicators of its presence, doctors had to detect insanity by observing the functional "derangements of intellect, sensations and motions" that it produced. As Brigham loosely defined them, symptoms consisted of either "derangement of the intellectual faculties, or prolonged changes of the feelings, affections, and habits of an individual." Diagnosis thus rested upon the generally accepted cultural standards that physicians used to distinguish sane from insane behavior. As long as no disagreement existed about these standards, the asylum doctors could easily rationalize their determination of an individual's sanity. But if any challenge arose, they had grave difficulties in producing scientific proof that their diagnosis was correct.[90]

Too much should not be made of the weakness of the asylum doctors' diagnostic abilities, however, for the medical system they developed commanded respect for several decades. In essence, the superintendents had devised a commonsense psychological medicine not unlike the commonsense philosophy of the time.[91] Their definition of insanity reflected popular beliefs about right behavior so widely held that they needed little confirmation. In addition, the asylum doctors' formulations provided a scientific explanation for the causes and treatment of insanity that served a variety of purposes for the larger society as well as for their own specialty. The strength of moral treatment, as its advocates interpreted it, lay not in its intellectual invincibility but in its ability to harmonize with the social needs of the period.

The superintendents' commonsense psychological medicine had an inherent appeal to a culture undergoing the rapid changes caused by economic growth and social dislocation. First, it reassured people that insanity, as well as all the signs of social disintegration they saw about them, was a natural result of progress. The increase in mental disease could be interpreted as a flattering tribute to the progressive character of American life. At the same time, the medical theory of insanity presented a scientific rationale for the ethic of self-control that so many looked to as a bulwark against social chaos. As Isaac Ray wrote, "if men were always correct in their ways, manners and habits, physical and moral, we should have little insanity." By forming good habits, individuals could avoid mental disorders. For those who refused to abide by the natural laws of human organization, the frightening prospect of insanity might be invoked as an incentive to reform. Thus, in a general sense, the medical model of insanity gave a scientific basis to the widespread emphasis on individual morality and self-control.[92]

The moral overtones of early asylum medicine reflected the tenuous balance between scientific and religious imperatives characteristic of mid-nineteenth-century medical thought. The superintendents were not unique in their tendency to conflate social and scientific truths; many physicians, as well as ministers and scientists, assumed a unity between natural and divine law.[93] Moreover, in a time of rapid social change, when many traditional forms of authority appeared to be faltering, health concerns became a logical focus for moral reform. Not all citizens went to church, but they all had bodies, which presumably they wished to maintain. Thus, appealing to the individual's desire for physical and mental well-being seemed an immediate, effective means to improve society.

By equating personal morality with health, reform-minded doctors hoped to create a universal moral code, shorn of theological issues that led to religious conflict, yet still suffused with divine authority. Subsequent generations found this blend of scientific and religious concerns unbearably sentimental or unscientific. But in their own time, the mid-century physicians' formulations seemed quite convincing.

For the asylum doctors, the task of setting a scientific imprimatur on traditional moral certainties had particular urgency. Although denouncing religious enthusiasm, they still appreciated the general desire for spiritual direction that prompted the religious ferment of the time. More importantly, the families of the insane often had an especially pressing need for reassurance and consolation. Because insanity struck at the very essence of the individual, destroying the personality and warping the moral sense, its onset, not surprisingly, prompted considerable soul searching and reflection by the family. To comfort them, asylum doctors had to address spiritual as well as scientific questions concerning the nature of insanity. As we shall see in Chapter 4, the superintendents' theories were well suited to offer this kind of reassurance.

By the 1840s, the first generation of asylum superintendents had devised a medical system to explain and treat insanity that nicely harmonized with the cultural preoccupations and conflicts of their time. They had also shown a precocious appreciation of the benefits to be gained by professional association. But the appeal of early asylum medicine, as demonstrated by the mental hospital's rapid growth between 1810 and 1850, can hardly be attributed to the strength of the superintendents' professional organization, the force of their intellectual formulations, or the originality of their social thought. Other mid-century reform movements – the utopian communities and the health reformers, for example – presented an equally relevant social commentary without achieving the institutional supremacy sought by this small group of physicians. However bold, the medical men's bid for authority had no automatic guarantee of success.

The asylum doctors succeeded in their bid for power largely because they devised an institution capable of meeting a deeply felt social need: the demand for a morally acceptable, humane alternate to family care of the insane. From this perspective, the elaborate structure of asylum medicine can best be understood as a post hoc rationale for the hospital's social utility. In other words, the superintendents' medical system *justified* rather than *created* a growing demand for institutional care. The specialty's real genius consisted not in their intellectual formulations or professional solidarity but in their ability, as moral entrepreneurs, to accommodate and legitimate the social forces impelling the insane out of the household and community. By providing a convincing medical rationale for asylum treatment, the asylum doctors forged a necessary link between general cultural concerns and specific institutional measures and, more importantly, between individual families and the hospital.

3

The burden of being their keepers

If asked where the best medical care in their community might be obtained, few of Thomas Story Kirkbride's contemporaries would have answered: the hospital. To the average citizen of the nineteenth century, good medical care was synonymous with *home* medical care. When stricken by a serious illness or injury, artisan and bank president alike hoped to be attended by their private physician and nursed by their female relatives, all within the familiar confines of home. The stage of medical knowledge at this time was such that the highest-quality care could as easily be provided there as anywhere else. Moreover, at the same time that hospitals offered no particular advantages in treatment, they exposed the sick to a far greater risk of infection and contagion. For the most part, institutional medical care fulfilled a charitable rather than a medical purpose; the general hospital existed primarily to provide care for those who lacked the money or family resources to be treated at home. The only sick people who immediately thought of hospitalization as a prospect, and hardly an attractive one, were either poor, friendless, or far from home.[1]

The success of nineteenth-century asylum treatment represented a radical departure from traditional attitudes toward the hospital. Many decades before the new surgery began to draw the comfortable classes into the private wards of late nineteenth-century general hospitals, mental institutions attracted patrons from every level of society.[2] In increasing numbers, families who could afford to provide private nursing and medical attendance for insane relatives chose to hospitalize them instead. Few made the decision without great reluctance and guilt, as we shall see; resistance to institutionalization remained very strong throughout this period. But other considerations eventually overcame the family's distrust or dislike of institutional care and persuaded them to patronize establishments such as the Pennsylvania Hospital for the Insane. Thus, the rise of moral treatment must be seen not only as a development in medical thought and practice but also as a significant change in lay conceptions of the hospital.

As might be expected, Kirkbride and his fellow superintendents were eager to encourage a more positive attitude toward hospitalization. The success of their professional enterprise depended largely upon their ability to overcome the family's distrust of institutional care. Of all the early asylum doctors, Kirkbride appears to have been the most sensitive to this dimension of the specialty's mission. In his relationship with the patients' families can be seen the genesis of Kirkbride's concern with institutional forms, a concern that dominated not only his own professional career but also the direction of the specialty itself for most of the nineteenth century.

Kirkbride's extensive correspondence with his asylum patrons reveals the changing lay attitudes toward insanity that prompted the nineteenth-century expansion of asylum treatment.[3] At the time of admission, relatives supplied an account of the patient's past history, including the onset of the illness, at Kirkbride's request. They often followed up these informal case histories with inquiries concerning the patient's progress and requests for special treatment. As a relative neared discharge, families sought Kirkbride's advice about post-hospital care; once the patient had gone home, they continued to report on his or her mental condition. From this voluminous correspondence can be documented the asylum patrons' conception of insanity and its causes; the circumstances leading to commitment, including prior treatment; and the dynamics of the doctor–patron relationship. Their accounts provide insight not only into the patrons' influence on Kirkbride's medical practice but also the social process of defining insanity.

The Pennsylvania Hospital for the Insane drew its patrons from every sector of society. A small sample of patient "securities," or individuals held responsible for board payments, matched with the 1870 manuscript census returns for Philadelphia reveals the following distribution of wealth: 19 percent listed no real estate or personal wealth; 27 percent had combined assets of less than $5,000; 24 percent had between $5,000 and $20,000; and 30 percent had more than $20,000. (The wealthiest patron in the sample possessed a fortune of more than $1,000,000.)[4] The structure of board rates provides another gauge of the patrons' financial status. Although the hospital maintained an average of 15 percent of its patients on the "free list," the vast majority of its clientele made some payment for treatment. Using 1855 as a representative year, we find 30 percent of the patients boarded for $3.50 per week or less; 42 percent paying $4.00–$5.00; 12 percent paying $6.00–$9.00; and 16 percent paying $10.00–$20.00. Assuming a rough correspondence between a family's assets and the assessment of board rates, this distribution confirms that a broad range of income groups utilized the corporate asylum, with the preponderance coming from the top half of society.[5]

LAY CONCEPTS OF INSANITY

Unfortunately, the hospital records do not provide enough information to distinguish among the specific concepts of insanity held by patrons of different social classes.[6] At best, relying on the internal evidence in the letters themselves, some crude generalizations about class and concepts of insanity can be drawn. Those patrons who, by the style of their correspondence, seem to have been well educated and affluent naturally demonstrated the greatest familiarity with prevailing medical concepts of insanity. A number were physicians themselves, and thus able to give detailed medical histories of their relatives. At the other extreme, Kirkbride's poor, barely literate correspondents, many from rural backgrounds, lacked sophisticated concepts or terms with which to describe mental disorders. Yet, regardless of their varying levels of sophistication, the patrons all employed the same basic language of disease: Individuals were spoken of as "sick" or "well," "disordered" or "cured," and their behaviors were referred to as "symptoms" or "manifestations" of disease. As the lowest common denominator of belief, Kirkbride's clientele possessed a rudimentary conception of insanity as a disease and believed it to have both physical and psychological origins.[7]

Those patrons who ventured an opinion on the disease's etiology usually implicated the nervous system. Only a few, echoing Benjamin Rush's line of reasoning, blamed the blood "rushing to the head" or "pressing on the brain" for derangement.[8] The majority considered "disordered" or "irritated" nerves to be the root cause of insanity. As the patrons crudely conceived it, the nervous system transmitted the shock of a stressful event to the brain, leaving it debilitated. Depending on the individual's personality, stress might depress the intellect and emotions, producing stupor or melancholia, or cause a maniacal outburst, or excitement. Although formulated in very simplistic terms, the patrons' understanding of the nervous system's role in producing insanity was easily compatible with more sophisticated medical concepts of the disease.

Asylum patrons apparently had little difficulty in regarding insanity as a physical malady. Like medical men, they saw the mind and body as inextricably linked and believed that a disturbance in one inevitably affected the other. In accounting for the onset of a relative's insanity, patrons mentioned a host of physical ills, including rheumatism, inflammation of the lungs, and fevers of all varieties. Uterine disease was cited in some women's cases. In several instances, family members asked that a female relative be given a gynecological examination on admission to the hospital to discover if "derangement of the womb" had caused her mental disease. Patrons also mentioned physical shocks to the body, such as falls, tooth extraction, overexposure, and sudden changes of temperature. In a typical letter, a woman trying to account for her husband's derangement recalled that after taking a night ride in the wind and rain, he complained of a "coldness" in his head; therefore, she deduced that "some chilling or stunning effect of the rain" had produced his "painful excitement."[9]

Along with physical disease and trauma, patrons often cited disturbances in normal bodily functions as causes of mental instability. Many lay accounts mentioned the "morbid state of the bowels," as manifested in constipation or diarrhea. A husband attributed his wife's attack of excitement to "her having been eating heavily for over two days and having nothing pass her bowels." Similarly, a man attributed his brother's derangement to "suppression of hemorrhoidal discharge." With women patients, lay explanations for insanity frequently involved the menses. Some patrons related the disorder to a suppression of the menstrual flow; others noted that it grew more violent during the "courses." Menopause, or, as one correspondent described it, "the period of life which is so critical with most women," was often linked with insanity in middle-aged females. The cessation of his wife's menses, a man confidently told Kirkbride, had been the "one great cause of the derangement of her nervous system."[10]

Some correspondents associated the habitual use of tobacco,

liquor, and drugs with the onset of insanity. "He has been in the habit of using tobacco, which is thought to affect his nervous system very much," reported one such account. In similar language, a patron stated that a relative's "continual use of strong drink for some years past has...weakened his mind." Although these statements referred in part to the corrosive effect of stimulants on the individual's moral sensibilities, they also implied that the substances damaged the nervous system itself.[11]

The asylum patrons' belief that insanity had a physical basis received reinforcement from the general physical debility of the insane. The headaches, dizziness, and pains their deranged relatives complained of were perceived as physical concomitants of mental disease. A patron noted, for example, that her daughter "often presses her hands upon her head, and otherwise indicates that the seat of her suffering is there." Whether seen as symptoms or causes of the mental disorders, the patients' many physical ailments reinforced the notion that mind and body were closely linked in insanity and must be treated simultaneously.[12]

Although often citing physical causes and symptoms of derangement, asylum patrons wrote more extensively and fluently about the psychological origins of insanity. No doubt, as lay people they found it easier to explain a relative's mental distress in terms of personal disappointments or anxieties rather than more obscure physiological changes. In accounting for insanity, patrons cited the same psychological factors recognized by asylum doctors: grief, anxiety over the sick, business losses, intense application to work or study, unrequited love, and the like. In most cases, family members conceived of the damage done to the patient's mind by these mental stresses as gradual and cumulative in nature. In a typical account, a wife explained to Kirkbride that after suffering financial reverses several years ago, her husband had "applied himself so closely to business as to injure his general health and nervous system." More rarely, patrons attributed a relative's derangement to a single grave emotional trauma. In one instance, a woman explained that her uncle had been at Ford's Theater the night Lincoln was shot and never recovered from that "great shock." The notion that a single, overpowering experience could permanently affect the mind had the appeal of providing a simple, immediate explanation for a relative's behavior. By this line of reasoning, a patron blamed a young man's insanity on a single visit to an "anatomical museum," or pornography shop, which made "an impression which I fear resulted in the ruin of his mind."[13]

However dramatic or even plausible the asylum patrons' etiological conjectures might seem, they still represented no more than post hoc justifications of a relative's mental state. Faced with a distressing change in a loved one's behavior and personality, family members cast about for a reassuring explanation of its origins, and had little difficulty in finding some physical or psychological disturbance in the individual's recent past to serve as a plausible cause. The list of questions concerning the patient's mental and physical condition before the disorder's onset, which Kirkbride included with the admission forms, no doubt helped the family discover an explanation. The imprecision or implausibility of their conclusions mattered little, since the patrons' etiological conjectures served only to confirm a judgment arrived at on other grounds. As their letters make evident, asylum patrons had decided that a relative was insane long before they began to speculate on the disorder's origins or even to think of consulting a doctor. As a result, they could give fuller and more precise accounts of the characteristics that led them to define an individual as insane. In retrospect, the standards or symptoms that lay people used to distinguish sane from insane behavior form a more consistent pattern than their attempts to locate the psychological or physical origins of mental disease.[14]

A patron's account of his son's mental deterioration, as copied into a hospital casebook, nicely illustrates the kinds of distinctions lay observers used to identify insanity. According to the youth's father, George had returned home from law school in a melancholy mood. "At this period, for the first time, some peculiarity was observed in his manners and habits – he became irritable and cross, but this was attributed merely to bad temper," the father recalled. Then George's appetite began to increase alarmingly; he would go out into the fields nightly and eat raw corn and cabbage, "declaring as a reason for it that his hunger was so excessive that night after night he was unable to close his eyes in sleep." At this point, his parents began to doubt that George suffered solely from bad temper; yet, they resisted the idea that he was insane because he continued to care for himself, do errands, and read occasionally. Then George began to talk to himself, refused to wear clothes, and burned his books, saying that his younger brothers "should not have a chance to pore over them as he had done." Over the past year, the youth had become dull and incoherent. His parents now believed George to be insane, but sought hospital treatment only after he had had a "fit of some kind" in addition to his other symptoms.[15]

By specifying the behaviors that led relatives to conclude that an individual had "lost his reason," as patrons often put it, accounts such as George's history provide insight into the social definition of insanity. To begin with, the letters from lay persons furnish a descriptive survey of the *range* of behaviors recognized as indications of mental aberration. Although conveying little sense of the dynamic process by which certain individuals became identified as mentally disturbed, a catalog of the symptoms mentioned in the patrons' accounts allows us to map the broad distinctions between sanity and insanity as recognized in the mid-nineteenth century. Imposing a minimum of order on the patrons' accounts, the characteristics repeatedly cited in lay definitions of insanity can be grouped roughly into four categories: loss of cognitive faculties, disturbances in basic living habits, debilitating mental states or moods, and delusions or bizarre beliefs.[16]

Asylum patrons frequently associated insanity with an inability to think and speak coherently. When deranged, their relatives could not express connected thoughts or even form complete sentences. Some patients had lost their memory, could no longer give a correct account of past events, or could not recognize old acquaintances. In a typical letter, a patron described his insane brother as "at a loss to articulate" and unable to name "his most intimate friends." Similarly, an aged insane woman appeared "much confused about places, persons and dates," her brother wrote, "and thinks those living long since dead."[17]

Second, lay accounts often cited extreme or abrupt changes in a person's living habits as symptoms of mental derangement. Some patrons described insane relatives who slept only a few minutes or hours at a time, or who lost several nights' sleep in succession. At the opposite extreme, individuals who "lay in bed I think quite too much," as a farmer wrote of his wife, concerned other patrons. The same extremes figured in observations about eating patterns. "She has no appetite for her food, eats very little, scarcely one spoonful at a meal" was a common complaint. Conversely, patients gave "evidences of a diseased mind" by developing "a morbid appetite that no reasonable amount of food could satisfy."

Mental distress altered work habits, relatives observed. The disturbed individual might have begun to labor more obsessively; a patron decided that her sister was "not right," for example, when she began "to commence her washing at night...wash all night and next night iron." Other patients forgot how to perform simple tasks. A husband, in describing his wife's symptoms, noted that she still sewed and knitted, but "as often did both wrong as right." Some patrons expressed concern because a relative had ceased to work entirely, as in the case of a farmer's son who would not do his chores because they "worried" him. A man noted of his wife, "As her work accumulates or any extended amount of it presents itself, she yields to feelings and thoughts and loses perseverance to accomplish it." Many letters mentioned an unusual restlessness among the insane. "In her uneasiness," wrote a patron of her deranged daughter, she "moves about the house a great deal in the course of the day." Conversely, other patrons worried about relatives who sat silent and motionless for hours on end. A woman so stricken told her husband that she could hardly move, "her trouble [was] so great."[18]

Asylum patrons often linked such disturbances in living habits with a third category of symptoms, the debilitating mental states or moods suffered by the insane. Their descriptions suggest at least three distinct states lay people associated with derangement: excitement, melancholy, and irritability. Lay observers used the word "excitement" to signify violent periods of agitation or turmoil. When excited, an individual would become very distressed or angry, talk loudly or irrationally, have "attacks of crying," and even attempt violence against bystanders. In one case, a woman's excitement had become so violent that two people had "to sit or stand by her, to prevent injury from being inflicted upon her own person, and upon her attendant....She cannot sleep, talks nearly all the time, and is made worse by the presence of her husband." Such violent "paroxysms" or "ebullitions of passion," as various accounts termed them, usually alternated with spells of calmness and lucidity. The rapidity and severity of the alterations in mood made excitement all the more frightening a symptom. As a mother described it, her daughter was transformed into a stranger, hurling "furious imprecating curses on everybody," attempting to "hurt those who approach her, wishing everybody dead, and sometimes threatening to kill herself."[19]

A less furious but equally distressing mental state was characterized by constant, severe depression, variously described by lay observers as "despondency," "gloom," and "melancholy." Relatives often bemoaned formerly cheerful individuals who now viewed everything "through the darkest medium." One patron relayed her husband's own eloquent description of his depression: "I don't know what it is but I feel something, a cloud, a sort of fatality, weaving, weaving, weaving, itself around me." When left alone he "walks and weeps and moans incessantly," the wife noted. Vocal expressions of melancholy often gave way to "silent agony," as another observer described it; her relative would sit, "her frame being more or less convulsed, her lips firmly compressed and her eyes staring and motionless."[20]

Besides excitement and depression, patrons described several less extreme mental states characteristic of insanity. Many disturbed patients, according to relatives, suffered from nervous irritability. A woman termed "exceedingly nervous and sensitive to opposition" was "much annoyed by any sudden noise, as the harsh closing of doors and the like," her family noted, "and when thus excited is quite irritable." The insane also exhibited an unhealthy state of mind by being "very much disturbed at times . . . by trifles which would not cost a strong healthy person a thought," as one patron put it. "The most trivial accident," complained another woman, caused her sister to make "unnaturally pitiful lamentations." A disordered mind sometimes produced extreme states of anxiety, seemingly unrelated to real probabilities. In one case, a woman's "constant dread of being torn to pieces by dogs" kept her from sleeping at night. Another patient had a terrible fear of death; "she wants to ride in the carriage and not die, but when riding, she wants to go home and not die – her desire for the change being evidently founded in an apprehension of danger and a hope of security," a relative reported.[21]

Although loss of cognitive faculties, disturbances in living habits, and debilitating mental states all figure prominently in the patrons' descriptions of insanity, delusions remained the most distinctive trait of the disorder, as far as they were concerned. In other words, this category of symptoms seemed the most compelling in forcing relatives to designate an individual's mental distress as insanity rather than mere eccentricity or bad temper. The bizarre beliefs that engrossed their deranged relatives held a peculiar fascination for Kirkbride's correspondents. Many letters described the "singular ideas" expressed by the insane in some detail. A carpenter's "notion of a gas rising from his abdomen and issuing out of his ear with a wurring noise" seemed incontrovertible proof to his family that the man was insane, despite his rationality on all other subjects. Similarly, a doctor described the unusual delusion of a mother of six who "supposes everything is more or less touched with or stained with sperm or adamantine – one drop or speck is as bad as a larger quantity," so she believed; "she is perfectly sane on all subjects but sperm." The delusions mentioned by the asylum patrons covered a wide variety of topics: the patient's own identity, persecution by organized conspiracies, possession by supernatural forces, convictions of religious damnation, and prejudices against family members. The patrons' remarks on delusional thinking are especially interesting for what they indicate about the limits of "right belief" on such topics as religion and family relationships in the mid-nineteenth century.[22]

At a time when universal salvation, the innate goodness of human nature, and the harmony between spiritual and secular concerns were becoming dominant themes in mainstream American Protestantism, the patrons' definition of religious delusions, not surprisingly, centered on too pessimistic or otherworldly beliefs. Family members frequently mentioned unwarranted convictions of sin and damnation as symptoms of insanity. To stop eating because as a transgressor one deserved no food, or to interpret one's mental anguish as God's punishment for a sinful life were simply not acceptable religious beliefs by many patrons' standards. They also mentioned overzealous religious practices, such as excessive Bible reading, too exacting observance of Lent, and adoption of old-style Quaker dress as signs of mental instability. Spiritually induced withdrawals from the world were viewed with disapproval. A father described his son's inclination to "dwell upon the millennium, spiritual changes, [and] destruction of the world" as "injurious to his mind." Similarly, a husband gave as an example of his wife's delusional state the conviction that, "believing all mankind but herself under condemnation," she had come to "refuse all intercourse with the world."[23]

Asylum patrons also made frequent reference to delusions concerning animal magnetism, spiritualism, and mesmerism. A man specified as a symptom of his sister's disease her belief that "she has charge of a set of spirits which she calls, translates and talks to and of...as she would a family of small children." Another woman, "insane upon the subject of magnetism," refused to take responsibility for her misbehavior, claiming that "a certain set of persons" had the "power over her to will her to do acts." The loss of individual volition inherent in such delusions seemed particularly distressing to relatives. At times, the patient's thinking shaded into a belief in demonic possession, as in the case of a farmer who claimed that the devil "kept coming up through his throat trying to choke him."[24]

Significantly, asylum patrons used the term "delusion" to denote not only bizarre beliefs such as these but also expressions of hostility or indifference toward family members. In fact, delusions or "perverted feelings," as one observer termed them, concerning relatives were among the most commonly cited symptoms of insanity. In describing the onset of the illness, patrons often noted that their relatives had been "devotedly attached" to the family until disease set them against their "nearest and dearest friends." A man cited his brother's loss of interest in their mother as a sign of insanity: "Since this mental disease came upon him, he has not noticed her in any way." Concerning his brother, the patron concluded, "so long as he desires to go to California and avoid his kindred, his disease is in full force." A husband found it quite unnatural that after a long absence, his wife "did not appear to be at all affected by the meeting with her children and friends." A lack of balance in familial affections also figured in descriptions of the insane. A man gave as a conclusive example of his sister's "great eccentricity" the fact that she refused to let one particular relative come near her. In another case, relatives complained about a woman who was "ruining" her son by sleeping with him rather than her husband; in addition, she so completely centered her "maternal affections" on the boy that her daughter suffered from neglect.[25]

A husband's account of his bride's "morbid notions" about marriage offers an interesting perspective on marital expectations. The patron committed his bride of a few months as the first step in obtaining an annulment. To secure Kirkbride's assistance in the suit, the disgruntled groom gave a lengthy account of the woman's insane "delusions" about marriage. She felt "the absence of any conscious feeling of affection" for him, he wrote, although she "invariably spoke of me in the highest terms." Other symptoms included an "intense dread of child bearing" and a "morbid abhorrence of and disgust at the idea of conjugal cohabitation." The wife attributed all her mental "troubles," the man concluded, to the "fact that she was a married woman, and as such, had assumed responsibilities to which she imagined herself constitutionally unequal." The husband's willingness to sue for annulment on these grounds suggests that lack of affection and extreme sexual frigidity fell outside the bounds of normal marriage even in Victorian times.[26]

A catalog of the delusions and other traits identified by asylum patrons as manifestations of madness provides some sense of the boundaries between sane and insane behavior in the mid-nineteenth century. But simply listing the symptoms cited in the accounts gives little insight into the *dynamic* process by which individuals became identified as deranged. In themselves, none of the symptoms described above constituted insanity. In other words, someone could be incoherent, depressed, or hostile toward kinfolk without being categorized as insane. The *severity* and *context* of the abnormal behaviors played a crucial role in distinguishing that special state lay observers classified as mental illness.[27]

First, the insane described in lay accounts almost always suffered from multiple symptoms, including loss of cognitive faculties, disruptions in living habits, debilitating mental states, and delusions. Their aberrations had persisted for months, even years, and had severely incapacitated them. Insanity, as opposed to mere eccentricity or ill temper, a distinction many observers drew, always involved a crippling degree of dysfunction, including an inability to perform the simplest tasks necessary for survival, unresponsiveness to human contact, and an almost complete withdrawal from the circumstances considered to be reality by the rest of society.

Second, the asylum patrons distinguished insanity from other states having similar symptoms by the *context* of the unusual behavior. If present from birth, an inability to form connected thoughts would be termed "idiocy"; if apparent only during a fever, it would be called "delirium." Insomnia and lack of appetite soon after a loved one's death would be viewed as normal concomitants of grief. A conviction of damnation developed during a revival meeting might be seen as a sign of religious awakening. The interpretation of the unusual behavior clearly depended upon its appropriateness in relation to both the individual's recent experience and the prevailing social custom.

In sum, insanity, as the asylum patrons defined it, represented a "great change in natural disposition and bearing" rather than a fixed set of symptoms. Lay observers identified mental disease by the radical, often lasting transformation it wreaked on a familiar personality; the element of sudden change, not a particular behavior or delusion, struck the family most forcefully in their perception of insanity. As one patron said of her son's disorder, "the sudden change from being lovely and amiable to opposite habits I scarcely can realize as true." A girl "naturally of a cheerful, gay and child-like disposition,...seldom even...serious or melancholy" became deeply depressed. A young man "fond of company and much disposed to indulge in debate, fun, etc." suddenly began to "seclude himself from society." In such a way, patrons identified insanity as a disease that turned its victim into a different sort of person.[28]

Of course, in some cases patrons acknowledged that the individual's disposition had always been difficult or unpleasant. Some patients were described as "naturally imperious or dictatorial," "highly nervous," or simply "perverse" since childhood. A man wrote of his insane daughter that her "eccentricity in many respects...became marked at the time of puberty." Among her early peculiarities, he noted, were "hostility to all real and true friends" (i.e., her family), "enthusiastic devotion to strangers," and "unsteady pursuit of objects of excitement, first books, then visiting...to the neglect of all else." A man described his brother in similar terms: "From a very small child he has seemed to be different from other persons, being moody, apparently melancholy, associating scarcely at all with other boys nor seeming to mingle with and enjoy their sports, ungovernable at home and entirely impatient of parental authority and control." The line between eccentricity and insanity was very indefinite in such cases. Often, the distinction consisted of nothing more than the family's reluctance to acknowledge the severity of the disorder. In the last mentioned case, the patron recalled, "the family were unwilling to believe him unsound in his mind though they could not but fear that it might be so." Only when the youth suffered "a real period of complete derangement," in which he was "unable to care for self, unconscious of all," did his relatives give up the hope that his problems were "only eccentricity."[29]

Despite the uncertain boundary between the two states, asylum patrons did recognize a fundamental difference between eccentricity and insanity. The latter, more serious disorder involved an otherness, a total alienation from self and society, not to be found in the eccentric. Those who had completely lost their minds had a strangeness, an unquiet about them that their families found extremely disturbing. In part, the patrons' uneasiness must have stemmed from a deep-seated fear of the unpredictable and sometimes violent nature of insanity. The recognition that none of the usual assumptions governing human interactions could be relied upon in their dealings with an insane relative no doubt contributed to the patrons' anxiety. Although their sentiments were less obvious than the instincts that brought their eighteenth-century forebears to "gaze unfeelingly" on the hospital lunatics, the patrons' letters nonetheless conveyed the same mixture of fearfulness and curiosity in contemplating the insane.[30]

Given the stigma attached to insanity, it is hardly surprising that relatives proved reluctant to acknowledge the severity of a relative's aberration. Quite understandably, they preferred to explain strange behaviors as signs of ill temper or eccentricity as long as they could. Not infrequently, patrons mentioned that someone outside the household had first recognized the patient's apparent derangement. A man writing to Kirkbride concerning his wife noted that his neighbors had first told him that "something was wrong with her mind." After they made this observation, he wrote, "I watched her very closely and, for some time, I could not say that I thought so." She had headaches, seemed unnecessarily quiet, and often sat with her head in her hands, the husband noted, but did not seem deranged to him. Not until she "got worse" and began to "talk foolish" did he see that his neighbors had been right.[31]

TREATMENT CHOICES BEFORE COMMITMENT

Once convinced that a relative was truly insane, families did not necessarily seek asylum treatment immediately. Most arrived at the decision to commit with the same reluctance they had shown in recognizing the disorder in the first place. As Kirkbride's patrons freely admitted to him, they had exhausted all alternative forms of treatment before even thinking of his institution. Only after the measures short of institutionalization had failed to alleviate the disorder's severity did the patients' families seriously contemplate the asylum as a "last resort."[32]

In the early stages of insanity, family members often attempted to reason with or scold a relative into behaving more acceptably. A man responded to his wife's growing melancholy, he wrote Kirkbride, by portraying her woes as "only supposed difficulties." When she professed to be too depressed by her "sad thoughts" to do housework, he sought "to erase these ideas by suggesting indolence as the cause, and "scolded and entreated but never openly sympathized – endeavoring to eradicate them as foolish imaginations." In addition, relatives devised activities, such as light physical exercise, music, and handicrafts, to distract or soothe the sufferer. They often passed on the results of these efforts to help Kirkbride in planning the patient's hospital regimen. "Our home experience," noted one patron, "has been that she was always much better after a long drive." When necessary, relatives took turns keeping a deranged family member "under our observation continually by day and by night," as a relative wrote, to guard against violent or suicidal propensities. Those families who could afford it often hired a private nurse to attend and amuse the patient.[33]

If an individual's mental aberration persisted, relatives turned to their family doctor for assistance. As with a purely physical disorder, they thought of home treatment for insanity as the first and most desirable form of medical intervention. The patrons' accounts, along with the letters written to Kirkbride by the physicians themselves, indicate that general practitioners in both the city and the countryside treated a substantial number of mental cases and played a crucial role in referring patients to the mental hospital.

By and large, private practitioners confined their medical attention to the physical imbalance that they believed to be the cause of the mental derangement. The majority presumed that "too much determination of blood to the brain" produced insanity, and bled their patients accordingly. Although the old-fashioned among them continued to use the lancet, most doctors relied on local depletion by cups or leeches applied to the temples. Blisters were frequently applied to the patient's neck as a means of counterirritation. Along with bleeding and blisters, general practitioners prescribed medicines to correct disorders of the stomach and bowels that they frequently thought to be a source of insanity. Calomel and croton oil seemed "well suited" to the disease, opined one doctor, and could be administered easily. Similarly, physicians valued purgatives and emetics for their ability to keep the "system in proper condition" and change "the character of the secretions." To calm excited or sleepless patients, many gave narcotics, most commonly morphine or hyoscamus. Overall, home medical treatment aimed, as one physician succinctly stated, at "restoring secretion of urine, regulating the bowels, procuring sleep and giving 'tone' to the nervous and muscular system."[34]

Only a few general practitioners professed therapeutic nihilism when confronted with a case of insanity. It was a rare doctor who admitted that "I am giving her no medicine." As one physician concluded, "some physicians in these cases blister and bleed, to be doing something, but I choose to let her alone." After bleeding, purging, and blistering a deranged man without success, another doctor tried moral measures. "I recommended mild management and deportment towards him and endeavored to gain his confidence so as to converse freely about the subjects on which his mind was deranged," he informed Kirkbride. For a time, this plan had proven "most efficacious," the doctor concluded, but the patient eventually grew worse.[35]

General practitioners often mentioned the difficulties they encountered in home medical management of insanity. Since most had urged the family to commit an insane relative (or else they would not be writing to the superintendent), they willingly admitted that their own efforts to control the patient had proved ineffective. Usually, the general practitioner had failed to control the violent excitements of insanity. One provided Kirkbride with a long list of drugs with which he had unsuccessfully tried to overcome a female patient's fit: musk, camphor, asafetida, ammonia, ether, warm pedilura with mustard, and morphine. When the morphine failed to calm her, the physician recommended asylum treatment. Another doctor reached the same conclusion after repeated inhalations of chloroform allowed his patient to sleep only ten to twenty-five minutes at a time. "Our stock of chloroform is running low," he concluded, so the hospital seemed the only answer.[36]

Doctors also complained that a proper regimen could not be maintained in the home. "Having entire control of herself," commented a physician on a difficult patient, she "has indulged her appetite with everything she desired, mostly fruits and confectionary and thus made herself much worse." Lack of control over the patient proved especially troublesome in cases involving drug or alcohol abuse. Wrote a doctor of an opium addict, "you must be aware of the great disadvantage we labor under in the management of such a case in private practice, when the patient is accustomed to [being] indulged with everything his disordered imagination may suggest to him, while at the same time he is annoyed constantly with the visits of his kind, but too officious friends."[37]

Having encountered such problems in private practice, physicians could better appreciate the advantages of asylum care. "The facilities afforded for treatment in such an institution are so superior to any in private practice," said one doctor in recommending a patient, "that no conscientious physician should hesitate in his advice." Kirkbride's physician correspondents also stressed the value of specialization in medical care of mental disease. Wrote a Baltimore doctor, "I myself have seen very little of insanity," and thus preferred to send his patient to a physician with "ample and wide experience. . . in the treatment and management of the insane among the better classes." General practitioners believed that the asylum had additional assets for addicts; "compulsory privation of drink, therapeutic remedies, moral enlightenment and encouragement with mental recreation and physical employment, all of which a Hospital like yours alone affords," seemed to them excellent treatment for alcoholism.[38]

General practitioners, if properly convinced of asylum medicine's merit, thus became an invaluable source of referrals for Kirkbride. With their more direct, intimate contact with the families of the insane, they became some of the Pennsylvania Hospital for the Insane's most effective ambassadors. A family physician's counsel often played a crucial role in convincing patrons to consider asylum treatment. Coming from a trusted medical man, the opinion that "but little benefit would arise from treatment at home," as one doctor put it, had considerable weight with the family. For this reason, Kirkbride greatly valued his contacts with his "professional brethren," as he referred to general practitioners. The more doctors who knew about his hospital, the better they could combat the "false imaginations most fertile regarding the inhuman treatment" of patients, fears that delayed many commitments. To cultivate his referral system, Kirkbride circulated his annual reports to local physicians, arranged asylum tours for local medical societies, and campaigned for the inclusion of lectures on asylum medicine in medical school curricula. As he wrote in his *Report* for 1846, "the judicious counsel given to their friends, by the family physician, contributes most essentially to the comfort of the physician of a hospital for the insane – to the success of his treatment, and to the character of the institution with which he is connected."[39]

In the 1870s, the pattern of referrals from the general practitioner to the asylum doctor was somewhat complicated by the rise of neurology. A medical specialty devoted to the study and treatment of both organic and functional nervous disorders, neurology represented a serious challenge to the asylum doctors' jurisdiction over insanity. (The conflict between the two specialities will be discussed in more detail in Chapter 6.) Criticizing asylum medicine on both scientific and administrative grounds, neurologists offered new extramural alternatives to the mental hospital: office or hospital outpatient treatment involving elaborate electrical devices, and a regimen of total bed rest and special diet that could be provided either in the patient's home or the physician's private clinic. For families anxious to avoid the stigma of institutionalization, the neurologists' treatment had obvious appeal. By the last decade of Kirkbride's career, his wealthier patients often came to him only after seeing a specialist in nervous diseases, such as Silas Weir Mitchell. Mitchell's lectures and writings on nervous disorders, among them the popular works *Wear and Tear* and *Fat and Blood*, gained him national recognition as a leading neurologist, as well as an extensive private practice.[40]

Despite their evident differences with the asylum superintendents, Philadelphia neurologists did not take an irrevocably hostile stance toward Kirkbride and his institution. When patients seemed too violently disturbed to be treated by their methods, neurologists referred them to the Pennsylvania Hospital for the Insane. Although an outspoken critic of asylum medicine, Mitchell himself maintained an apparently cordial relationship with his father's old friend, and occasionally sent Kirkbride patients. In one case, he referred an affluent young man with a history of "mental oddities" who compulsively committed small thefts. Mitchell believed that the youth suffered from "moral insanity," that is, derangement of the moral or emotional faculties without intellectual impairment, and asked Kirkbride "to take charge of him for a brief period until the effect of a stern naval discipline can be tried."[41]

Whether recommended by a neurologist or a general practitioner, the necessity of asylum treatment still proved difficult for many families to accept. As a halfway measure, they often sent their mentally deranged relatives to a spa or health resort. The numerous health-care establishments available in the mid-nineteenth century offered a variety of therapies that were mostly dependent upon mineral water baths and drinks, plain diet, and light exercise. Less regimented and forbidding than an asylum, such resorts had an obvious appeal to affluent clients suffering from nervous disorders. Many patients came to the asylum only after a resort stay had failed to help them. One patron noted that a prolonged residence in an "institution for cold water treatment" had improved his brother's "liver complaint" and general health, but not his insanity, "for which their treatment is not adapted."[42]

Rather than patronize the more public and less regimented facilities of a spa, some families tried boarding insane relatives in private asylums run either by laymen or doctors. Although less common than in England, small private asylums existed throughout the United States. Several of the better-known establishments, such as Sanford Hall in Flushing, New York, and the Woodbrook Retreat outside Philadelphia, were run by former asylum doctors. Affluent families found the privacy, security, and comfort of these small establishments well worth the price; yet, like the spas, they had their limitations. Some asylum keepers refused to take difficult or dangerous patients. A man boarding his wife in a private home wrote to Kirkbride, asking the superintendent to commit her because "the persons with whom she is living are so much terrified with her threats to kill them and to burn the house that they will keep her no longer." Private asylums could also prove ephemeral. Patrons of a small Cincinnati establishment wrote to Kirkbride concerning the transfer of an "unmanageable and even dangerous relative" after the doctor had to close it, "for want of means as he has to pay a large rent and has but a few patients."[43]

THE COMMITMENT DECISION

As their search for alternatives demonstrates, the families of the insane followed a very torturous pathway to the mental hospital in the mid-nineteenth century. After deciding that an individual was suffering from true insanity, a long process in itself, relatives exhausted every form of extramural treatment they could afford. Even when other measures proved ineffective, patrons waited for months, sometimes years, before applying to the asylum as a last resort. In most cases, their decision to commit came only after a prolonged period of escalating tension and desperation culminated in a crisis; some event or situation that could be neither ignored nor tolerated finally tipped the balance of considerations in favor of the asylum.[44]

The case of Mrs. R, a patient admitted in 1879, illustrates the complex dynamics often involved in the commitment process. Her mother had inquired about committing the widowed Mrs. R soon after her mental disorder became apparent. But other relatives proved "so averse to placing her in an asylum" that they sent her to a spa for the water cure instead. Mrs. R remained there for a year without benefit, returning home only to grow worse. Her relatives next took her to see several noted neurologists, who pronounced her case hopeless. Again the subject of commitment came up, but as the mother wrote, "we could not make up our minds to do so, as she was so intelligent on some subjects, read, painted, played on the piano, and took an interest in many things." Then one of Mrs. R's sons died. She showed no grief, yet her delusions became more "fixed." Believing herself "persecuted by spiritualists, who are always talking to her," she carried on conversations with imaginary persons, "asking and answering questions in a loud agitated voice," day and night. Mrs. R's relatives finally decided to commit her to the Pennsylvania Hospital for the Insane because her behavior had clearly begun to affect her two young sons.[45]

Like Mrs. R's mother, patrons frequently explained to Kirkbride why they had been forced to place a relative in his care, almost as if seeking absolution for the act. Their accounts of the circumstances leading to commitment help to reveal the interplay between the patient's condition and the family's choice of treatment, as well as suggesting the limits of tolerance to certain kinds of disruptive behavior. By presenting their justifications for the commitment decision, the patrons' letters pinpoint the factors that tended to eliminate the preference for household care of the insane.

Outbreaks or threats of violence most quickly overcame the

family's resistance to asylum treatment. The fits of excitement often characteristic of the disorder rendered an insane relative "dangerous at times and alarming to his family," as one letter put it. Prospective patrons often regarded commitment as conditional upon their ability to control the patient. "If he should become so violent [that] we could not keep him at home," one woman wrote of her husband, then the family would need Kirkbride's services. In a typical case, a man brought to the asylum had shown marked symptoms of insanity for more than a year, but only recently had become violent. "As he is now," a neighbor wrote Kirkbride, "it is necessary to keep him bound, for he is constantly seeking an opportunity to kill his wife and children."[46]

Patrons worried about their relatives' self-destructive tendencies as well as their outwardly directed violence. Suicidal attempts or intentions prompted many admissions to Kirkbride's mental hospital. An individual might suffer for months from depression or "distressed feelings" without being considered a fit candidate for the asylum, but let family members detect preparation for suicide, and commitment would swiftly follow. Likewise, a relative's persistent refusal to eat or sleep, if potentially life-threatening, spurred intervention. A man whose wife had not eaten for three days brought her to the hospital when her countenance "showed the marks of her abstinence," hoping that "some means may be found to force her to take nourishment immediately." In a similar case, the family realized that a relative who would not sleep "must surely sink from exhaustion." Some patrons grew apprehensive when disturbed individuals were in any way liable to injure themselves, even unintentionally. One young man "much inclined to ramble away" had recently endangered his life on impromptu jaunts, once by starting an unattended locomotive and another time by trying to swim a broad river. Confinement, it seemed obvious, was the only way to prevent the youth from inadvertently doing away with himself.[47]

At the same time that patrons feared a relative's capacity for violence or self-injury, they were very reluctant to adopt extreme measures, such as straitjackets or muffs, to secure the patient in the home. Quite understandably, the prospect of keeping a loved one permanently confined or secluded horrified them. Thus, once an individual was "obliged to be confined," as a patron put it, the family considered commitment much more seriously. Faced with a choice between two unpleasant measures, physical restraint in the home or commitment to the asylum, patrons came to decide that the latter was less offensive to their sensibilities. Rather than have a "madwoman in the attic," they chose to brave the "horrors of the madhouse."[48]

Although violence and self-destructiveness often prompted action, asylum patrons had other, less dramatic reasons for seeking hospital treatment as well. Sometimes the behavior of the deranged relative was simply so disruptive that the family could no longer tolerate his or her presence in the household. Fear of public embarrassment contributed in no small part to the family's lessening tolerance. When a relative's behavior could no longer be controlled, humiliating incidents inevitably occurred. For example, a woman described these events leading up to her daughter's commitment: The girl had gone to the home of a neighbor whom she felt to be a special friend. When no one answered her knock, "she would not be moved from the door but continued knocking until her sister at last got her home." The same scene took place several times a day until, "finding we could do nothing with her," her mother brought her to the asylum. Another deranged young woman meant to leave home and marry a man her family believed she hardly knew. They saw commitment as the only way to prevent her from "taking a step" that would cause a "scandal" for all concerned. In a parallel case, a father worried about his daughter's desire to run away from home and pursue a theatrical career. "I dare not indulge her idea of wandering about to support herself – she would be ruined, as under such excitement she often forgot the proprieties of life," he concluded. Although often presented as watchful concern for the insane person's well-being, such arguments for commitment also reflected a desire to protect the family's reputation.[49]

More frequently, asylum patrons justified commitment on the grounds that a relative's insanity endangered the physical or mental well-being of the whole household. As a patron wrote of a relative, "he has attempted no violence but eats and sleeps very little, is very noisy and difficult to manage, and always interfering with the conduct of the farm and household affairs, to the great detriment of both." Sometimes, the person's disruptive behavior actually threatened the family's economic livelihood. A woman whose husband had suffered "pecuniary losses" needed to take in boarders to supplement the family income; as a result, she felt compelled to hospitalize her insane mother, for "it would be folly in me to attempt such a thing while my dear mother is with me." Many patrons simply mentioned the grave psychological strain of living with and caring for a seriously disturbed relative. A woman stated that her daughter's mind had been "affected" for more than a year, but only recently had she been unable to sleep at night. "This change has so worn her friends" (i.e., her family), she concluded, that the family doctor had convinced her to commit her child. "I dare not keep her at home," wrote another patron of an insane daughter; "she would hurry her mother and sister to a premature grave." Patrons complained that the insane made the domestic environment unbearable by their profane or lewd behavior. "It is destructive of all family comforts to keep a man about a private family, in his condition," wrote a man about his father's filthy habits. In the same vein, a husband complained that his wife continually disturbed the "peace of the family" by "using all sorts of filthy language."[50]

Of course, tolerance for insane behavior varied considerably from family to family, for reasons impossible to determine solely from their letters. Some relatives seemed very anxious to reach an accommodation with the insane, so long as the patient's behavior remained within certain bounds. One patron who had lived for many years with an insane son sent him to the asylum only when an illness confined her to bed and he became restless at night. As soon as she recovered, she wanted him back, for as another son wrote, "she is lonely without Fred K and would rather have him at home if he is not noisy." In a similar case, a young woman, "although far from well," appeared to her brothers "so much better as to be within their control at home" that they decided against sending her to Kirkbride. As a friend explained, "it is their choice to take care of her themselves if they can do so, and hope for her recovery."[51]

On the other hand, by the mid-nineteenth century, it was not unusual for families to commit relatives described as "harmless" or "inoffensive," on the grounds that they might be cured or simply made more comfortable in the asylum. For example, in 1863 a man sought treatment for his young sister after she had manifested these relatively mild symptoms for only a few weeks:

She is perfectly inoffensive but much of her time is spent through the day muttering inaudibly. She has no appetite for her food, eats very little, scarcely one spoonful at a meal, but sleeps tolerably well at night, and exhibits great restlessness all day, constantly expressing a wish to go out somewhere and take a walk. Her pulse is regular and she makes no complaint except she sometimes complains of cobwebs being around her head and brain.

This patron committed his sister not because she had become uncontrollable, but because he knew of a neighbor's son who had been cured at the Pennsylvania Hospital for the Insane and hoped that his sister might be "equally fortunate." Usually, such relatively mild cases brought to the asylum were young people. But occasionally, relatives sought a more convenient arrangement for an elderly individual they believed to be incurable. A man wrote asking admission for an aged sister who had lost her memory and picked sores on her face, but was otherwise inoffensive, on the grounds that "she might find increased comfort and happiness in your institution" for the duration of her "second childhood."[52]

Obviously, some families utilized the asylum more readily and optimistically than others. But for the average patron, the decision to commit a relative invariably involved some anguish and guilt. Indeed, most arrived at the Pennsylvania Hospital for the Insane in a state of "depression and hopelessness," as Kirkbride described them. For months, even years, the family had tried to keep the patient at home and avoid the shame, guilt, and expense of institutionalizaton. At last, desperate and exhausted, they had concluded that they had no choice but to consign a relative to Kirkbride's care. However inescapable commitment appeared, it still seemed "as if I was resigning her to the grave," to use one patron's words.[53]

EXPECTATIONS OF HOSPITAL TREATMENT

Although distraught, Kirkbride's patrons were hardly passive or bewildered in their dealings with him. Precisely because commitment came after such long, anguished consideration, patrons tended to approach hospital treatment better informed than they might have been about a less radical medical procedure. In some cases, they had already gotten information concerning the asylum from an annual report or a family doctor. More generally, the family's own experience in caring for the insane shaped their demands of Kirkbride. Having attempted home treatment of insanity and found it wanting, patrons expected the asylum to provide a degree of privacy, regimentation, and coercion that had eluded their own efforts. By expressing these expectations, the patrons could not help but exercise a subtle influence on the superintendent's conception of treatment.

First and foremost, patrons valued the privacy afforded by institutionalization. By commitment, they expected to put an end to embarrassing public displays and discussions of their relative's insanity. For this reason, when choosing an institution, families looked for "as private a situation as possible." If they could afford it, many selected an asylum away from their home town or even home state. A New York family wrote Kirkbride about transferring a relative from the Bloomingdale Asylum, because the patient himself objected to the institution "as being too near home and shrinks from the notoriety of it in his case." Sometimes commitment allowed the family to deny the patient's existence entirely. In 1868, a South Carolina man wrote Kirkbride concerning a long-time resident of the hospital: "It is due you to state that Mrs. M's grandchildren were brought up in entire ignorance of her existence." Most patrons simply expected Kirkbride to protect the family and the patient from the undesirable "publicity," as one person termed it. More specifically, they wanted the superintendent to regulate the patient's visitors and correspondence. In a typical request, a man asked that visitors to his wife be discouraged, "fearing that some of her incoherent expressions might be repeated, and might lead to unpleasant gossip." In a similar manner, a patron wanted his mother prevented from writing to certain friends, "who are either disposed to be officious or are extremely indelicate, and by their use of the letters, subject our family to annoyances."[54]

Since loss of control over the patient's behavior prompted most commitments, patrons naturally looked to the asylum to supervise the insane very closely. At the most elemental level, this supervision meant providing physical security for the inmates. Maniacal outbursts had to be subdued, suicidal patients constantly observed, and peripatetic individuals kept from wandering off. The family of the young man who started up railroad engines and swam rivers logically wanted to know "if there is a good enclosure around the premises, which would prevent him from roaming off." The patrons' expectation that the asylum would restrain the insane went far beyond mere physical confinement, however. In placing a relative in the hospital, they sought, as one correspondent wrote, "a positive control which he can neither oppose or resist." The control patrons envisioned included a psychological constraint that treatment would inculcate in the inmates themselves. A woman returning her sister after a relapse wrote, "I am of the opinion that what she needs is the restraining influence of your asylum, the remembrance of which has now considerably worn away, to keep her within bounds."[55]

By restoring a positive authority over the patient, patrons believed that the superintendent could better direct medical measures to eliminate the physical aspects of the disorder. Since so many lay people thought that a physical imbalance had produced a relative's insanity, they valued the asylum's provision for systematic and constant medical attendance. In a hospital, patients could be more easily "made to take such medicine and yield to such regimen" as their situations required. A number of patrons even mentioned specific remedies they wanted administered to a relative. A man convinced that disordered reproductive organs had caused his wife's insanity suggested a "simple medicine" to act on her ovaries and "adjacent parts." Another husband wanted his wife given "purgative pills, to keep her system open." Yet another relative, expressing her faith in "Moffit's pills and bitters," wrote, "If my son would take them, they might cause a change in his system which might cast off the gloom in his spirits, and his mind then become strengthened." For patients addicted to alcohol or drug use, the asylum had the added benefit of enforcing abstinence. Patrons hoped that the addict, "restrained from his indulgence," would be "led...to see the danger into which he has plunged himself."[56]

Having usually sought medical treatment before bringing a relative to the asylum, few patrons expected Kirkbride's medical therapeutics alone to effect a cure. On the whole, they expressed higher expectations of the hospital's moral regimen. A man committing a female relative who "gives way at times to great violence" stated his conviction that "if she was placed under some restraint and compelled to conform to certain rules...she could be cured." Patrons believed that the hospital routine could counteract the irregularity of thought and behavior so characteristic of insanity; the "regular and systematic life" imposed on the patients would encourage "stability of mind and habits."[57]

Kirkbride's patrons regarded the varied amusements and occupations incorporated into the hospital routine as particularly valuable for their afflicted relatives. Easily associating certain activities with desirable changes in the patient's behavior, they made many requests concerning specific amusements. For example, a husband asked that his depressed wife be supplied with entertaining novels, to "take her mind from herself and thus relieve her." Books, lectures, handiwork, and games all struck patrons as sensible ways to divert a troubled relative. "Please set pen and ink and paper before him, and see what ideas he would express on paper," advised a mother in her son's case. Some families suggested a demanding course of study as a means to strengthen a patient's mind. One man wanted his nephew to study medicine as "something to occupy his mind." An equally ambitious woman wanted her son and daughter, who were hospitalized at the same time, to be made into "scholars" during their asylum stay. Exercise was yet another aspect of moral treatment popular among the patrons. For female patients, relatives requested carriage rides and scenic walks; one patron regarded daily rides as "an absolute necessity" in his daughter's treatment. For male patients, relatives approved of light manual labor as a logical means to overcome "want of energy" or "lethargy."[58]

Of course, not all features of asylum life gained the patrons' approbation. Many retained the apprehensions concerning institutional care that had led them to delay commitment in the first place. Despite Kirkbride's efforts, the hospital building struck some visitors as far from homelike. Complained a woman of her sister's room, "it had a gloomy look and I was fearful it was damp and too near the ground to be healthy." Although desiring that their relatives be confined, other patrons found the hospital too prisonlike. "I consider it quite important," stated a patron, "that the other patients in whose company he may be should be well behaved, cleanly, and not disagreeable." Patrons often asked that a relative be segregated from noisy inmates; as one letter politely requested, "should it be practicable and not infringing on your rules," the family would be glad "if you will let her rooms be out of hearing of any shrieking you may have."[59]

The quality of attendants was another focus of the patrons'

anxieties. On the one hand, an expectation of watchful care had convinced many families to try asylum treatment. A man wrote of his daughter that a good attendant was a sine qua non of her commitment; "her mother and sisters, who felt that they could hardly part with her, could not endure the thought of her being left for a moment without someone to watch over her with care and kindness, as they had done." On the other hand, families had grave doubts about the type of individuals serving as asylum attendants. "Such folks as nurses are not always the tenderest," opined one patron. Relatives were particularly fearful that undue force might be used to control unruly patients, and often insisted that "kindness and forbearance" be shown them. Many patrons echoed the sentiment expressed by one that "more could be effected by kindness and patience than by irritating and crossing her feelings."[60]

Ultimately, the patrons centered both their expectations and anxieties about asylum treatment on the personality of Kirkbride himself. Their acceptance of his special jurisdiction over the insane informed the patrons' whole conception of hospital care. In Kirkbride's authority as a Christian and physician, families sought a replacement for their own lapsed influence over an insane relative. "Dr. Kirkbride will understand me," wrote an unhappy mother of her insane daughter; she had "lost ... authority over her" and needed the doctor to tell the girl "what to take and how to act." Patrons believed that with his special tact and expertise, Kirkbride's efforts to modify the patient's behavior might succeed where theirs had failed. "You must in some way make him take the medicine and do everything to effect his cure, but you will know how to manage it," concluded a patron. Kirkbride, it was assumed, had a peculiar ability to rid the insane of their delusions. A husband expressed his conviction that Kirkbride's "good advice and sound reasoning" would "drive out" his wife's "false notions." A farmer specified in his father's case, "Try and persuade him out of that notion that the folks cough and spit in his presence to be as scoffs and sneers to him."[61]

At best, patrons hoped that the combination of "positive control," ordered regimen, and parental authority offered by the asylum would effect a cure. Some aimed for nothing less than a "total change...morally and physically and mentally." But others viewed the hospital only as a means to avoid "the burden of being his keeper," as one relative put it. Wrote a patron committing a supposedly incurable individual, "your tact in caring for his fancies and indulging him in desserts, etc., may give him such an attachment to the place that he will remain willingly and thus relieve us from much trouble and anxiety." For both the hopeful and the pessimistic, the asylum had become a morally defensible means of ridding the household of an admittedly difficult resident. At the same time that commitment relieved tension within the home, it could be justified as the most therapeutic solution for the individual's problem. Thus, the asylum promised both a respite and a remedy, a potent combination for the families of the insane.[62]

TENSIONS IN THE COMMITMENT PROCESS

Once family members, by using such justifications, had overcome their reluctance to seek hospital treatment for an insane relative, they found the commitment process itself relatively simple. The Pennsylvania Hospital for the Insane, like all mid-nineteenth-century mental hospitals, required no formal legal proceedings for involuntary confinement. Recognizing that the family found institutionalization extremely painful, hospital authorities sought to make the act as quiet and private as possible. From its earliest days, the Pennsylvania Hospital had required only that the committing party supply one physician's certificate testifying to the individual's insanity before accepting a patient. Kirkbride found this long-standing tradition entirely adequate for the Pennsylvania Hospital for the Insane. When in 1867 the hospital attorney suggested that the asylum begin asking for two doctors' certificates (presumably as insurance against lawsuits), Kirkbride replied, "I do not think any special advantage would result from it, while very often it would seem to the friends, as giving them an unnecessary degree of trouble, annoyance and expense." The prevailing system, he concluded, had been in practice for 115 years without, to his knowledge, wrongfully confining a patient. The 1869 passage of a state law making two certificates mandatory for commitment to all Pennsylvania mental hospitals struck Kirkbride as a gratuitous insult to the physician's judgment of insanity. By his estimation, the law's only real benefit lay in the added protection from meddlesome lawsuits it afforded the asylum.[63]

Yet, changing patterns of utilizing the asylum made the old, informal commitment procedure increasingly subject to conflict. To begin with, the nineteenth-century asylum, as compared to its eighteenth-century predecessor, clearly admitted individuals suffering from a broader range of mental disability. As a result, some patients showed more equivocal symptoms of insanity, and their suitability for commitment could more easily be disputed. Admitting patients with a wider range of disorders without tightening admissions criteria inevitably created more commitment controversies. The increasing number of patients involuntarily confined for treatment of drug- or alcohol-related problems is a case in point. While under the influence of the addictive substance, individuals displayed enough symptoms of insanity, including violent excitement and delusions, to make their sanity questionable. But as soon as the addicts sobered up – a process greatly expedited by the enforced abstinence of hospitalization – most of them could give very convincing displays of rationality. Kirkbride, like many physicians of his time, willingly accepted the family's judgment that the addiction itself constituted a mental disorder. But the equation of alcoholism and addiction with insanity did not have widespread public acceptance in the mid-nineteenth century, and as we shall see in Chapter 5, commitment controversies involving alcoholic patients became more frequent.

Second, as patrons increasingly cited "perverted" feelings toward relatives as symptoms of insanity, and made preservation of domestic order a motive for institutionalization, the family's intentions in seeking commitment naturally became more suspect. As domestic life became more private in the nineteenth century, neighbors or friends less often had an opportunity to observe and verify an individual's aberrations. If the person's major symptom consisted of a settled dislike of a relative, or manifested itself only within the domestic circle, the family constituted the sole authority for establishing the existence of insanity. Patrons frequently complained about the dissembling appearances their insane relatives could maintain in public. "She can deceive anybody living without you could see her in those capers," a man claimed of his wife. Similarly, a private nurse told Kirkbride of an insane woman, "There's a *strange deception* about her, for it is one thing to see her with company and another thing to see her in domestic circles." But observations of this sort could not easily be verified by outsiders. Given the selfish or malicious sentiments one relative might entertain toward another, commitments based primarily upon family testimony, not surprisingly, raised serious questions about the proper definition of sanity.[64]

In the more subtle cases of mental aberration, the burden of judging the individual's sanity initially fell not on the asylum doctor, who rarely saw a patient before commitment, but on the general practitioner, who had to supply the certificate of insanity. If a medical man had known the family for some years, he usually felt confident in accepting their judgments. But when asked to rule on a person's sanity after only a short acquaintance with either family or patient, doctors sometimes felt uneasy. Without detailed knowledge of the individual's past history, even the most perceptive physicians had difficulty in distinguishing between a rational and an irrational dislike of one's relatives. A local doctor described the dilemma he faced when asked to provide a certificate for a woman he had seen only a few times: "Certainly I did not observe enough about her to warrant me in believing that she is insane – as I do not know whether her motives concerning her family history and relations are correct or otherwise, I am not sure but that she has an *external* foundation for her emphatic opposition to the wishes of her family." He concluded, "Without a more complete knowledge of her previous history than the patient herself has given me, I am not able to decide whether her mind is sound or unsound."[65]

General practitioners often characterized cases they found difficult to diagnose as moral insanity. Unlike the medicolegal experts of the day, who limited that diagnosis to derangements of the emotional or moral faculties without apparent intellectual impairment, the average medical man employed it to designate "those troublesome cases...in which the real condition of the patient might not be recognized at first unless under some special excitement." For the general practitioner, moral insanity served as a convenient label for those individuals whose symptoms of aberration were either muted or transitory. One physician applied the term to a wild but charming young man who could "talk down a steamboat." Another used it to characterize an alcoholic, writing, "There might be some question as to his insanity, but in my opinion such cases should be deemed moral derangement and fit subjects for an asylum." Yet a third meaning for moral insanity emerged in a physician's account of a man who had only briefly on two occasions displayed the "wild appearance," unconsciousness, and violence of a "true madman." The doctor wrote to Kirkbride, "there is not one here ever thinks of him being insane, indeed I scarcely think so myself – but his constant thought of it, is enough to render him so. He talks as sensibly as ever – it is impossible to notice anything which would lead you to suspect insanity except in the two instances referred to."[66]

As long as the doctor and the family agreed upon the verdict of insanity, the difficulties inherent in judging borderline cases rarely led to public controversy. The only party likely to challenge the doctor–family consensus, that is, the patient, had little power to dispute the decision. Only in a few instances, as will be seen in Chapter 5, did asylum inmates succeed in obtaining legal hearings on the subject of their sanity. Far more often, disputes arose among different members of the same family concerning the propriety of a commitment. An 1858 battle between a patient's husband and father well illustrates the problems created by a family's lack of agreement concerning commitment. According to the husband, the woman had suffered from insanity, chiefly manifested in her "perverted feelings toward him," for some time. He blamed her "badly balanced mind" on "very faulty" training and indulgence at the hands of her father. The father's account of the case, needless to say, differed on every point. The husband, he declared, had caused his daughter's mental distress, and if separated from him, she would be perfectly well. Due to the difference of opinion within the family, the husband felt that he had to "await such developments as would fully satisfy the public mind, if not the parties making active opposition to her being placed in a Hospital," before committing her. Eventually, the woman behaved so outrageously in public that other relatives used "decided pressure" to overcome the father's opposition. Even after his daughter's commitment, the old man kept up his campaign on her behalf, using his letters and visits to strengthen her resolve to leave the asylum as soon as possible. Unfortunately, Kirkbride could not avoid getting caught in the controversy. All the parties involved – the husband, the father, and the patient – besieged him with complaints about the other two and resented his efforts to maintain a neutral position. Although seemingly most sympathetic to the husband, Kirkbride nonetheless refused to withhold the father's letters or forbid his visits to his daughter, a refusal that infuriated the former.[67]

However Kirkbride resolved such family disputes, they caused him immense concern, for his practice of asylum medicine depended heavily on the therapeutic alliance between physician and patron. The treatment of insanity, like any medical regimen in the mid-nineteenth century, was built upon a set of shared ideas about the nature of mental disease. As the lay descriptions of the insane suggest, patron and doctor defined mental aberration in very similar terms. The family's standards for distinguishing insanity seem remarkably like those laid out by Amariah Brigham in 1844: Insanity consisted of the "derangement of the intellectual faculties or prolonged changes of the feelings, affections and habits of an individual." Although possessing more sophisticated medical conceptions of insanity, asylum doctors rarely played an active role in either the initial recognition or diagnosis of mental disease or the decision to commit a patient to the hospital; relatives decided that an individual was insane and needed institutional care long before they ever consulted the superintendent. Because asylum doctors encountered the insane at such a late stage of development, their work was necessarily dependent upon the multiplicity of social judgments involved in the commitment process. By *incorporating* rather than *contradicting* the family's perception of mental illness, physicians gave their theoretical formulations about treatment a force that would have otherwise been lacking.[68]

Yet, the congruence between medical definitions and cultural values concerning insanity created liabilities as well as strengths for asylum medicine. The very agreement between lay and medical judgments became a drawback when the social consensus about an individual's sanity came into dispute. As long as the physician confirmed an uncontested commitment, his etiological ability would not be called into question. But let the public, particularly members of the patient's family, disagree about the necessity for commitment, and the superintendent's theoretical formulations could lose much of their force. Lacking any quick, reliable test for insanity other than the commonsense standards employed by the patrons, asylum doctors found their diagnostic judgments very vulnerable, especially in a court of law. Critics could fairly say that physicians had no more scientific means to identify insanity than the intelligent lay person.

In the long run, however, the high degree of consensus between lay and medical concepts of insanity aided the new specialty. Asylum medicine found its strength not so much in the doctors' etiological or diagnostic skills as in their ability to meet the patrons' demand for a morally defensible form of institutional treatment. As a result, the early superintendents did not greatly concern themselves with setting exact boundaries between sane and insane behavior or devising a complicated etiological system; instead, they concentrated on developing a medically sanctioned institutional solution to the problems involved in home care of the insane. And in stressing the benefits of a strict regimen, varied employments and amusements, and the physician's parental authority, asylum doctors responded very effectively to lay expectations of medical treatment.

To argue that the family's needs influenced the direction of early asylum medicine does not necessarily mean that the patrons determined the physicians' intellectual interests in a simple, direct fashion. Kirkbride did not blindly follow the family's preferences in order to secure a lucrative practice. Rather, asylum medicine reflected a shared consensus regarding the origins and treatment of mental disorders. Agreed upon the definition of insanity and aware of the problems involved in its treatment at home, doctor and patron sought a mutually agreeable concept of treatment. Within the intellectual and practical bounds of his medical training, Kirkbride chose a therapeutic method that appealed to his lay clientele. Their preferences reinforced his commitment to certain features of moral treatment, such as building design and amusements. Although retaining the dominant authority in the interaction, the physician was nonetheless never isolated from or unaware of his patrons' perspective. Insofar as the patrons' attitudes dictated the *types* of patients he saw, the stage of the disorder at which he became involved with the patient, and the family's disposition to cooperate with him, Kirkbride's intellectual judgment about insanity could not help but be influenced by them.

As will become evident in the following chapter, the asylum patrons' fears and expectations of institutional treatment had a profound influence on Kirkbride's medical practice. But before we move on to a detailed consideration of his asylum philosophy, it is necessary to place the composite portrait of the asylum patron presented here within a broader framework. For the family's motivation in seeking asylum care is of interest to the historian not only as a factor shaping the internal dynamics of the mental hospital but also as a reflection of changing cultural values. What, then, can we deduce from the asylum patrons' accounts about the long-term processes underlying the nineteenth-century discovery of the asylum?

To begin with, if we compare the patrons of the Pennsylvania Hospital for the Insane with the clientele of the old general hospital, it is evident that throughout the period from 1750 to 1880, families confined the insane for the same types of behaviors: violence to self or others, destructiveness and extreme troublesomeness. In justifying their decision to commit a family member, eighteenth- and nineteenth-century patrons invoked similar themes: hope for cure, inability to control the patient's behavior, and concern about the deleterious effect of insanity on the household. And for all its new attractions, the nineteenth-century mental hospital retained many negative associations so that its patrons still came to it as a last resort. Even over the course of a century, commitment had not become an easy matter.

The continuity in certain lay attitudes toward the mental hospital should not blind us to the larger parameters of change, however. Families remained reluctant to commit relatives, but the fact remains that they did so in ever larger numbers. The increasing number of hospitals that treated the insane, from 18 in 1840 to almost 140 in 1880, reflected not only population growth but also a greater demand for the asylum's services. The ratio of hospital beds for the insane to the adult population grew dramatically, from 1 for every 6,000 persons over age fifteen in 1800 to 1 for every 750 persons in 1880. When compared with the best estimates of insanity's prevalence during the same period, these figures suggest that the percentage of the insane in hospitals rose from less than 3 percent in 1840 to almost 20 percent in 1880. As the reformers of the time well knew, demand so far outstripped construction of new facilities that overcrowding was a serious problem, especially in municipal institutions, for most of the century; as a result, many insane persons were sent to almshouses and jails, much to the reformers' dismay. Overall, the pace of nineteenth-century institutional growth confirms the observation that hospitalization steadily gained favor among all sectors of society.[69]

Kirkbride's correspondence with his patrons suggests that this shift from home to hospital care depended upon several key changes in the lay person's view of the asylum. In part, the growing acceptance of the asylum alternative stemmed from a popular appreciation of moral treatment as an innovative therapy. Much as anesthesia and the X-ray attracted later generations of patients to the general hospital's surgical wards, moral treatment brought new patrons to the asylum because it seemed a markedly more effective and humane approach to insanity. The precocious growth of the mental hospital also reflected the peculiar strains that caring for the insane placed upon the household. By its very nature, mental disease created a level of disruption uncommon in other disorders. And for whatever reasons, families became more loath to use physical restraint or isolation as methods to control the insane at home. Thus, commitment was justifiable on two grounds: that it might cure the individual at the same time as it relieved the family of a burdensome responsibility.

As might be expected, changing perceptions of the hospital resulted in a broader range of disorders being considered appropriate for institutional treatment. True, the majority of families continued to resist commitment until, by their judgment, the patient had become too violent or uncontrollable to be kept at home. But the *level* of violence, disruptiveness, or intellectual impairment deemed necessary to merit confinement had certainly fallen since the eighteenth century. Increasingly, families sought asylum care for patients who could still be managed at home without resorting to extreme measures. Although probably only a small percentage of the total admissions, the number of insane persons described as harmless or inoffensive whom Kirkbride received at the Pennsylvania Hospital for the Insane indicates a broadening of the criteria for commitment. It is certainly difficult to imagine such relatively "mild" cases finding a place in the old Pennsylvania Hospital.

Thus, the evolution of the Pennsylvania Hospital from the eighteenth to the nineteenth centuries reveals a broadening of the asylum's function, not only in the numbers of patrons it attracted but also in the types of mental disorders considered suitable for treatment. It remains to be seen whether or not these trends signified a decreasing tolerance for insanity, as many scholars have been tempted to conclude. The argument is a problematic one, since eighteenth-century families had economic constraints on their choice of treatment alternatives that nineteenth-century families did not. Until the late 1700s, one might argue that the American economy was too undeveloped to finance expensive institutional alternatives to home care. Therefore, families had little choice but to take care of deranged relatives and control them as best they could. Simply because the insane remained in the home, we cannot conclude that their presence was any more acceptable to those around them than it was in the nineteenth century.[70]

An economic parallel suggests a more useful way to envision the growth in demand for asylum treatment. To explain the rise of a mass market for consumer goods between 1780 and 1830, economic historians point to a cycle of increasing demand, production, and innovation: Greater demand for goods due to population growth led to innovations in production methods, which eventually lowered the price of manufactured items; reduced prices stimulated more demand, thereby encouraging further innovation, and so on. In a similar fashion, we might hypothesize that population growth placed pressure on those few eighteenth-century institutions capable of confining violent lunatics. In the Pennsylvania Hospital, where strong scientific and humanitarian traditions prevailed, overcrowding stimulated a disposition to experiment with new types of treatment. The more attractive institutional regimen that resulted brought more patrons to the asylum, thereby keeping the pressure to innovate relatively constant. Such a process might have resulted in an expansion of the asylum's facilities, as well as its clientele, even if tolerance for insanity had remained exactly the same.[71]

But there is also some reason to believe that a stronger push out of the household coincided with the pull toward the asylum created by moral treatment. Scholars have long posited a relationship between the more exacting standards of personal behavior required in a complex modern society and decreasing tolerance for insanity. Certainly, the period from 1750 to 1850, during which the asylum first emerged, saw an ever-increasing emphasis on internalized forms of self-discipline as population growth, economic development, and geographic expansion eroded old forms of authority. Movements for popular education, moral purity, health reform, and temperance all represented different facets of the drive to reorder instincts and behaviors into more regular, productive patterns. In a society striving mightily to regulate itself, so the argument goes, the insane naturally became more threatening. Their irregularity, unpredictability, "impure habits," and lack of self-control ran counter to the most basic premises of the new modern society. The asylum patrons' litany of complaints about the incoherence, unsystematic habits, unstable moods, and irrational beliefs of the mentally deranged certainly suggests their internalization of an exacting personal code. Patrons looked to the asylum to inculcate the same code – the regular habits, stability of the mind, and self-restraint – in its patients.[72]

An even stronger case can be made for a connection between the asylum and a more specific dimension of social change: the family. Between 1750 and 1850, as manufacturing moved out of the household, the family's educational and emotional functions achieved new significance. A "cult of domesticity," popularized in novels and advice literature, assigned middle-class women new responsibilities for the moral and emotional caliber of family life. The "true woman" was supposed to uplift and comfort her husband and inculcate habits of industry and self-discipline in her children. This new conception of domesticity not only gave the economically disenfranchised woman a compensatory moral power within the home, but also served to make the family an oasis of stability, a "haven in the heartless world," within a rapidly changing, increasingly fluid industrial society.[73]

The asylum patrons' accounts suggest that the greater emphasis upon the family as an affective and educational unit may have changed popular attitudes toward home care of the insane. As more significance came to be attached to the quality of emotional relationships, the "perversions" of the familial affections found in insanity became more ominous. Increased expectations of the intimacy and moral uplift of domestic life as a counter to the materialistic world of work reduced the family's willingness to tolerate lewd, noisy, profane behavior. The more social and moral education for children became identified with individual success and social stability, the more pernicious became the disruptive example set by the insane. Perhaps in the concern for children lies the link between the larger process of modernization and the rise of the asylum. Given its responsibility for instilling habits of industry, regularity, and moderation in the young, the family had all the more reason to expel the insane from the home.[74]

Given what little we know about eighteenth-century attitudes toward insanity, the argument that rising standards of family life decreased the willingness to keep the insane in the household can never be conclusively proved. But there can be little doubt that the asylum's success heralded a new alliance between the family and the asylum. Clearly, the nineteenth-century mental hospital resolved a deeply felt social problem by providing an institutional solution to a painful domestic situation. The strength of the new asylum specialty rested squarely on its ability to legitimate the family's commitment decision in both moral and medical terms.

Thomas Story Kirkbride understood that the success of his asylum practice, as well as the specialty of asylum medicine, depended upon the correspondence between the family's needs and the institutional provisions the asylum offered. From his earliest years as an asylum doctor, he aimed at combining his medical knowledge with an appreciation of his patrons' desperation to produce a "persuasive" institution: a hospital whose form and function would assuage the family's guilt about committing a relative and heighten their confidence in his healing powers. His efforts to relieve the family of the "burden of being their keepers" produced not only the Pennsylvania Hospital for the Insane, the leading corporate hospital of its day, but also a blueprint for the ideal mental hospital, a hospital design that would have a lasting influence on the development of American psychiatry.

4

The persuasive institution

Upon arriving at the Pennsylvania Hospital after a long carriage ride from the city, the families of prospective patients beheld an institution quite unlike the horrible madhouse they had feared. Its secluded rural location promised the protection from public notoriety they desired, and the pleasant, even luxurious appearance of the building and grounds belied grim preconceptions of institutional life. Wherever the patrons looked, from the ten-pin bowling alley to the reading room, they saw evidence of the efforts made to watch over and amuse the patients, efforts far more extensive and well organized than their own home regimen. Meeting the asylum superintendent, who spoke to them with a blend of paternal concern and scientific authority, the family found themselves further comforted. From first to last, every aspect of the asylum's appearance and organization seemed designed expressly to relieve and reassure them. The institution and, more importantly, the physician at its head held out to the family the promise of a benign control, a persuasive influence, that would rid insanity of its horrors.

The impressions created by the Pennsylvania Hospital for the Insane were hardly effortless or unpremeditated. The reassuring details of its regimen and appearance reflected Thomas Story Kirkbride's painstaking labor. From his earliest years as superintendent, he made the creation and maintenance of the asylum's therapeutic image his central professional concern. Personal factors, including his father's pursuit of agricultural improvements and his own practical bent, so early manifested in the love of surgery, contributed to Kirkbride's interest in asylum construction. His devotion to the Friends' principles no doubt made him particularly sensitive to the sufferings caused by insanity and desirous of relieving them. All these predilections found expression in Kirkbride's philosophy of asylum medicine, which made hospital design and administration central to its practice. This philosophy, first enunciated in an 1847 article in the *American Journal of Medical Science* and then amplified in his 1854 book, *On the Construction, Management, and General Arrangements of Hospitals for the Insane*, not only guided Kirkbride's own practice at the Pennsylvania Hospital for the Insane but became the dominant credo for the whole American specialty.[1]

More than any of his contemporaries, Kirkbride divined the importance of institutional forms to the profession's success. The moral architecture and moral order of the new hospital, he realized, were the most powerful means physicians possessed to summon up belief in the new asylum treatment. The asylum doctors' reputation as healers of mental disease depended almost entirely on their ability to inspire faith in this, their most impressive asset: the mental hospital. To extend medical jurisdiction over insanity, Kirkbride developed an asylum philosophy designed to control the hospital environment completely. Every detail, from the design of the window frames to the table settings in the ward dining rooms, had to be arranged to sustain the impression that here was an institution where patients received kind and competent care. The result, Kirkbride believed, would be that after one visit to his carefully managed institution, his patrons could not fail "to see that neither labor nor expense is spared to promote the happiness of the patients"; they would thus be led "to have a generous confidence in those to whose care their friends have been entrusted and readiness to give a steady support to a liberal course of treatment."[2] By providing patrons with a persuasive institution, he hoped firmly to establish the physician's authority over insanity.

Kirkbride's institutional philosophy was by no means unique to him. His contributions to medical practice were those of a rationalizer rather than an innovator. From his own hospital experience, Kirkbride developed a keen insight into the dynamics of asylum medicine, particularly the patrons' needs and the efforts required of the superintendent to meet them. In his professional writings, he did little more than develop practical guidelines aimed at helping his fellow asylum doctors make a success of their institutions. Far from being radical or innovative, his formulations simply articulated and attempted to refine a system of asylum medicine already well established. Kirkbride's stance appealed to the brethren, as we shall see in Chapter 6, precisely because he addressed so ably problems they all shared.

Similarly, Kirkbride's preoccupation with building design and administration was not an obsession unique to him as an asylum doctor. In expecting institutional forms to promote specific therapeutic aims, he had much in common with other nineteenth-century reformers. During this period, a wide spectrum of social groups used architecture to embody and advance their collective ideals. Utopian sects such as the Shakers and John Humphrey Noyes's Oneida community paid careful attention to their building plans and arrangements. More closely aligned with Kirkbride's own moderate political views, advocates of prison reform and public education took an intense interest in "moral architecture." So, in expecting spatial and organizational arrangements profoundly to affect his patrons and patients, Kirkbride exhibited a characteristic nineteenth-century belief in the power of carefully designed institutions to effect social change.[3]

Kirkbride's attention to asylum architecture also paralleled an increasing interest in hospital design. Soon after his book on asylum construction and management appeared, Florence Nightingale published her influential essay, *Notes on Hospitals*, a powerful argument for sanitary reform through better hospital design. Nightingale's hygienic concerns led her to focus on many of the same mundane subjects, that is, ventilation, plumbing, and the like that Kirkbride found so engrossing. Nightingale's work presaged a lively medical debate over the sanitary merits of various hospital plans. Thus, works on asylum construction such as Kirkbride's were but one category of a growing medical literature on hospital design.[4]

In common with these other medical and social reformers, Kirkbride took an interest in building design and management that went far beyond simple architectural issues. Although he was often concerned with very prosaic details, his institutional philosophy was not bureaucratic in spirit. Historians have been misled by a too literal reading of his discussions on furnaces and window fixtures, concluding that he and his brethren were mere managers. But as we shall see in this chapter, underlying Kirkbride's practical advice concerning asylum fixtures was a visionary ideal of the hospital society: a therapeutic community modeled on the outside world, yet operating according to hygienic principles. In its ward arrangements and governance, the "great whole," as Kirkbride liked to call the asylum society, re-created the social environment patients came from, yet recast its features in therapeutic terms.

When viewed from this perspective, one is struck not by the mundane quality of Kirkbride's thinking but by the highly idealized vision of the mental hospital it encompassed.[5]

To comprehend the full import of Kirkbride's asylum philosophy and practice, we must first examine the set of beliefs about the mental hospital that he sought to project to his lay clientele. The first section of this chapter discusses the perceptions of insanity and its proper treatment, which Kirkbride developed for patrons in his *Reports*. The next section analyzes Kirkbride's professional writings on asylum construction and design as efforts to resolve certain "design dilemmas" inherent in his asylum persuasion.[6] The second half of the chapter contrasts Kirkbride's ideal asylum to his own experience at the Pennsylvania Hospital for the Insane, suggesting the genesis of his asylum philosophy as well as illustrating the basic strengths and weaknesses of moral treatment.

THE IDEAL ASYLUM

Kirkbride first began to cultivate his patrons' generous confidence by supplying them with a comforting, easily understood set of beliefs about insanity and the mental hospital. Building upon lay persons' rather crude concepts of disease, as discussed in the last chapter, the asylum doctor provided a more elaborate but still comprehensible medical rationale for the institutional treatment of mental disorders. Central to all of Kirkbride's explanations for the patrons was a nonjudgmental view of insanity and its causes joined with a benign vision of the asylum. In such terms, Kirkbride's therapeutic persuasion articulated the consensus between doctor and patron that was to guide the patient's treatment.

The asylum persuasion

The dominant elements of Kirkbride's therapeutic persuasion can be traced most clearly in his *Reports of the Pennsylvania Hospital for the Insane*, which he published annually. Although written for several audiences, including his managers, professional brethren, and potential contributors, Kirkbride's *Reports* functioned primarily as brochures designed to attract and inform readers who might be considering asylum treatment for an insane relative or friend. He received frequent requests for copies from prospective patrons and patients' families alike, and composed his discussions of insanity and its treatment with them in mind. Reserving issues of any complexity for professional journals, Kirkbride aimed his *Reports* at "those interested in knowing the character of our hospitals, and desirous of learning something of the general principles of treatment now adopted." He particularly wanted to reach the intelligent but uninformed people he frequently encountered among his patients' families. The relatives of the insane often came to him, he wrote, "for counsel, with feelings of depression and utter hopelessness, far beyond what are commonly connected with the occurrence of any ordinary malady." He observed that "while prepared to make every sacrifice to secure the restoration of the patient, before doing so, they very properly desire some explanation of the nature of the disease, the chances of a recovery and the reasons for plans of treatment so different from what are commonly adopted in the management of ordinary sickness." In his *Reports*, Kirkbride provided general answers to all these questions and attempted to overcome, point by point, the most common reservations about hospital treatment.[7]

In format, the *Reports of the Pennsylvania Hospital for the Insane* covered many of the same topics every year: the cause and nature of insanity, improvements to the building and grounds, amusements, restraint, classification, care of the chronic insane, a short financial statement, and statistical tables describing the patient population. From the superintendent's repetitive discussions of these topics emerge a clearly articulated set of beliefs and attitudes. The image of the asylum that Kirkbride sought to project in these discussions bears closer inspection, since it formed the goal of both his practice and his philosophy of asylum design.

At the simplest level, the *Reports* provided basic information on the admission of patients. Each copy included admissions forms that explained the types of cases accepted at the Pennsylvania Hospital for the Insane. The reader learned that the hospital took no "idiots," or persons with congenital mental defects, and received epileptics only by special arrangement. Cases of "mania-a-potu," or delirium tremens, were to be taken to the Eighth Street hospital. The forms also made clear that the hospital *did* accept incurable cases. In order to admit a patient, friends and relatives were told to submit one or, after 1869, two certificates of the patient's insanity from "respectable graduates of medicine." The rate of board would then be determined according to the patient's financial resources and the accommodations desired. "Large chambers and private attendants" might be obtained if the family so wished. The forms included questions to be answered in the "full and detailed history" that Kirkbride wanted to accompany each patient, giving details of previous treatment, suicidal propensities, and duration of symptoms.[8]

In addition to spelling out the terms of admission to the Pennsylvania Hospital for the Insane, the *Reports* provided elementary information about the nature of insanity. Kirkbride defined insanity simply as a "functional disease of the brain" and offered no detailed discussion of its pathology, preferring instead to elaborate on the proper attitude to be taken toward the disease. Couched in soothing, nonjudgmental terms, his explanations presented insanity as a disease that might affect anyone. "Insanity is truly the great leveler of all the artificial distinctions of society," he frequently told his readers. He minimized the sufferer's personal responsibility for the disease, characterizing it as "an accident... to which we are all liable, and especially, if without any direct agency of our own, or certainly without anything on our part that was dishonorable or criminal... no reproach to anyone." (Note the use of the inclusive pronoun.) Although "prudence and a good constitution" might successfully ward off mental disease, even respectable, morally irreproachable people might be stricken with it; "it is found among the purest and the best of all dwellers upon earth, as well as those who are far from being models of excellence," he wrote. Kirkbride also denied that heredity played a major role in most mental disease. Feeling that medical and lay thinking accorded too much importance to hereditary propensities, he urged the families of the insane not to scrutinize anxiously all their relatives for signs of some ancestral taint.[9]

Kirkbride seemed particularly concerned to present insanity as a disease that did not spare the educated or wealthy. Although rarely making special reference in his *Reports* to patients on the free list, he frequently mentioned the number of "persons of cultivated and refined minds" in the hospital. He cautioned his readers that "high social position, exalted intellectual endowment, [and] the most abundant wealth" were no guarantee against insanity. On the contrary, he explained, some forms of mental disease particularly affected the better classes. For example, the neglect of physical exercise by many "studious men and women, and...others with different sedentary occupations" often led to a "variety of nervous affections." He concluded that a "high state of civilization, with all its benefits, is...likely to bring in its train a host of ailments...serious and distressing in their character." The superintendent thus implied to his readers that the more cultured an individual, the more vulnerable he or she would be to mental disease. He also gave the impression that the hospital was patronized by the best sort of people, thereby making it more acceptable to both the wealthy and their less fortunate neighbors.[10]

Having reassured prospective patrons that insanity did not necessarily result from wrongdoing and affected the most civilized classes, Kirkbride still had to provide some explanation for its onset. As stated in the last chapter, patrons needed to make sense of the unexpected and often disruptive mental illness of a friend or relation. Therefore, Kirkbride frequently enumerated what he believed to be the principal causes of insanity: ill health (which he said accounted for the majority of cases), loss of property, unemployment, grief, intense application to study or business, disappointed expectations, "mental anxiety" (such as arose in nursing the sick), intemperance, and masturbation. With the exception of the last two, none of these explanations for the disease implied any reproach to the patient or family. Within such a broad framework, insanity could be accounted for in relatively comprehensive terms; few individuals could have avoided at least one of these stresses before developing a mental disturbance, thus providing all concerned with a convenient explanation for its onset.[11]

The most difficult and demanding portion of Kirkbride's arguments sought to convince the family that insanity must be treated in the hospital rather than in the home. Acknowledging that most families found the decision to commit a relative very difficult, he continually tried to allay their anxiety and sense of guilt by providing arguments to justify the action and refute the objections he knew "misguided friends" would make. First, Kirkbride assured his readers that home treatment never benefited the insane, however kind and competent their care. "All the devotion of the tenderest friendship and everything that wealth can furnish," he told them, "are often powerless to afford relief." Without ever implying that the family situation itself might be exacerbating the patient's symptoms, he stated that "simple removal from familiar scenes and associations, with changed habits of life, is often, of itself, sufficient to modify favorably the diseased manifestations." Although acknowledging the prevalent belief that "the friends of the insane are disposed unnecessarily to remove them from home and place them in institutions," he insisted that the opposite was, in fact, true; families usually waited too long to commit a patient to the asylum, thus missing the opportunity to arrest the disease in its early stages. Kirkbride also attacked the notion that families frequently acted from improper motives in committing relatives. Regarding the widely held belief that people sent family members to asylums in order to steal their fortunes or obstruct their happiness, he insisted that "as far as my knowledge extends, nothing of the kind has ever been attempted here." Absolved of accusations of undue haste or selfish considerations, his readers could begin to consider hospital treatment seriously.[12]

Having attempted to persuade his prospective patrons that hospital treatment for insanity represented the family's wisest, most benevolent course, Kirkbride discussed the prognosis of the disease. The reward for prompt action, he assured them, might very well be a complete recovery. His experience had shown that 80 percent of all recent cases of insanity recovered in the asylum. The longer the disease had been established, the longer a cure might take; cases of long standing often proved incurable. For recent and chronic cases alike, Kirkbride alerted his prospective patrons that the patient's hospital stay might be a long one. The family must possess "a determination to persevere in the treatment when once commenced, even under what seems to be the most discouraging circumstances." He condemned any "vacillating course of treatment" that might weaken the patient's cooperation with the hospital regimen. "Let no temporary discouragement, no suggestions of officious friends, no histories of wonderful recoveries by marvelous appliances, no importunities from the patients themselves," he warned, "lead to the suspension of a course deliberately adopted, till after a fair and full trial."[13]

At the same time, Kirkbride's remarks on the chronic insane made clear to his audience that should a relative's disease prove incurable, he or she would still receive kind and competent care. His *Reports* continually presented the presence of the chronic cases as an asset to the institution; anyone familiar with the wards, he would aver, knew that persons with chronic disease were among the most intelligent and agreeable in the asylum, exercising a "beneficial influence" on all their fellow patients. As long as they could "conduct [themselves] with propriety," they had all the privileges of the institution. Yet, Kirkbride did not advise removing them from the asylum. No case was absolutely incurable, he argued; seemingly chronic cases had been known to recover after years of treatment. If removed from the hospital uncured, the patient might quickly deteriorate and again become a burden to the family. Thus, Kirkbride encouraged families with incurable relations to give them a trial at the hospital and let them remain, even when the case looked hopeless. Although few chronic patients may have exercised the beneficial influence Kirkbride claimed for them, he obviously wanted to make the incurable patient's situation appear as attractive as possible.[14]

Yet, the superintendent could not leave prospective patrons with the impression that recent and chronic patients lived side by side in the hospital. He knew that many families' objections to institutional care arose from their fear that in the hospital, "all classes of invalids are mingled together." They had to be convinced that "a thorough separation of the different classes of patients might be effected." Kirkbride's regular discussions of classification reassured patrons that their relative would not have a room next door to a shrieking, filthy lunatic. He explained to his readers that he assigned patients to the wards on the basis of mental condition and "social traits"; in other words, both the degree of the patient's disorder and his or her class affiliation were taken into account. Wealth alone would not entitle a disagreeable or "repulsive" patient to a room on the best ward, he stated. Kirkbride developed several analogies to explain hospital classification convincingly. The hospital, he often said, resembled "a community made up of distinct and congenial families." Each ward resembled a family, "select in itself." Although enjoying the benefits of properly selected acquaintances, a patient was not obliged to associate with undesirable individuals outside the ward. Like families of different status living on a city block, Kirkbride explained, "in walking along the streets, it is their own fault, if their attention is directed especially to what is unpleasant rather than to the agreeable sights that are constantly before them."[15]

Kirkbride had another common prejudice to overcome: Many people could not see the benefit to be obtained by gathering all the insane into one institution, when it seemed only logical that they would make each other worse. He insisted that this was not the case. Patients had such varied symptoms that no process of emulation or imitation took place. Instead, he claimed, they helped one another to recognize their own delusions. "Every one who has been much about institutions for the insane," Kirkbride wrote, "will acknowledge that certain patients are constantly exercising the most beneficial influence on others." Again, as in his characterization of chronic cases, the superintendent emphasized the salutary effect certain patients had on others. He mentioned, for example, the increasing number of voluntarily admitted patients, who as "intelligent, sympathizing" persons led others "to take views of their own cases which had not before occurred to them." He assured his readers that a "real interest in the troubles and sorrows" of fellow patients often became an individual's "best means of getting rid of [his] own."[16]

Yet, this beneficial patient interaction did not extend to relations with the opposite sex. After early experiments with social events involving the two sexes, Kirkbride abandoned them on the grounds that they exercised a poor influence on both patients and attendants. He characterized as "among the sacred things confided" to him as the hospital's chief physician, the duty to see that patients "be prevented from forming' while there, any acquaintances...with the opposite sex, that would be unpleasant to their friends, and after recovery, no less so to themselves." The only "true mode of securing the male patients, the humanizing influence of female society," he concluded, was to have, as female attendants, "ladies of suitable age and character with cultivated minds and attractive manners."[17]

When it came to presenting the patients' accommodations themselves, Kirkbride strove to describe the asylum in the most attractive terms. He well understood the importance of first impressions in securing a patient's confidence and willingness to submit to the hospital regimen, and continually worked to give the buildings "a pleasant and cheerful" character. To this end, he regarded "all the aids of external improvements, a certain degree of architectural embellishment, spacious halls, large and well-furnished parlors, and comfortable chambers" as among the "legitimate objects" of his expenditures. Each *Report* invariably included some pleasant description of the building or the pleasure grounds surrounding it, which Kirkbride repeatedly characterized as "highly cultivated and improved." One early *Report*, for example, lovingly detailed the ornamental trees, shrubs, flower borders, and walks surrounding the hospital. "These walks," Kirkbride elaborated, "have been so located as to embrace our finest and most diversified views, to wind through the woods and clumps of trees which are scattered through the enclosure."[18]

Having sketched in the hospital's comfortable accommodations, Kirkbride reassured his prospective patrons that the patients were kept ceaselessly amused. Every *Report* included a list of their entertainments, which grew longer and longer each year. Outdoor exercise and games, excursions to the city, teas and dinner parties, and church services were all detailed in such a way that the reader would have difficulty imagining a patient ever being bored or unoccupied. One memorable year, Kirkbride listed more than fifty different activities available to the patients, ranging from light gymnastics to "fancywork." The centerpiece of the hospital's offerings was its celebrated lecture series and magic lantern displays, given by a succession of assistant physicians. Reading the list of topics covered, including scenes of foreign countries, demonstrations in the natural sciences, and illustrations of new inventions such as the telegraph and steam engine, families would be convinced that hospital treatment included the equivalent of a lyceum series.[19]

Kirkbride gave an equally encouraging impression of the constant attention patients received from their attendants. Readers learned of the high standards he used in selecting these members of his staff, who, as he pointed out, spent the most time with the patients. The perfect attendant, according to Kirkbride, possessed "a pleasant expression of face, gentleness of tone, speech and manner, a fair amount of mental cultivation, imperturbable good temper, patience under the most trying provocation, coolness and courage in times of danger, cheerfulness without frivolity, industry, activity, and fertility of resources in unexpected emergencies." Such individuals would be "able to act as the guide and counsellor and friend of all the patients in their varying conditions." Despite their excellent personal qualities, however, the regular attendants could not be expected to engage the intellectual and artistic interests of the more cultivated patients. To fill this need, the patients enjoyed the services of companions or teachers, "intelligent and educated individuals with courteous manners, and refined feelings, genuine Christians" who encouraged reading, music, and handiwork in the wards. Never hinting that he might have difficulty hiring attendants or companions of such saintlike virtue, Kirkbride left his audience with the impression that the hospital's attendants conformed to the high standards set for them.[20]

Kirkbride insisted that his attendants used only kindness and persuasion in controlling the patients, and repeatedly expressed in the *Reports* his aversion to any form of physical restraint. He warned prospective patrons that he could not dispense with it altogether, however, for at times patients became violent with others or tried to harm themselves. To ensure that restraint was used only when all other methods had failed, Kirkbride told his readers that he kept the restraining devices in his office and always supervised their use himself. "I do not approve of a great variety of apparatus being kept in the wards of a hospital," he stated, for the constant presence of the "strong chair, muffs and other fixtures of the kind" has an "unpleasant influence" on both the patients and their attendants. Kirkbride felt that the free use of restraint encouraged the attendants to "think of their own ease, rather than the welfare of the patients," a tendency not to be countenanced in his hospital.[21]

Through his discussions of such topics as restraint, classification, and attendants, Kirkbride projected a reassuring set of beliefs about insanity and hospital treatment, beliefs that helped families and friends make sense of the disease and encouraged their patronage of the hospital. Kirkbride had to do more than simply explain these truths in the *Reports*, however. The asylum itself had to confirm his arguments whenever family members came to commit a patient or returned to visit. By comparing the image of the hospital created in his *Reports* with his professional writings on asylum construction and management, it becomes clear how the desire to impress and reassure his lay patrons shaped Kirkbride's professional priorities. From the perspective of his lay clientele, his attention to particular aspects of the hospital's appearance and function takes on new significance. One can begin to see how he worked to have the building's design and organization reinforce his patrons' beliefs about the hospital and eliminate certain realities of institutional life that might potentially undermine such confidence.

This was no easy task, for as his *Reports* make clear, Kirkbride promised his patrons a great deal. His asylum persuasion addressed a very complex and somewhat contradictory set of expectations. His patrons wanted the hospital environment to be homelike, yet exert a powerful influence over the insane; desired their sick relatives to be secluded and restrained without making the hospital look or feel like a prison; and expected patients to be classified by social and mental condition without neglecting the poorer or incurable ones in any way. To meet these expectations, Kirkbride had to strike a delicate balance between restraint and comfort, awesomeness and cheerfulness, class distinctions and egalitarianism. Resolving these design dilemmas required much of his professional energy. From this perspective, Kirkbride's careful attention to certain aspects of hospital design and management takes on more meaning.

The asylum blueprint

Kirkbride's concern with asylum construction began literally from the ground up, with the choice of a good site. He advised that the hospital be located outside a city of some size, and easily accessible by train and good roads. Such a location would ensure plentiful supplies and employees, as well as varied excursions for the patients. The hospital itself, he instructed, should be in a secluded area to ensure complete privacy. The soil had to be easily tilled, so that the farm and gardens would produce food for the patients' table and the area around the hospital itself could be extensively improved. "The surrounding scenery should be of a varied and attractive kind, and the neighborhood should possess numerous objects of an agreeable and interesting character," he wrote. The building itself should be placed so that the views from every window, especially the parlors and rooms occupied during the day, had pleasant prospects and "exhibit[ed] life in its active forms." The choice of a good site thus determined some of the hospital's most desirable features in its patrons' eyes: its accessibility, attractiveness, and supply of fresh food.[22]

The advantages of a good site had to be complemented by a sound building design. The general layout of the hospital determined two vital aspects of institutional life: the internal environment of the building, particularly its lighting and ventilation, and the proper classification of patients. The linear, or Kirkbride, plan,

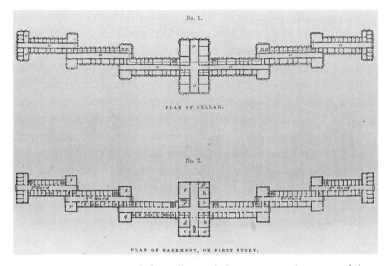

Figure 2. Linear plan of the cellar and first story as it appeared in Thomas Story Kirkbride, *On the Construction, Organization, and General Arrangements of Hospitals for the Insane* (Philadelphia, 1854), opposite p. 30.

as set forth in his 1854 treatise, emphasized several important features as fundamental to a good building plan. It had wings radiating off the center section (see Figure 2), so that each ward had proper ventilation and an unobstructed view of the grounds. By leaving open spaces at the end of each wing, "the darkest, most cheerless and worst ventilated parts" of the hospital could be eliminated, Kirkbride explained. He also advised inserting bay windows in the long halls, so that more light and air could enter. If the wings were not close together, there was "less opportunity for patients on opposite sides seeing or calling to each other, and less probability of the quiet patients being disturbed by those who are noisy." The linear plan also allowed for the maximum separation of the wards, so that the undesirable mingling of the patients might be prevented. Male and female patients had entirely separate wings. Within the wing, each ward had its own staircase, so that the patients might proceed directly outside to the pleasure grounds or to the center building without marching through another ward. Eight wards, the minimum Kirkbride felt desirable, could be established in each wing. He advised that the worst patients be confined in the ground-floor wards farthest from the center building and the best patients in the top-floor wards closer to the center.

"A classification that admits of no greater mingling of patients than this," Kirkbride concluded, "is quite rigid for all practical purposes."[23]

The style as well as the layout of the building had to be carefully considered. "Although it is not desirable to have an elaborate or costly style of architecture," Kirkbride wrote, "it is, nevertheless, really important that the building should be in good taste, and that it should impress favorably not only the patients, but their friends and others who may visit it." Any resemblance to a prison had to be carefully avoided. "The means of effecting the proper degree of security should be masked," he advised, and the building's custodial appearance camouflaged by ornamenting its grounds with gardens, fountains, and summer houses. These external improvements cost a considerable amount of money, Kirkbride acknowledged, but played such an important role in convincing patients and their families to support the institution that they could not be neglected. Every detail made a difference, he warned, for "no one can tell how important all these may prove in the treatment of patients, nor what good effects may result from first impressions thus made upon an invalid on reaching a hospital."[24]

The good impression made by the building's exterior arrangements had to be sustained by the appearance and practicality of its interior. "No desire to make a beautiful and picturesque exterior should ever be allowed to interfere with the internal arrangements," Kirkbride wrote. The interior had to sustain the cheerfulness of its exterior; as he advised one asylum superintendent, "have your parlors and rooms large and airy, with high ceilings, your corridors wide," and the overall good impression of the building would be sustained.[25]

Balancing the need to make the building appear as inviting as possible with the imperative to provide adequate restraint for its inmates posed the most difficult challenge Kirkbride faced in asylum design. Security measures inevitably detracted from the attractive image Kirkbride wished the hospital to have; yet, he felt that patient safety had to be the chief priority in its arrangements. As he wrote to Dorothea Dix in 1856, "The death of a single patient in ten years, or the escape and public suffering of one insane man or woman, would be a greater evil, than all the properly constructed window guards to be found about a well arranged Hospital."[26] Only by painstaking attention to details, Kirkbride believed, could the asylum be made secure without taking on the features of a prison. To this end, he showed considerable ingenuity in making the asylum's measures of restraint as unobtrusive as possible.

For example, Kirkbride believed that a mental hospital had to have a high wall around it to keep patients from escaping; at the same time, he did not want an obtrusive enclosure that would constantly remind visitors and patients of its confining purpose. As a compromise, Kirkbride proposed putting the wall as far from the building as possible, even sinking it in a trench, "to prevent its being an unpleasant feature, or to give the idea of a prison enclosure." He also attempted to soften the forbidding aspects of the wall by pointing out that it sheltered as well as confined the patients "by keeping improper persons out, by securing complete privacy to the institution," and by "protecting [patients] while out of the wards from the unfeeling gaze and remarks of passers by."[27]

Careful construction of the building's interior further minimized the potential for disruptive events in the hospital. Many of Kirkbride's detailed designs for ward fixtures reveal his underlying concern with the prevention of destruction, violence, suicide, and escape. Doors should always be made to open into the hallway, he advised, "as great annoyance and no little danger frequently results from patients barricading their doors from the inside, so as to render it almost impossible to get access to them." "Wickets" should be put in the doors so that patients could be observed or given food "when it might not be prudent for a single individual to enter the room." In constructing windows, the lower sash should be protected by a wrought iron window guard, so that it could be opened to admit air without allowing the patient to escape. This guard, "if properly made, and painted a white color, will not prove unsightly," unlike a cast iron sash, which, when raised, gave the appearance of "two sets of iron bars." A window guard "of tasteful pattern and neatly made" appeared no more forbidding than the devices used in the front windows "of some of the best houses in our large cities," Kirkbride claimed.[28]

Kirkbride's attention to doors and windows also reflected his fear of suicide, an event that inevitably contradicted the impression of constant watchfulness and protection he wished to project. For example, he gave explicit instructions for the construction of inside window screens, which prevented the patients from breaking the windows and using the glass for violent purposes. At the same time, the screen's frame had to be carefully fastened or it too would be used by patients determined to hang themselves. Other details had to be considered in order to make the hospital as injury-proof as possible. Kirkbride advised buying furniture that had no projections, sharp corners, or "other facilities for self-injury." In his directions for bathing facilities, he directed that the water handles be inaccessible to the patient, so that "improper use," presumably suicide by drowning, could not be made of the tub.[29]

If security was Kirkbride's primary concern in designing hospital fixtures, the general appearance of the building easily ranked as his next priority. "The process of wear and tear, and even of decay," he noted, occurred more quickly in a hospital for the insane than in an ordinary building. In order to "patient-proof" the building against its most destructive inmates, he suggested a few simple expedients. Plastering should be given "a hard finish...calculated for being scrubbed" in rooms "likely to be much abused by patients." When the floors of patients' rooms might be expected to need frequent washing, he suggested that they be inclined slightly toward the door.[30]

In the section of the building designed for less destructive patients, Kirkbride concentrated on making the wards as attractive and comfortable as possible. In order to convince patients and their families that hospital treatment involved no hardships, the wards had to appear homelike. The inevitable smells of an institution formed one of the biggest obstacles in this respect. Kirkbride's concern with ventilation originated in this practical problem. A good system of forced-air ventilation was "indispensable to give purity to the air of a hospital for the insane," he felt. A large section of his book was devoted to directions for the most effective form of heating and ventilation; he advocated using steam to heat outside air and circulate it through an extensive system of flues. In his directions for locating the flues, Kirkbride anticipated certain problems that might have spoiled their good effect; for example, he suggested that the hot air flues be placed near the ceiling in the ward rooms to prevent patients from "congregating around the hot air openings and using the flue as a spittoon." This plan, he added, "effectually secures the wards from all the offensive odors with which it is frequently filled from articles thrown through the registers."[31]

The toilet and cleaning facilities posed another threat to the hospital's appearance of good order. Kirkbride characterized water closets as the most unsatisfactory arrangement in most hospitals; their primitive design made them "a constant source of complaint, and a perfect nuisance in every part of the building where they are found." Yet, proper design might eliminate the unsavory aspects of this indispensable facility. Kirkbride explained that toilets constructed to provide a strong downward ventilation made "unpleasant odors in the wards...scarcely possible." All the fixtures of bathrooms, water closets, and sink rooms should be "left open and exposed to view" so that they provided "no harbour for vermin of any kind, no confined spot for foul air, or the deposit of filth." Another frequent nuisance "familiar to all who spend much time in the wards" was the "annoyance and unpleasant odors" coming from the wet cloths and brushes constantly used by the attendants. Along with his designs for the toilet facilities, Kirkbride included a detailed plan for a ward drying room, which would eliminate this problem.[32]

These examples demonstrate the ways in which Kirkbride related design and construction details to the asylum image he created in the *Reports*. In a properly constructed hospital, so he hoped, no escapes, suicides, and offensive smells would disturb either the patients or their families. But the building itself was only the foundation of the proper institutional order. The hospital structure had to be maintained by a cooperative staff, who would help manage the asylum pleasantly and efficiently. Thus, along with his suggestion for hospital construction, Kirkbride included an administrative plan that he felt would effectively complement his building design.

The essential prerequisite for proper hospital management was the complete authority of the chief physician. To divide his responsibility with any other officer made as little sense as to expect a "proper discipline" and "good order" from a ship with two captains or an army with two generals, Kirkbride felt. Every fixture of the hospital, "its farms and garden, its pleasure grounds and its means of amusement, no less than its varied internal arrangements, its furniture, its table service and the food, the mode in which its domestic concerns are carried on," he wrote, "everything connected with it, indeed, are parts of the great whole; and in order to secure harmony, economy and successful results, every one of them must be under the same control." This control, he argued, had to exist in an insane hospital, because its arrangements had an influence on the patients "not readily appreciated by a careless observer."[33]

In order to ensure the proper order of the great whole, the asylum superintendent had to have complete authority over his staff, for in a mental hospital, divisions among employees had potentially disastrous results. Personnel conflicts destroyed the "active and unceasing vigilance, joined with gentleness and firmness," needed to care properly for the patients. The superintendent prevented disruption of discipline not by constantly exercising his absolute power but simply by having it; "the simple possession of adequate authority...often prevents the necessity for its being exercised," Kirkbride wrote. His authority might be "unseen and unfelt and yet a knowledge of its existence, will often alone prevent wrangling and difficulties in the household, and secure regularity, good order and an efficient discipline about the whole establishment."[34]

Kirkbride's insistence on one-man rule in the asylum represented a departure from the usual practice in general hospitals, as he well knew from his own service at the old Pennsylvania Hospital. He justified the unusual amount of power given to asylum superintendents on the grounds that the asylum had to maintain a higher level of discipline and cleanliness than did the general hospital. Unlike critics of the asylum who came to view the superintendents' managerial duties as a source of the specialty's weakness, Kirkbride thought this fusion of medical and administrative authority highly desirable. Any asylum superintendent who voluntarily confined himself to the "mere medical direction" of his patients had a "very imperfect appreciation of his true position, or of the important trust confided in him," he wrote. Such an officer would be regarded by all concerned with the hospital as secondary or subordinate. Under such an arrangement, Kirkbride warned, no institution could obtain a "permanently high character."[35]

Effective management depended upon a carefully devised organizational plan, which ensured that the staff reinforced rather than countermanded the superintendent's authority. To secure the chief physician's dominance, Kirkbride outlined a suitably hierarchical scheme of management for the asylum. Under this plan, the assistant physician served as a less powerful version of the chief physician, with the same responsibility but limited authority.

Kirkbride specified that assistants had to be men of "such character and general qualifications as will render them respected by the patients and their friends" and able to "perform efficiently" in the superintendent's absence. The steward and matron had a less critical role in the asylum; they attended to the practical duties necessary for its cleanliness and good order. If their duties were "precisely defined" and their "subordination to the principal...well understood," their contribution to hospital discipline would be ensured. The attendants in many ways had the most critical functions in the asylum. As Kirkbride noted, their "presence and watchfulness" in the wards had to be the superintendent's "grand reliance." To ensure proper performance, he advised that attendants be carefully selected and constantly supervised.[36]

As the only authority superior to the superintendent, the Board of Managers played a particularly delicate role in Kirkbride's scheme of hospital organization. The managers had to possess sufficient authority to act as an ultimate check on the asylum superintendent without actually interfering with his administration of the asylum. Kirkbride realized that the community would ask for some assurance that the absolute power held by the asylum head was not misused. Therefore, the managers had to be men who "possess the public confidence," with a reputation for "liberality, intelligence...active benevolence," and "business habits," so that they could properly attend to the hospital's financial affairs and enhance its public reputation. He believed that a weekly visit from two managers would furnish enough supervision to convince the public that no abuse or neglect could occur. At the same time, the managers had to maintain a proper disinterestedness. They could not have any contracts for the hospital's supplies or show a "personal interest" in any of its subordinates; otherwise, people might question the institution's nonprofit nature. The managers also had to be careful not to "weaken the authority of the principal of the institution." Kirkbride warned that the managers should "most carefully avoid any interference with what is delegated to others, or meddling with the direction of details for which others are responsible."[37]

From the judicious choice of a site to the proper management of managers, Thomas Story Kirkbride provided the blueprint for the ideal asylum. His plans for the hospital's building and administration translated the principles of asylum medicine outlined in the *Reports* into concrete form. As the basis of his medical practice, Kirkbride articulated a therapeutic persuasion that insisted that insanity was curable, especially when treated promptly; that hospital treatment was far superior to home care; that patients could be effectively classified and amused according to their social class and degree of illness; and that the asylum staff provided constant, humane care for their charges. Having encouraged these beliefs, Kirkbride then had to maintain his asylum as a visible confirmation of his therapeutic claims. Only by keeping the reality of institutional life as close to his patrons' expectations as possible could Kirkbride ensure their generous confidence in his medical authority.

THE HISTORIC ASYLUM

Despite their pragmatism and ingenuity, Kirkbride's directives concerning asylum design and management were by no means easily implemented. The supervision of the great whole, as Kirkbride envisioned it, obviously placed tremendous demands on the superintendent. Not only did the asylum doctor's success depend upon taxing his own physical and mental resources to the limit; it also required extensive cooperation from managers and employees, generous financial support, and more than a little good luck. The administrative career of Kirkbride himself, by all accounts one of the most successful nineteenth-century superintendents and his generation's acknowledged authority on hospital construction and management, nicely illustrates the challenges of asylum work. The contrasts between Kirkbride's ideal asylum and realities at the Pennsylvania Hospital for the Insane suggest some of the institutional tensions inherent in the practice of moral treatment.

The original hospital building

Kirkbride's challenge, like his injunctions on hospital design, began with the original building of the Pennsylvania Hospital for the Insane. Since he was hired only shortly before the hospital opened, Kirkbride played no part in the preliminary planning for the institution, a circumstance he deeply regretted. His emphatic advice that no hospital plan should ever be implemented without prior inspection and approval "of some one or more physicians who have had a large practical acquaintance with the insane...as well as with the advantages and defects of existing hospitals" reflected his own bitter experience.[38]

The hospital site, Kirkbride had to acknowledge, was excellent. The 111-acre farm purchased by the managers had fertile soil and a good water supply. Forty-one acres had been enclosed by a 10.5-foot wall to form the asylum pleasure grounds; the remaining 70 acres comprised the hospital farm. Surrounded by lightly wooded, gently rolling hills, the building had attractive vistas from its windows. Although sufficiently remote to ensure complete privacy, the asylum had all the advantages of being close to Philadelphia, with its markets, shops, and services, as well as the small community of Blockley, where the convalescent patients often went to attend church services.[39]

Kirkbride thought the original hospital building, designed by the English architect Isaac Holden, far less desirable than its site. It comprised a basement and two stories, all of stone (refer to Figure 1). The upper stories of the center section housed the officers' rooms, business office, apothecary, parlors, and visitors' rooms. In the basement were the servants' rooms, laundry, kitchen, and furnaces. Two wings extended north and south of the center, every floor forming a ward with twenty patients' rooms, each eight by ten feet in size, ranged on both sides of a twelve-foot corridor. Perpendicular to these wings stood two end buildings, called the *return wings*, containing wards made up of eight rooms, measuring eight by eleven feet, and three larger rooms, thirteen by eleven feet. All the wards had their own parlor, bathroom, and water closet. In all, the hospital had the capacity to house 160 patients.[40]

Kirkbride found the design and construction of the original hospital building deficient on several counts. First, the division of the wards allowed for only four groupings of each sex, an arrangement he found seriously inadequate. After patients had occupied the hospital for only four months, the superintendent asked the managers to authorize additional accommodations for the "noisy, violent and habitually filthy," to be built some distance from the main building. This class of patients had been living in the already crowded lower wards of the return wings, where their noise disturbed the other patients. The managers approved the construction of two lodges, located next to the return wings but facing away from the hospital. Each new lodge had twenty rooms ranged along three sides of a square; the fourth side was left open, but was protected by an iron palisade fence.[41]

In the late 1840s, Kirkbride expanded these outlying buildings to provide more wards. First, he filled in the area from the return wing to the lodge with an infirmary and a seclusion ward. On the far side of the lodge, he built another section with an "associated dormitory," or open ward, for ten chronic cases. These additions increased the hospital's capacity to 250 patients and gave Kirkbride eight wards in each wing to classify them properly. He housed the upper-class patients in the first and second wards on the top floors of the main building; the wealthiest patients had the larger rooms on the second ward of the return wing. In the third and fourth wards on the ground floor of the main building, he placed the moderately excited recent patients; the worst-behaved members of this group had the fourth ward in the return wing. The fifth ward provided an infirmary for patients with acute physical ailments. The old lodges constituted the sixth and seventh wards, for noisy or violent patients. The quiet chronic patients occupied the eighth ward.[42]

In 1847, Kirkbride had constructed another type of accommodation, a secluded, elegant little "cottage" paid for by the relatives of a wealthy woman patient. This small, one-story Italianate house could hold one or two patients, along with their attendants. "The whole is furnished in good style, and has the air of a neat and comfortable private residence," Kirkbride informed his readers in the *Report* for 1847. Intending originally to build more small residences for rich patients, Kirkbride eventually abandoned the plan when he realized that the cottage's separation from the main building made it more difficult to supervise, and turned his attention instead to improving the accommodations in the better wards.[43]

Often stymied in his attempts to remake the hospital building, Kirkbride found it much easier to turn the pleasure grounds into a showcase. In the hospital's first decade, he had dry walks and extensive flower gardens laid out, and built a greenhouse to furnish flowers for the wards and serve as "an attractive object for daily visits at a little distance from the Hospital." A museum and reading room, funded by donations and constructed in 1851, provided another location where "the more highly cultivated class of patients" might go to read and talk. The museum also housed the hospital's constantly growing collection of stuffed birds, minerals, and other curios. A "calistheneum," erected in 1852, was used for tenpins and other forms of light exercise. Additional small improvements completed the ornamental aspects of the hospital grounds; a walk from the return wing built in the 1850s conducted the patients past the cottage, summerhouse, swing, "pleasure railroad" (a miniature ride for the patients), calistheneum, "mound" (a terraced garden), and pigeonhouse.[44]

Although Kirkbride succeeded in improving and expanding the original building and grounds in some respects, basic defects in the hospital's design remained. The ventilation system could not produce the purity of air he desired, because it lacked the means to force the air to circulate, and the flues provided for heating and ventilating the rooms were much too small. "In close rooms constantly occupied by patients or even temporarily by those of filthy habits," Kirkbride complained to the managers, "it is often extremely difficult to remove the impure air." In the lodge, he tried using a portable fan, or "ventilator," to freshen the air, noting approvingly that one "individual who has caused the necessity for the ventilator has been induced to work it," but soon felt dissatisfied with such a piecemeal solution. The patients were not always the source of hospital smells; the latrines located in the yard adjacent to the seventh ward filled it with "an unpleasant odor...the credit of which is generally given to the patients," Kirkbride pointed out to the managers. Unfortunately, the superintendent could not easily convince the managers that a new ventilation and plumbing system was a pressing necessity in a building hardly a decade old.[45]

The baseboard and walls of the new asylum were soon infested with insects and rodents. Kirkbride informed the managers in 1854 that the kitchen had become such a "harbor for vermin" that he could no longer take visitors there. Mice in the wards caused complaints from both the patients and their families. Kirkbride had to be summoned from his bed late one night to soothe a woman patient who, after seeing a mouse in her room, threatened to stand on a chair all night if forced to sleep there. The rodent problem caused another, more serious incident that illustrates the damaging effect such nuisances could have on the hospital's reputation. In 1850, the body of a male patient who had just died of a chronic disease was left in his room for several hours. When the attendants came to take the corpse to the "dead house," they saw (as Kirkbride later reported to the managers) that a "portion of the cartilage of his nose had been destroyed, how they were unable to say, but it is supposed by a mouse or a rat." The assistant physician tried to repair the damage as best he could, but the patient's family and friends demanded a coroner's inquest. After hearing testimony from the steward, wing supervisor, and attendants, the coroner found no evidence of wrongdoing by the hospital. Still, some of the patient's friends "thought it necessary to talk in a strain of considerable exaggeration about a very simple matter," Kirkbride reported, and the episode caused the institution a good deal of embarrassment.[46]

In light of such incidents, Kirkbride's concern with seemingly trivial details of hospital construction appears more understandable. The smallest flaws in a building's design, whether poorly constructed toilets or baseboard havens for vermin, could create vexing problems for the asylum superintendent. Naturally, Kirkbride regretted his lack of involvement in the planning of the Pennsylvania Hospital for the Insane, for the building's features, both good and bad, deeply affected his asylum work, yet he had had no role in determining its structure. A few years' experience gave him many practical insights into the art of designing asylums, knowledge that he attempted to pass on in his professional writings and consultations. But as a young superintendent, Kirkbride never expected to be able to apply his expertise to the construction of his own hospital. Writing to Amariah Brigham in 1844, he confessed, "I cannot help envying you, who have the building to suit yourself – it is one of the things I should like exceedingly to be allowed to undertake, but our arrangements are now so far completed, that it is hardly possible that I shall ever have a chance to do more than make alterations in what we already have."[47]

The male department, 1859

Eventually, the asylum's growth did make it possible for Kirkbride to build a hospital to suit himself. As so frequently had occurred in the old Eighth Street hospital, overcrowding once again became a catalyst for innovation. A steady increase in admissions, from 238 in 1842 to more than 400 in 1852, began to place severe strains on the asylum's resources in the early 1850s. Caring for an average of 230 patients required "an unusual amount of vigilance, anxiety and labor" on the staff's part, as Kirkbride reported in 1855. With the hospital so crowded, he felt compelled to turn away even patients whom he knew required immediate attention. The consequence of this situation, as the superintendent stated dramatically in his 1854 *Report*, formed "a sad story of grievous sufferings unrelieved, of mental darkness perpetuated, of family griefs unassuaged, and of a whole community exposed, in a greater or less extent, to the mischievous or dangerous propensities of irresponsible individuals."[48]

Appealing to the civic pride and benevolence of Pennsylvanians, Kirkbride used the problem of overcrowding to promote a plan he had long had in mind: the construction of an entirely new asylum, the same size as the old, on the grounds of the hospital farm. The original building would become the Female Department, the new building the Male Department. Such a plan would appeal greatly to the asylum's patrons, Kirkbride argued, because it would provide both sexes with a "greater degree of liberty...with more privacy." It also conformed to Kirkbride's experience that there were no advantages and many disadvantages attendant upon treating men and women in the same building.[49]

The managers approved Kirkbride's scheme and commissioned him to raise the necessary funds for the new hospital. The Male Department, which cost approximately $350,000 to construct, was begun in 1856 and completed in 1859 on a site less than one mile from the original hospital (see Figure 3). Its design conformed closely to the linear plan Kirkbride had formulated in his 1854 book on asylum construction, although modified, due to the size of the lot, so that the wings did not lie at such a distance from the center building. The new hospital differed from the old in several respects, having three stories instead of two and including one-story buildings at the end of the return wings that served the same function as the old lodges. The building's proportions had been increased as well; the rooms were larger (8 × 11 feet), the halls wider (14 feet), and the ceilings higher. The new wards also had more elaborate facilities, including parlors, dining rooms, bathrooms, water closets, and storerooms, and could more effectively be isolated from each other. In many important details, such as the window construction, ventilation system, and vermin-proof baseboards, the new hospital conformed to Kirkbride's ideal asylum. The Male Department became his showpiece; Kirkbride used

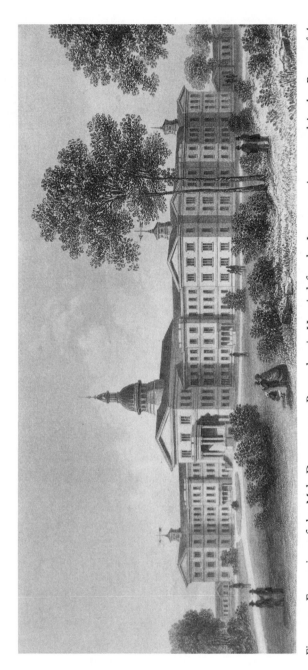

Figure 3. Engraving of the Male Department, Pennsylvania Hospital for the Insane, as it appeared in the *Report of the Pennsylvania Hospital for the Insane for 1859*, the year the new hospital opened.

its architectural plans as the frontispiece for the second edition of his book on asylum construction and frequently entertained his professional friends in its spacious public rooms. "The whole building inside and out, gives one an impression of strength, endurance, good taste and some elegance," observed his friend and fellow superintendent, Isaac Ray.[50]

Once the new asylum was finished, Kirkbride turned his attention to the original hospital building. To be brought up to the Male Department's standards, the Female Department gradually had its wards replastered and repainted and its ventilation, toilet, and bathing facilities overhauled. In the 1860s and 1870s, Kirkbride undertook fundraising drives to finance further expansion of and improvements in the women's accommodations. With this money, two infirmary wards were constructed in 1868 and 1873, and the Mary Shields Building (for the upper-class female patients) was finished in 1880. The two hospitals each had a capacity for 250 patients, with greatly expanded facilities for classification.[51]

Improving the physical foundation of his asylum practice necessitated not only a great deal of Kirkbride's efforts but also the active support of the hospital's Board of Managers. Before the superintendent could consider how to design and implement desirable improvements, he had to secure their approval. Preserving an amicable relationship with the board depended first upon satisfying the attending managers, who visited the asylum once a week to record the number of admissions and discharges, examine the steward's accounts, and inquire into the general state of institutional affairs. More serious business between the superintendent and the managers was transacted at the monthly board meetings held at the Eighth Street hospital. From Kirkbride's written reports for these sessions emerges a sense of his relations with the managers and the strategies he used to gain support for his proposed improvements.[52]

The superintendent and his managers

The Pennsylvania Hospital's managers were precisely the sort of benevolent, wealthy, well-respected men that Kirkbride thought made for an ideal governing body. They all held important positions as financiers, manufacturers, and merchants in the Philadelphia business community. With their connections to iron and steel manufactories, railroad companies, and import–export firms, the managers had access to the wealth being generated by the city's economic growth. They also played an active role in the burgeoning field of urban philanthropy; besides their work at the Pennsylvania Hospital, the managers involved themselves in numerous other humanitarian and civic organizations, including the newly established institutions for the blind, deaf and dumb, and feebleminded. The fact that the majority were Orthodox Friends like himself also contributed to the harmony of interest between doctor and managers. Throughout his tenure of office, Kirkbride seems to have maintained an excellent working relationship with the Pennsylvania Hospital's board.[53]

The managers displayed a consistent but not overbearing interest in the asylum's affairs. As Kirkbride was fond of boasting, the attending managers never missed their weekly visit to the West Philadelphia branch of the hospital. Over the years, some managers had developed a particularly intense interest in the asylum. Samuel Welsh, who served on the board from 1856 to 1890, and William Biddle, who served from 1847 to 1888, were two of the managers most actively concerned with the mental department of the Pennsylvania Hospital. Welsh frequently visited the asylum, getting to know individual patients and making a special effort to acquire novelties for their amusement. On a trip to Europe in 1859, Welsh toured a number of insane asylums in order to get new ideas for his own institution. "You have been much in our minds and conversations," he wrote to Kirkbride from Scotland. William Biddle was also an enthusiastic manager with a special fondness for Kirkbride. "The twenty-four years I have been associated with thee," he wrote to Kirkbride in 1873, "have been to me truly an interesting portion of my life, and I can look back to none of my associations with more pleasure."[54]

However intense their concern with the hospital's welfare, the managers usually expressed their interest in ways that did not infringe upon Kirkbride's institutional authority. As a body, the board rarely interfered with the superintendent's day-to-day management of the asylum. Occasionally, a committee might be convened to look into a special matter, such as a patient complaint; but these investigations served more to protect the hospital against legal action than to question Kirkbride's handling of the matter. When individual managers had some specific task they wished accomplished at the asylum, they consulted with rather than commanded the superintendent to obey their wishes. For example, managers frequently recommended cases in which they felt a personal interest for admission on the poor list or at a reduced rate of board. Although possessed of the power to issue the order themselves, the managers always asked Kirkbride's permission first (requests with which he invariably complied). Managers also avoided calling at the asylum or bringing visitors without informing Kirkbride beforehand. What suggestions concerning the details of hospital management the managers did occasionally venture reflected their solicitude for the institution. After getting his feet wet on a rainy day, Caleb Cope wrote to Kirkbride, "Surely we are not so poor but that we might afford a few boards to extend our dry walk in the direction referred to." Having broached the subject of improvements, Cope went on to suggest that Kirkbride dismantle the "rabbit domicile," a structure that Cope felt detracted from "the beauty of the ground." Even if Kirkbride resented Cope's interference, he could not help but appreciate the manager's concern for the asylum.[55]

Although the managers exercised commendable restraint in regard to the asylum's domestic affairs, they took a far less detached view of its financial administration. Their primary role as governors of the hospital, so they believed, was to conserve its fiscal resources rather than oversee its daily operation. As a result, the board required a more detailed accounting of Kirkbride's expenditures than they asked for in other aspects of his asylum work. However much they respected his medical and administrative talents, their final approval of Kirkbride rested primarily on his financial skills. First and foremost, the managers wanted the superintendent to make the hospital self-supporting: "What I wish," the president of the board stated unequivocally in 1880, "is that our Insane Department may be able to pay its own expenses." Unfortunately, Kirkbride rarely met this expectation. In only thirteen of his forty-three years as head of the Pennsylvania Hospital for the Insane did he manage to balance expenditures with receipts or end the year with a small surplus. More often than not, Kirkbride had to request a sum that ranged from $500 to $5,000 to be advanced from the Pennsylvania Hospital's general funds. Compared to the state mental hospitals, which during these same decades were requiring between $10,000 and $20,000 in appropriations each year, Kirkbride's financial record appears quite sound. But to the managers, who naturally grew alarmed at any diminution of the hospital's assets, the superintendent had to justify his requests very carefully.[56]

In large part, as the managers realized, Kirkbride's financial embarrassments stemmed from economic conditions over which he had no control. The asylum experienced its worst fiscal crises in the 1860s and again in the late 1870s, when inflation caused ruinous price increases for supplies at the same time that economic uncertainty diminished the patrons' ability to meet board payments. During the Civil War, the Pennsylvania Hospital for the Insane suffered a loss of almost $38,000 in board from southerners, always a sizable contingent among its patrons. "The affairs of the Hospital occupy my mind very much of late," Caleb Cope confided to Kirkbride in 1866. "The question [of] how it is to be maintained is a very embarrassing one." By a public appeal for funds, the asylum managed to survive the wartime difficulties. But again in the late 1870s, the institution's financial position became precarious as depression cut deeply into the patrons' capacity to make board payments. William Biddle, a longtime manager, observed in 1880, "There certainly never before since I was a Manager of the Board, have been so many applications for a reduction [of board] as during the last year or two."[57]

All too aware of the external factors involved in the asylum's financial problems, the managers never accused Kirkbride of mismanagement during these worrisome times. On the contrary, they often praised the superintendent's judicious administration of the asylum. Samuel Welsh, congratulating Kirkbride on collecting so many subscriptions for the new hospital after the Panic of 1859, wrote, "You have shown yourself to be a capital financier in raising so much money during the crisis." Yet, a chronic lack of funds still placed Kirkbride in a vulnerable position with his managers. Every time he wished to introduce a new improvement, he had to wage a determined campaign to convince the managers that the expenditure represented a wise investment. The larger the deficit at the end of the fiscal year, the harder he found it to secure their support. To overcome this disadvantage, Kirkbride had to develop tactics not unlike those he pursued with his patrons in the *Reports*. But rather than expound the principles of moral treatment, Kirkbride used his Monthly Reports to the managers to develop a persuasive theory of hospital economics.[58]

Kirkbride's periodic fiscal reports to the managers constantly reminded them that improvements in the building and grounds brought a better class of patrons to the asylum. "True economy," as he wrote in one Monthly Report, "I conceive to consist in the smallest possible expenditure of money that will enable us to maintain a high character for the institution and to secure at least a share of that class of patients who are able and willing to pay liberally for their accommodations." Affluent patrons could afford to send an insane relative to almost any asylum they liked, so Kirkbride reasoned; naturally, the quality of an institution's fixtures had a significant bearing on their decision. If the Pennsylvania Hospital for the Insane were to remain equal with its competitors, the managers had to make generous outlays on the building and grounds. To drive his point home, Kirkbride often marshalled statistics and observations about the McLean, Butler, and Bloomingdale hospitals, that is, the other corporate institutions with which the Pennsylvania Hospital for the Insane competed for wealthy patrons. In 1863, after returning from a visit to eight northern hospitals, Kirkbride warned the managers, "no hospital can long keep in advance of others without steadily elevating its system of treatment, and increasing its means for promoting the general health, and the occupations and amusements of its patients." Stating that the Pennsylvania Hospital for the Insane compared unfavorably with its rival institutions only in its furnishings and dining arrangements, Kirkbride proceeded to outline improvements needed in these two areas. Unless the managers cooperated, he implied, the Pennsylvania Hospital might slip from the "first rank" of mental hospitals and so lose its affluent patients to more "liberal institutions."[59]

Kirkbride reinforced these claims by demonstrating the asylum's financial dependence upon its wealthiest patrons. "Without our large list of $10, $15 and $20 patients," he pointed out, "we should not be able to get along without large demands on the Treasury." In fact, the 20–25 percent of the patrons paying the highest rates accounted for half of the hospital's income. Since almost half of the rich patients came from other states, they could indeed have gone to another institution with only a little more effort. Of the out-of-state clientele, more than half, including many of the very wealthiest, came from southern states. Although the Pennsylvania Hospital for the Insane was the closest and most prestigious corporate asylum available to the planter class, they could easily have sent their insane relatives farther north. Thus, the institution had to work to keep these patients by making it doubly attractive to them. "No fact is better established," Kirkbride wrote in 1859, "than that to enable us to secure the class of patients who are really profitable to the hospital and enable it to keep its free list – everything about it must be kept in the very best order, and the arrangements and accommodations must be of a liberal kind."[60]

As Kirkbride reminded the managers constantly, the patients' family found the quality of the hospital's accommodations, that is, the patients' rooms and furnishings, "much easier to appreciate than many other things connected with the medical and moral treatment of the patients." Yet, many patrons were also very sensitive, as their letters to him demonstrated, to less tangible features of hospital care. Referring to his ambitious program of evening entertainment, Kirkbride wrote in his Monthly Report for 1864, "I am having unmistakable evidences, that what we have been doing for the occupation and amusement of our patients is becoming known very generally, and in many quarters, that are important to our permanent success, is recognized as a proof, that we are at least in the front rank of [mental] institutions." In another instance, he asked the managers not to cut the attendants' salaries, on the grounds that "From the published reports of this hospital, the public has learned what we consider the requisite qualifications for attendants, and the details of our organization, and a knowledge of these, has in many instances, caused patients to be sent here, in preference to other institutions." In order to meet the expectations that Kirkbride had raised in his *Reports*, the asylum had to be kept as close to ideal conditions as possible, however expensive that might prove, for only by a generous outlay of funds could the patrons' generous confidence in the institution be maintained.[61]

Kirkbride's success in using these arguments with the board depended in large part upon his ability as a fund raiser. As long as the superintendent promised to raise the lion's share of the money needed to finance a particular project, the managers more than willingly agreed to his plans. Luckily, Kirkbride's talent for fundraising matched the scale of his ambitions. He had a clever way of soliciting funds by translating dollar amounts into visions of benevolence. An average gift of less than $75, he once explained to Dorothea Dix, "enables us to *cure* a patient." Therefore, any one "adding two thousand dollars to our capital would have the cheering reflection that through future years, there would always be ten under treatment from his fund, and that from it, 12 to 15 would every year be restored to health and society." Kirkbride, as his former assistant, John Curwen, once remarked to Dix, exercised the "faculty of begging...by persuading people that it was their distinguished privilege to give this or that." The funds for the women's infirmary wards were solicited in precisely that fashion, for, as Kirkbride explained to the managers, he sought (and found) a donor eager to accept the "privilege" of connecting his or her name "enduringly with a structure destined in all future time to prove of such inestimable benefit to a peculiarly interesting class of the afflicted."[62]

For all his evident ability in this aspect of asylum upkeep, Kirkbride occasionally complained of the effort he had to expend in persuading "benevolent old ladies and gentlemen...to allow the Managers and myself to have the privilege of using some of their superfluous funds." Yet, ambition made Kirkbride dependent upon such donors, for as he confided to Dorothea Dix, "I want everything magnificent and beautiful and useful that I can get for the Hospital, but I have become fully convinced that it is better to get such things as presents rather than buying them." The superintendent's "begging" produced handsome results, for the asylum regularly received large cash gifts and legacies. The huge sums needed to build the Male Department and renovate the Female Department were obtained entirely by his subscription campaign. In addition, supporters provided the many small embellishments and luxuries that the asylum boasted of, including the patient libraries, museum, reading room, calistheneum, and billiard hall. At the end of each *Report*, Kirkbride carefully noted the sums of money given, along with the numerous gifts of live and stuffed animals, mineral "cabinets," paintings, and exotic curios sent to the asylum each year, thereby expressing his gratitude while at the same time hinting at the desirability of further contributions.[63]

Kirkbride's prowess as a fund raiser undoubtedly mitigated the managers' concern about asylum finances. In the long run, they appear to have been persuaded by his argument about the true nature of hospital economy. A Committee of Managers reporting on the asylum in 1869 stated that "one of the prominent causes of our success in the treatment of disease as well as the general estimation in which we are held has long been owing to the great pains taken to vary both the day and evening amusements." Thanking Kirkbride for his devotion to the hospital, the managers concluded with the hope that he "may be long spared to us." The board expressed their confidence in Kirkbride in more concrete terms as well. His salary was among the highest paid to any asylum superintendent of the period: $3,000 per annum for the first decade and a half of his service, with raises to $4,000 in 1866, and $5,000 in 1871. In addition to his salary, Kirkbride lived rent-free in the mansion house on the Female Department grounds and, after 1855, had his expenses paid to the annual Association of Medical Superintendents' conventions. Declaring at the time of Kirkbride's last raise that their asylum was the "equal of any one in the country," the managers affirmed their belief that their institution's reputation was "attributable in a great measure to the untiring exertions of our Physician in Chief."[64] Through hard work and a talent for fundraising, Kirkbride sustained a good relationship with his managers. If not as easily acquired or generous as he might have liked, the managers' backing was reliable and consistent, enabling Kirkbride to maintain the asylum's accommodations at a high level. Kirkbride's advancement as an asylum superintendent depended in large part upon the cooperation he gained from both the managers and the contributors. Without their backing, he would have been unable to finance the modification and expansion of the hospital's physical accommodations, which he felt to be essential to its therapeutic purpose.

But on a day-to-day basis, Kirkbride's relations with the managers had a less decisive effect on the quality of his asylum practice than did his interactions with the asylum staff. Without their cooperation, the superintendent's efforts to improve the hospital's accommodations would have been in vain. The asylum's proper functioning required not only a well-designed, nicely appointed building, as Kirkbride observed in his professional writings, but also an administrative structure of considerable range and complexity. As its head, Kirkbride had to oversee the work of a varied work force, ranging from the apothecary to the gardener. Ultimately, the superintendent's ability to inspire loyalty and diligence in his employees determined the success of his asylum administration as much as his rapport with the managers and contributors. In a very real sense, the staff's strengths and weaknesses set the boundaries for the chief physician's accomplishments. Thus, the motivations and skills of Kirkbride's staff became a vital factor in the realization of his asylum philosophy.

With only one major alteration, the administrative structure of the Pennsylvania Hospital for the Insane remained unchanged throughout Kirkbride's tenure. The principal asylum staff consisted, in descending order of authority, of the assistant physician, steward and matron, wing supervisors, companions, and attendants. The hospital also employed a number of ancillary personnel, including domestics, cooks, farm laborers, engineers, gatekeepers, night watchers, and seamstresses. When the Male Department opened in 1859, the same staff structure was duplicated, with the addition of an extra assistant physician. In 1875, both branches of the hospital gained another physician, making the total number of assistants two at the Female Department and three at the Male Department. In theory, the hospital employees all reported directly to the superintendent; in practice, the steward and matron supervised the menial workers, including the cooks, domestics, and seamstresses. Although limited in his capacity to supervise the whole staff directly, the superintendent still maintained a commanding presence in every corner of the institution. "Dr. Kirkbride never fails to see when a counterpane is laid crooked on a bed," hospital rumor had it, and he was "sure to come where there was neglect of duty"[65] (see Figure 4).

The assistant physician

At the top of the staff hierarchy stood the assistant physician, who, in authority and responsibility, was second only to the superintendent. Depending on a "frank and confidential intercourse...in regard to patients and hospital matters" to ensure good service, Kirkbride allowed the assistants to perform the routine forms of medical and moral treatment without constant supervision. They had rooms in the asylum's center building, so that they might be on call twenty-four hours a day. The assistants' duties began early in the morning with ward rounds, which were often, but not always, made with the superintendent. During the morning visit, the assistants spoke to the patients, noted their mental and physical condition, and distributed the medicine prepared by the apothecary. Depending on an individual's behavior, they might order a change in ward assignment. Sometime during the day, the infor-

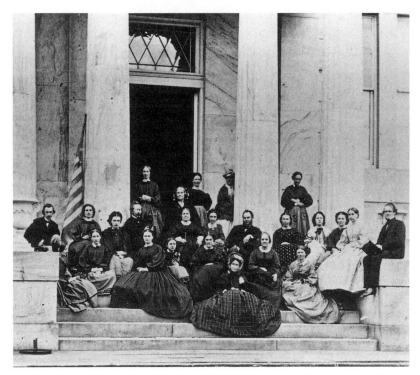

Figure 4. The hospital "family": Thomas Story Kirkbride and the employees of the Female Department. Photograph taken in the early 1860s. (Courtesy of the Historic Archives, Institute of the Pennsylvania Hospital.)

mation gathered on ward rounds had to be recorded in the case records, which the assistants wrote up as part of their duties. When visitors arrived to see patients, they would leave their work to see to the patrons' requests and conduct them about the asylum. Kirkbride considered patron management to be an essential aspect of the assistant's responsibilities. "It is especially important that you should see the friends of patients, and visitors promptly," he admonished Edward Smith, "so that there may be no complaints or useless detentions, waiting to see officers." The superintendent also liked his seconds-in-command to make a daily tour of the hospital's various departments. "This," as he told Smith, "would add to your own interest, and increase their respect for you, just as your frequent visits in the wards would secure the confidence of the attendants and patients." In what spare time they had left from all these duties, the assistants prepared the lectures and slides for the evening entertainment of the patients.[66]

The first assistant's position in the Male Department involved additional obligations. Kirkbride had originally asked the managers to appoint another physician to have complete, independent control over the new hospital, but the board preferred to have him continue as superintendent of both branches of the asylum. Kirkbride reluctantly consented to this arrangement, and gave the man hired as first assistant in the Male Department, S. Preston Jones, much more authority than he usually granted his assistants. The superintendent explained to the manager in 1862, when asking for an increase in Jones's salary, "His duties and responsibilities in his present position are greater than is common for Assistant Physicians, from the fact that a large portion of *my* time is unavoidably taken up by consultations in reference to the hospital and patients, by persons who come to the institution from various parts of the country." Although under the new arrangement Kirkbride felt that he spent his time in "the most profitable mode" possible, he regretted that his double duties prevented him from seeing the male patients "as frequently as I otherwise should." If his management of two hospitals was to work smoothly, Kirkbride argued, the managers had to realize "how important it is, that a man of some experience and of good ability should fill that post" in the Male Department, and that he be paid an appropriate salary. As Kirkbride grew older, he delegated even more authority to Jones. He wrote to the managers in 1881, "for several years past, I have gradually been allowing the care and responsibility of the Department of Males to fall more and more directly on Dr. Jones...in...whose competency, there can be no question." Until his death in 1883, Kirkbride continued to urge the managers to hire two chief physicians when he retired (advice the managers chose not to follow, as we shall see).[67]

Despite Jones's special position, Kirkbride still maintained a check on the younger doctor's authority, especially in patient-related matters. All information regarding the Male Department had to be funneled through Kirkbride's office, even though he frequently knew much less about its affairs than Jones did. When the superintendent received a letter asking about a particular male patient, for example, he would forward it to Jones, asking for a statement regarding the patient's condition; when he received the assistant's reply, Kirkbride would then write the letter himself. When a woman patron wrote directly to Jones asking for information, saying, "I have heard your visits to Mr. B [a patient] were more frequent than those of Dr. Kirkbride," she was told in no uncertain terms to communicate directly with the chief physician. Under this arrangement, Kirkbride probably received more credit than he deserved for Jones's work with the patients. Patrons often sent the older doctor grateful letters that referred to an assistant's competent treatment of a case, but thanked only the superintendent for its successful resolution. In some instances, patrons became angry when they realized that Kirkbride would not have immediate charge of their male relatives. A man declaring himself "perfectly satisfied of the skill and under obligation for the kind attention" of Dr. Jones nonetheless begged the superintendent to see his father, claiming that "when I placed him there, it was with the express understanding that you would see him and examine into his case." Jones's feelings about such incidents cannot be determined, but, as will be shown in Chapter 5, the "divided authority" at the Male Department led to some unpleasant publicity for the asylum during the commitment controversies of the 1860s and 1870s.[68]

Generally, Kirkbride's relations with his assistant physicians were marked by a curious mixture of deference and dependence. The complexities of their working relationships were most fully revealed in the letters they exchanged during Kirkbride's annual absence at the AMSAII convention. In their missives, the younger doctors gave a detailed report on hospital events, calling particular attention to those situations that might prove troublesome. For example, they mentioned patients who had to be restrained, force-fed, or given chloral hydrate, a relatively new drug that Kirkbride experimented with hesitantly in the 1870s. In a somewhat more defensive tone, the assistants reported on escapes and suicide attempts. S. Preston Jones, informing Kirkbride of a patient's attempt to kill himself by pitching himself head first from a toilet seat, obviously felt that he had to account for the man's being left unattended. "We knew he was suicidal," Jones explained, "but did not imagine he was so desperately determined to make away with himself." Similarly, Edward Smith emphasized his diligent attempts to recover an escaped patient: "Upon finding he had gone, we scoured the grounds, but I could think of no other proceedings in regard to him until your return." Assistants not infrequently ran into difficulties with the patients' relatives, which they dutifully reported to the superintendent. J. Edwards Lee recounted an unpleasant interview with a patron who wanted to take his niece on a trip that Lee thought ill-advised. After arguing with the uncle, Lee refused to let the patient go until Kirkbride returned. "I write this to give you a correct idea of our interview," he concluded, knowing full well that the uncle would pursue the matter when Kirkbride came back from his trip. Problems with attendants also figured in the assistants' letters. Smith wrote agitatedly that an attendant had been arrested for stealing hospital supplies. "I can hardly make up my mind that it is our Charley and until tomorrow will not believe it," he lamented. William Moon interceded for an attendant in precarious health, writing to Kirkbride, "I promised to ask your consideration of her case as among the first to have her vacation."[69]

A few notes written to summon the superintendent's aid when an assistant faced an urgent problem on the ward further suggest the limits of the younger doctors' equanimity and authority. Edward Smith's resourcefulness failed him when the female patient frightened by a mouse in her room threatened to stand all night on a chair. "Shall I try and persuade her or what course shall I take?" he wrote in a note sent to Kirkbride's home. The more experienced S. Preston Jones felt equally unnerved when one of Kirkbride's fellow superintendents arrived at the Male Department "considerably run down and...in quite low spirits." Asking that Kirkbride come to see the man the next day, Jones admitted, "I don't know what to do in the matter."[70]

Clearly, the assistant physicians' duties in the asylums were both onerous and tension-laden. On the one hand, they had unremitting contact with patients, attendants, and patrons, all of whom presented demands and problems for the younger doctors' arbitration. On the other hand, the assistants had only limited authority to deal with the domestic difficulties they frequently encountered. Because Kirkbride believed so completely in one-man rule, the assistant physicians had to seek his approval for any independent decision, however limited the superintendent's knowledge might be of the specific situation involved. In circumstances calling for a prompt response, the assistants' ambiguous position undoubtedly delayed their reactions, thereby complicating the resolution of ward problems.

The assistant physicians' salary did little to compensate them for the job's tensions. Assistants in the 1840s and 1850s received between $400 and $600 yearly. Although the managers proved sparing in pay raises over the next two decades, their salaries gradually increased to between $600 and $1,000, depending on prior experience. In the 1870s, second assistants started at $750.00 and first assistants at $1,000. S. Preston Jones, the highest-paid assistant, went from a salary of $800 in 1850 to $1,800 in 1872. On the whole, the assistants' recompense compared unfavorably to the amount an ambitious young doctor could make in an urban private practice. Kirkbride may well have had his own assistants in mind when he commented, "There is about as little [financial] inducement for medical men to take charge of the insane as is possible."[71]

The arduous labor and low pay associated with asylum work led most assistant physicians to discover relatively quickly whether or not they had a vocation for the profession. Of the nineteen assistants Kirkbride had in his tenure at the Pennsylvania Hospital, six resigned within the first two years. Some found their health impaired by the constant labor; others simply disliked asylum life. Thomas Mendenhall left after a year and a half, "circumstances having induced him to change his determination to devote himself to the treatment of insanity," as Kirkbride put it. At the time Mendenhall resigned, the superintendent noted his resolve to find an assistant "who in addition to the proper qualifications, intends to devote himself to the profession." John T. Wilson, a second assistant at the Male Department, left after one year, having received a "pecuniarily more advantageous" offer of an unspecified nature in the West. Wilson explained to the managers that although he had enjoyed his association with the asylum, "a position of this kind is necessarily attended with a certain degree of pain and sadness by being brought in constant contact with the sufferings of our unfortunate fellow mortals." Kirkbride persuaded, or rather pressured, Edward Smith into resigning because he had failed to perform his duties with enough vigor and enthusiasm. Given the assistants' many responsibilities, both superintendent and managers could not comprehend Smith's constant complaint that he had "nothing to do." He left the asylum to establish a private practice in Philadelphia.[72]

In spite of the difficulties inherent in the post, the majority of assistant physicians settled into asylum work to both their own and Kirkbride's satisfaction. Four of the assistants at the Pennsylvania Hospital for the Insane served for more than a decade; S. Preston Jones spent a record twenty-five years at the Department for Males. Kirkbride's successful assistants did not necessarily aspire to stay at the asylum, however; they viewed their work there as an apprenticeship that would prepare them for a superintendency of their own. But as competition for asylum posts became more and more fierce, their aspirations proved difficult to realize, as the careers of Kirkbride's most promising assistants demonstrate.

Robert Given, a young English physician who served as Kirkbride's assistant from 1841 to 1844, found his ambition to be an asylum superintendent frustrated by his foreign birth. After Given failed to get the superintendent's post at the new North Carolina asylum in 1849, Dorothea Dix informed Kirkbride, "I have found his foreign birth and education objected to very decidedly." Dix doubted, as did most people connected with asylums, that a foreigner knew enough of American society "to understand well the genius of the people" and be qualified to "treat the insane on correct principles." Although unable to get a regular hospital post, Given remained in asylum medicine by opening a private asylum outside Philadelphia in Delaware County.[73]

Given's successor, John Curwen, had no such obvious disadvantage as foreign birth, yet still encountered barriers to his pursuit of an asylum career. With Kirkbride's strong support, he left the Pennsylvania Hospital for the Insane in 1849 to look for a superintendent's post. Besides wanting to advance his career, Curwen desired a superior position so that he might marry; as he explained to Dorothea Dix, "it was out of my power to do so" as long as he remained an assistant. After several unsuccessful applications, Curwen was almost ready to leave the field of asylum medicine. He wrote to Dix in 1850, "Many of my friends are anxious that I should go into private practice and as no opening appears for me in a hospital, I am more than half-inclined to do so although my partialities are all for that branch of my profession in which I have been so long engaged." The only possibility left, he concluded, was the superintendency of the new Pennsylvania State Lunatic Asylum at Harrisburg. "For that," wrote Curwen, "I have no particular liking for reasons I have not room now to detail and do not think I will take that if I can do better." Evidently, Curwen's other prospects failed, for he accepted the Harrisburg post in 1851, serving there until 1881. After dismissal from that position, he obtained the superintendency of the state hospital at Warren, Pennsylvania, where he remained until his retirement in 1900. Of all of Kirkbride's assistants, Curwen alone became an asylum superintendent and a professional leader in his own right, playing an active role in the AMSAII and lobbying for pro-asylum bills in the state legislature.[74] (His career will be looked at in more detail in Chapter 6.)

Curwen's success undoubtedly related to his relatively early entry into the profession, for as time went on, superintendents' posts became even harder to obtain. The career of J. Edwards Lee, another of Kirkbride's most promising assistants, well illustrates the personal consequences of the specialty's increasingly limited mobility. After serving for five years at the Pennsylvania Hospital for the Insane, Lee left in 1856 to find a better post, and three years later succeeded in obtaining the superintendency of the new Wisconsin State Mental Hospital at Madison. The competition for the job made Lee all too aware of the political considerations involved in appointing asylum superintendents. Only two of nine applicants had the "advantage of having had special Hospital experience," he told his fellow superintendent, Charles Nichols. The other seven tried to get the job by bringing "outside pressure" to bear on the trustees. Because of its political nature, Lee expected his new work "to have fully its share of troubles which do not legitimately belong to it." His fears proved well founded, for after serving only a year he lost his position to a Wisconsin-born doctor with better local connections. After failing to secure another post, Lee returned to the Pennsylvania Hospital for the Insane to act as a companion in the Male Department. As soon as Edward Smith resigned in 1862, Kirkbride appointed Lee to the assistant physician's post in the Female Department. After a long period of ill-health and "much mental depression," Lee died there in 1868. His last years evidently were very difficult, for Kirkbride informed the managers, "There is now little room to doubt but that the disease of the brain of which he died, had been gradually coming on for a long time, and that many things which had been by some attributed to other causes, were owing to this disordered condition of his health."[75]

Faced with the improbability of ever obtaining or keeping a superintendency, young physicians entering the specialty apparently lowered their expectations; they sought professional advancement primarily by moving horizontally from one institution to another, seeking to maximize the salary, responsibility, and status obtainable at the assistant's level. As asylums grew larger and more numerous, a hierarchy of assistantships developed within which ambitious doctors could rise by moving from second to first assistant, or from a state to a private hospital. After the 1840s, Kirkbride's assistants increasingly came to the Pennsylvania Hospital for the Insane after serving at state asylums. Lee had been at Utica, Smith at Worcester, and S. Preston Jones at Harrisburg and the Government Hospital in Washington. When Kirkbride offered Jones the first assistant's job in the Male Department, Charles Nichols, the superintendent of the Government Hospital, urged his younger colleague to accept the post, saying that Jones should not miss "an opportunity to improve his professional prospects" by moving to the Pennsylvania Hospital for the Insane.[76]

Although ambitious doctors might gratify a desire for advancement by seeking ever-better assistantships, others avoided moving up the asylum hierarchy precisely because they feared greater responsibility. The asylum career of Henry Nunemaker, an assistant at the Female Department from 1879 to 1908, well illustrates this phenomenon. Nunemaker came to the Pennsylvania Hospital after service at four asylums. Twice he changed positions in order to remain with his mentor, Richard Gundry, as the latter moved from one superintendency to another. Nunemaker might have succeeded to the chief physician's post in two of the asylums he left, Gundry informed Kirkbride, but he "wavered so" that the other candidates "carried it away." Gundry explained, "Knowing what you wish he goes straight forward unmoved, but when in my absence from home he was left in charge, his fear and anxiety lest anything amiss should happen were excessive." Gundry concluded of Nunemaker, "He feels happy as an Assistant physician; wishes to be, but fears to be a Superintendent." Undoubtedly, for some physicians, the limited opportunities for advancement in the asylum field afforded a welcome excuse for avoiding the rigors of a full-fledged superintendency.[77]

The anxieties and frustrations Kirkbride's assistants suffered in pursuit of their own independent careers could not help but spill over into their asylum work. Lee's depression and Nunemaker's timidity must have added little to their performance on the ward.

Even Edward Smith's despair at "having nothing to do" may have stemmed from his dissatisfaction with a perpetually subordinate position; certainly, when Kirkbride went on vacation, he seemed filled with a new enthusiasm, urging his chief to stay away longer. The sacrifices required of the assistant physicians were hardly compensated for by recognition within the specialty. Until 1893, only superintendents could belong to the AMSAII and attend its meetings. Thus, until the late nineteenth century, assistant physicians did not share in a wider intellectual exchange or professional comradeship that might have made their travails seem more meaningful.[78]

The only antidote to the assistant physicians' isolation came from their relationship with Kirkbride. Through him, and him alone, the younger doctors became part of a larger intellectual and professional brotherhood devoted to asylum medicine. For all his efforts to preserve a hierarchical upper hand in his day-to-day dealings with them, Kirkbride appears to have been quite devoted to his protégés. John Curwen maintained a long and intimate correspondence with his old mentor, often asking his advice on hospital and political matters. J. Edwards Lee regarded Kirkbride as a "counsellor wiser than myself" and wrote, when he took the Wisconsin job, that he wished "such a friend, as it was my privilege to be so long associated with could stand by my side." When Lee met with professional reverses, Kirkbride lent him money, offered him a place to live until he could find another post, and finally took him back as an assistant. After Lee's death, Kirkbride employed his widow, Harriet, as a wing supervisor. Even Edward Smith got to serve as Kirkbride's representative to the AMSAII convention in 1858 when the construction of the Male Department kept the superintendent close to home.[79]

Although secure in his own position as a superintendent, Kirkbride did not forget the professional disadvantages suffered by his younger colleagues. His understanding of their bleak situation certainly colored his strictures on asylum politics. Lee's experience at Wisconsin, for example, lent a special vehemence to Kirkbride's warnings about managers who took a "personal interest" in appointments. In a broader sense, his assistants' uneven careers contributed to Kirkbride's perception of the profession's precarious status, a perception that underlay his conservative positions on seemingly unrelated issues such as institutions for the chronic insane. In evaluating Kirkbride's stance on these topics (which will be discussed in more detail in Chapter 6), it is important to remember that his outlook reflected not only his own experience but also that of his assistants.

At the same time, however sympathetic Kirkbride was toward his young colleagues, he was in some ways responsible for their predicament. The assistant physicians' frustrations can be seen as the result, albeit an unintended one, of the specialty's insistence on one-man rule. The asylum hierarchy Kirkbride set up simply had no place for more than one independent physician; so, as the number of assistants outstripped the superintendent posts available to them, the aspirations of younger doctors were inevitably stymied. And as a consequence, asylum work attracted more and more individuals such as Nunemaker as the century progressed. The specialty's limited mobility, and the personal and professional casualties it produced, had a destructive effect not only on asylum practice but also on the development of the profession as a whole.[80]

Steward and matron

In contrast to his relations with the assistant physicians, Kirkbride enjoyed a more distant, serene association with the other hospital officers. Although the steward and matron occupied an important position in the asylum hierarchy, the more limited nature of their duties, which included less responsibility for patrons and patients, and their modest social backgrounds, which precluded professional aspirations, lessened the tensions inherent in their work. The steward acted as the hospital's business manager, purchasing all supplies, collecting board payments, keeping the accounts, hiring the household staff, and supervising the various service departments (farm and garden, engineering, laundry, and the like). He also purchased special food and toilet items for the patients at the patrons' request, adding the cost to the board bill. When the superintendent undertook any construction on the hospital grounds, the steward acted as foreman on the building crew. The matron, who was usually the steward's wife, attended to the housekeeping matters, including cleaning, cooking, washing, and sewing. Care of the patients' clothing consumed much of her attention, as did the provision of their meals. The hospital rules specifically charged the matron with seeing that the "supply [of food] is abundant, varied, well cooked, and neatly served." Both matron and steward were enjoined to check the tables during a meal in order to make sure that these standards were met. Unfortunately, the problems involved in feeding large numbers of insane patients quickly and appetizingly defeated the best of matrons, and the food service remained a weak point in the asylum's accommodations.[81]

The matron and steward only tangentially concerned themselves with patients. They had some responsibilities for "supervision and police" of the wards, particularly the dining rooms, and assisted the other staff in time of crisis. The steward occasionally handled emergencies, such as notifying a manager of a crisis or soothing a perturbed relative. The matron sometimes developed "considerable intercourse" with the female patients, allowing them to eat at her table or help with chores, although Kirkbride discouraged her from taking too independent a role in patient care. When a patron repeated some advice the matron had given him about removing his wife from the asylum, Kirkbride replied tartly, "I may just remark that neither the Matron or servants are supposed competent to give opinions on cases, nor are they consulted on the subject."[82]

Supervisors and companions

Supervisors, each having charge of one hospital wing, had the chief responsibility for the conduct of the patients and wards. They reported directly to Kirkbride and his assistant, serving as a "medium of communication" between the physicians and attendants. In order to see that ward work got done properly, the supervisors had the authority to change the attendants' ward assignments, allot duties for special watching or nursing, and discharge individuals who committed serious infractions of the rules, such as falling asleep on duty. In addition to overseeing the attendants' work, the supervisors had general responsibility for the "preservation of order and quiet in the house." More specifically, the hospital rules enjoined them to "aid and encourage the attendants in their efforts to interest, amuse and employ the patients" and "especially attend to the prevention of disturbances among the patients." In order to keep the physicians acquainted with events on the ward, Kirkbride had the supervisors maintain a daily journal of observations, which was to be turned in at his office every morning before rounds. By alerting him to marked changes in a patient's behavior, such as symptoms of physical illness or suicidal propensities, the wing supervisors acted as important sources of information about the patients as well as the attendants.[83]

In a more informal fashion, the wing supervisors served as a link between the asylum and its patrons by seeing that families' special wishes concerning the patients' comfort were carried out. The physicians, steward, and matron were far too busy to attend to the patrons' innumerable small requests, so it fell to the supervisors to see to the details of patient care that often mattered a great deal to their families. Not always confident of an attendant's honesty, patrons felt safer entrusting the supervisor with items of clothing or food for a relative. When plagued by anxieties about the patient's eating habits or personal hygiene, families often found it easier to seek reassurance from the supervisor than to bother the physicians. From references in the patrons' letters, it is evident that the wing supervisors sometimes wrote letters to relatives, reporting on the patient's condition as well as requesting needed clothing and toilet articles. In contrast to his policies in regard to the assistants and the matron, Kirkbride does not appear to have discouraged the supervisors from transmitting such information to the patrons. He may have condoned it when the family demanded a more frequent correspondence than he himself had time to undertake; short notes from the wing supervisor satisfied the relatives' need to hear from the asylum without challenging the superintendent's medical authority over the patient. Patrons often became very dependent on the wing supervisors, especially the more experienced ones, such as Mary Sharpless and Margaret Brennan. One man, barred from visiting his wife because his presence disturbed her, wrote plaintively to Kirkbride, "I see her through Mrs. Brennan's eyes." By their skill in handling the patrons, wing supervisors could achieve considerable presence within the asylum.[84]

The teacher or companion assigned to each wing played a similar, if less wide-ranging, role in ward affairs. Attendants of "higher grade than ordinary," these "lady and gentleman" companions circulated daily among the wards, organizing group activities and attempting to amuse individual patients. On Kirkbride's instructions, they took special pains with the newly admitted patients in order to give them "pleasant impressions of their new home and pave the way for a ready acquiescence" in treatment. Along with the wing supervisors, they kept a journal of observations on the patients. Companions also had the authority to "suggest" to the attendants "whatever they think will add to the comfort of the patients or the tranquility of the wards" and to report "any neglect or improper conduct that may come under their notice."[85]

A journal kept in 1870 by a companion named Lucy Rous illustrates the character of her duties. After breakfasting with the patients at 6:30 in the morning, Rous visited half of her assigned wards between 9:00 and 10:00 A.M., spending a "few minutes with one lady and a few with another." In the remaining two hours before dinner, she conversed and walked with those patients who seemed most receptive to her influence. After the main meal of the day, also taken with her charges, Rous made her rounds in the other half of her wards, again singling out the most promising patients for special attention. In the afternoon, she took turns visiting the different wards to read aloud stories about the "New Fashioned Girl" or "Ministering Children." On pleasant days, Rous accompanied small groups of patients on carriage rides about the hospital grounds or to nearby Fairmont Park. After tea at 6:00 P.M., she attended the evening amusement and then returned to the wards to prepare her charges for bed with prayer reading or hymn singing. Rous took her responsibilities very seriously, making careful notes of the amusements that appealed most to her "ladies." " 'Godey' is a great boon going around the wards," she noted, "pictures, reading, and music, something to suit nearly everyone." She also commented on the servants' performance: "This week our table has been remarkably pleasantly and attentively waited on," ran an entry, clearly hinting that such was not often the case. On another occasion, Rous asked the doctor to "please give the attendants a hint (if you think best) to be as quiet as possible with their work and movements during mealtimes, and ask Emma Otter and Hattie Mayne to try and cultivate rather a less curt, snappish tone of speaking to the ladies."[86]

Rous's diary suggests that the companions occupied a somewhat ambiguous position in the hospital hierarchy. Their duties aligned them most closely with the wing supervisors, yet their superior education and social standing appears to have weakened this natural alliance. By reporting the attendants' infractions to the physician, the companions hardly endeared themselves to their subordinates either. Effectively isolated from the asylum staff, the higher-grade attendants found some relief from their anomalous position through association with the superintendent's family. Lucy Rous and Agnes Turner, for example, developed close friendships with Kirkbride's second wife, Eliza.[87]

But by and large, the companions' satisfaction in asylum work depended primarily upon their involvement with the patients. Unlike the wing supervisors, who had only general responsibility for preserving order on the wards, the companions were immediately accountable for the patients' well-being. Their duties brought them into constant contact with their charges, even at mealtimes. The strain of "brightening" a difficult audience told on companions quickly. Elizabeth Bennett, confiding her anxieties about her influence on the patients, wrote to Kirkbride, "I have made so little progress compared with the anxious interested motives of action." Comparing herself unfavorably with Agnes Turner, whose "vivacity and natural disposition" made her a favorite with the patients, Bennett felt that she must be "deficient in some way or manner so that my usefulness and popularity are retarded." The companion concluded by asking Kirkbride, "If you have seen any conspicuous failings in me it would confer a lasting favor by making them known."[88]

Since their work involved direct responsibility for the patients' frame of mind, the companions inevitably felt less settled in their achievements than did the wing supervisors. Successful performance of their duties required great physical stamina and mental stability. Not many individuals were willing to take on such duties at a salary of $24 a month. As Kirkbride told the managers in 1864, when Agnes Turner had to leave the asylum due to ill health, "It is at all times difficult to find ladies of education and refinement of feeling, with the indispensable natural traits of character, to take such positions." The women who served as companions often felt some special vocation for work with the insane. Some, such as Elizabeth Bennett, viewed their labor as a religious duty. Others, such as Lucy Rous, had a relative afflicted by mental disease. Occasionally, Kirkbride recruited teachers from among recovered patients in need of work. A young woman grateful for the return of her sanity wrote to Kirkbride, "I have been thinking not a little of what you said to me about visiting or teaching among some of your good people, and feel strongly inclined to try and do what

I can." The most successful companions, as Kirkbride once remarked, had the "same qualities of mind and heart which win greatest success in missionary work."[89]

Attendants

In comparison to the companions, the attendants performed equally demanding work yet received fewer psychological or material rewards. Occupying the lowest rank of the hospital hierarchy (except for the domestics), they had the most extensive contact with the patients. Two attendants had charge of a ward, with a ratio of approximately 10 patients to one attendant. In terms of daily care, the attendants had by far the most significant impact on the patients' comfort. Whereas Kirkbride could conceivably have done without a supervisor or companion for a short period, he could not afford to leave a ward understaffed for a moment. The amount of space devoted to the various staff members in the 1850 rulebook well illustrates Kirkbride's dependence on his lowest-paid employees: He used one page each to outline the duties of the supervisor and companion and twenty pages on the attendant's responsibilities. To the attendant, then, the superintendent committed the most crucial details of asylum practice.[90]

In the first place, the attendants preserved the physical appearance of both the patients and the ward. Each day, their charges had to be "properly dressed, well-washed and...their hair and clothes neatly brushed." Once a week, the attendants gave the patients baths, including shaves and haircuts for the men. Although the hospital domestics did the heavy cleaning, the attendants handled the patient-related housekeeping chores: emptying their chamber pots in the morning, airing their bedding, and putting their rooms in order. When "unpleasant effluvium" appeared on the ward, the attendants had to find and remove the cause of the odor. If an inmate dirtied the parlor or halls during the day, they had to clean the area immediately. Soiled bedding had to be washed with boiling hot water and carefully dried. Finally, the ward had to be made tidy, with the halls and parlors swept, the furniture put in place, and the spittoons, water closets, and urinals "carefully watched, and prevented from impairing the purity of the air in the ward."[91]

At the same time they attended to all these chores, the attendants had to keep the patients from harm. They were expected to know exactly where their charges were at any time of the day or night. If patients stayed in their rooms, the attendants had to "find reasons for frequently calling to see how they are engaged." If the patients went outdoors for exercise, the attendants had to maintain a careful watch on them. "An attendant's eye should always be kept on a patient known to be disposed to escape," warned Kirkbride. At mealtimes, they counted the silverware to make sure that no potentially dangerous weapon found its way back to the ward. The attendants also had to make sure that patients took their medicine, using the "utmost gentleness" to induce them "to take it willingly."[92]

Preventing or containing patient violence constituted the most demanding portion of the attendants' duties. If an inmate became disruptive, they were expected to confine the malefactor in his or her room quickly, before any destruction or injury took place. This task was considerably complicated by Kirkbride's scruples concerning restraint. He insisted, for example, that patients should always be given an explanation for their confinement. After locking up an unruly inmate, the attendant was instructed to "sit down quietly by him, and calmly tell him why he [had] been placed there, and that he will be released as soon as he is able to control himself." In addition, no matter how violent the individual, an attendant could not apply a straitjacket or bedstraps without a physician's presence. Self-destructive cases involved further precautions. Rather than confine a potential suicide, Kirkbride had the attendants keep a twenty-four-hour watch to prevent any self-injury.[93]

The proper performance of all the attendants' duties required them to adhere to a strict discipline. As if aware that they could hardly remember all twenty pages of their responsibilities, Kirkbride had each attendant carry a rulebook at all times, to be presented once a week for inspection. He also defined the hospital etiquette that he expected them to observe. "Spend no unnecessary time in your rooms, at your own work," he instructed them; avoid visiting other wards and "talking in one ward of what is said and done in another." Attendants had to eschew any behavior "that might embarrass or annoy the patients, including all nicknames, undue familiarity, disrespectful remarks and especially repeating to other than the proper officers, the sayings and doings of patients, or even mentioning their names to persons outside or visitors." Finally, he enjoined the attendants to work in harmony with one another, for those "who quarrel with each other can never do justice to, or exercise the proper influence over the patients, and would do well to seek another occupation."[94]

Kirkbride stated in his *Reports* that he chose individuals for the onerous position of attendant according to high standards, including "proper mental and physical qualifications," temperance, and abstinence from the use of tobacco in any form (a particular obsession of Kirkbride's). But in practice, the superintendent found his high standards difficult to match, and, like most asylum superintendents, grumbled periodically about the shortage of good applicants. Yet, as head of a relatively affluent private hospital, Kirkbride probably saw a far better grade of attendants than most of his colleagues.[95]

The manuscript census schedules, which recorded the age and ethnic background of every employee at the Pennsylvania Hospital for the Insane, allow us to construct a general profile of the attendant class. As a group, they were dominated by the young and Irish: Roughly half of the attendants were between the ages of twenty and twenty-nine, and the Irish-born ranged from 27 to 63 percent of the total at different times. Attendants rarely made asylum service their lifetime work, for only a few individuals persisted from one decade to the next. Of fifty-four attendants employed in 1860, only five, one man and four women, remained in the hospital's employ in 1870. (No doubt women tended to stay longer because they had fewer alternative employment opportunities.) Overall, the census information suggests that asylum work primarily attracted young men and women looking for short-term employment before moving on to a more permanent occupation.[96]

Although the majority of Kirkbride's attendants were young and presumably unfamiliar with asylum work, some had prior experience in caring for the insane. Of the letters from prospective attendants preserved among Kirkbride's papers, fully one-half cited previous employment at mental institutions throughout the Northeast. Evidently, there existed a small but regular circulation of employees between asylums, as individuals left one hospital for another in search of new surroundings or better working conditions. One couple left the Utica, New York, asylum from "a desire to live further South." A male attendant left the Friends Asylum, according to his former employer, because he "got discouraged at the quantity of work required of him which was taking care of the Lodge," the worst ward in the hospital. A highly qualified English woman who had worked in private asylums wanted to find not only a better-paying position but also one in a more therapeutically oriented institution: "There is simply no treatment at all (where I have been working) and nothing special to do except attend to the housekeeping, the general wants, and be a little companionable to the inmates." She continued, "I hope and wish for a different life being *interested* in my work and looking upon it as a real profession." Whatever their motives for changing institutions, some attendants came as experienced workers rather than novices to asylum life. As one applicant told Kirkbride, "I understand the business well."[97]

A smaller number of applicants had pursued some other line of hospital or nursing work. Occasionally, attendants came from the Eighth Street general hospital or the nearby almshouse. Some had been private nurses for mental patients. One young woman had lived with her brother, a doctor, and tended two of his insane patients, one suicidal and the other "rather idiotic...violent, obstinate at all times." Although unfamiliar with the specific regimen of a mental hospital, such applicants still had a general familiarity with hospitals or mental patients that must have smoothed their transition to asylum life.[98]

Even the attendants who applied for a post without having any prior experience seemed, at least from their personal histories, to represent a respectable class of young workers. Some male applicants had looked for work out West, but found it inhospitable. An Irish attendant who had tried farming in Illinois said that he "found their way of living so unneat and rough" that he could not remain there. Another youth sought asylum work after his father's death as a means to support his mother and siblings. Female applicants were also young, single, or widowed and "thrown upon their own resources," as they put it. Some had been teachers or seamstresses before trying asylum work. "It is not pleasant living alone," wrote a former seamstress, "and I would rather be engaged in some more active life than sewing." Another young woman preferred steady employment "not so public as clerking or anything of the kind." And of course, asylum work offered opportunities for a woman described as knowing "nothing by which she can support herself except domestic concerns, at which she is very good."[99]

Applicants produced testimonials to their moral condition as well as their willingness to work. Most simply gave references affirming that they were "honorable, reliable and pious." Obviously hoping to curry Kirkbride's favor, a young man gave his moral qualifications in more detail: "I am an American, 24 years old, do not chew or smoke tobacco, drink any liquor, nor do I even use any profane language." Some female applicants professed to have a special talent for helping the insane, or "turning their gloom into cheerfulness," as one put it. A young woman who had "been with the insane considerably" told Kirkbride, "I like to be with them, to cheer and console them and to do all I can for them." In more eloquent language, an applicant assured the superintendent that the sacrifices entailed in asylum work would be compensated for by "sharing the sympathies or alleviating the sufferings of a portion of our fellow creatures."[100]

At least in superficial respects, the asylum's attendants hardly conformed to the image of the unskilled, insensitive, morally depraved drudge who figured so prominently in the asylum exposés of the period. Although few could match Kirkbride's demanding specifications, they did not come from the lowest ranks of urban society. In fact, a certain level of quality was ensured by the relative attractions of asylum work in the mid-nineteenth-century job market. Unlike the many seasonal or irregular types of work available, being an attendant was "steady and sure," as one applicant described it. Along with a decent wage came room and board, as well as the sociability of a large institution. Although the work certainly had its unpleasant aspects, it did not involve constant, backbreaking physical labor. Given the hardships endured by most unskilled laborers in the nineteenth century, these were considerable assets ensuring a surplus of applicants. In 1870, for example, advertisements for a few posts available at the Male Department brought between thirty and fifty inquiries. Not forced by desperation to take any and all prospects, Kirkbride could afford to be somewhat discriminating in his choice of attendants.[101]

Notwithstanding their overall quality, however, the attendants' performance of their many and difficult duties remained the single most vulnerable aspect of Kirkbride's asylum practice. Their problems resulted not so much from personal inadequacies as the force of inexorable institutional pressures. Even a cursory performance of the tasks outlined for the attendants quickly filled a working day. Continually overworked and pressed by the patients' demands, the least disturbances of ward routine could seem an intolerable burden to them. Personal animosities toward patients or other staff members inevitably developed, creating more tension. Not surprisingly, the attendants proved to be the most disputatious faction among the hospital family.

Attendants complained chiefly about the distribution of work and privileges. Considering the labor entailed in caring for a suicidal, violent, or filthy patient, they often protested the assignment of difficult individuals to their wards. Lee told Kirkbride, for example, that he had placed a "nervous and restless and somewhat suicidal" patient on the fourth ward, much to the attendants' "discomfort." An attendant on a lower ward asked to be moved, "partly because I am not stout enough to control the patients and partly because my fellow attendant and myself do not work harmoniously together." Quarrels often centered on the distribution of privileges or "liberties" among the attendants. Kirkbride received an indignant letter from an attendant named Andrews, claiming that a fellow worker had made an "incredible number of visits to the storeroom." The other attendants feared to expose Reilly's petty thefts, but Andrews refused to "pull this mess behind the screen." He told Kirkbride, "I know that bowing, scraping and a kind of humility will not pass with an enlightened gentleman for more than it is worth."[102]

The attendants' relations with the patients were even more difficult. They often faced physical danger from their charges, especially on the male wards, where attacks occurred frequently. One attendant lost his position due to head, shoulder, and leg injuries inflicted by a violent patient. Sometimes the attack was unprovoked, but as often as not, the attendant's own lapse brought about the assault. An assistant physician's journal recorded a typical incident that escalated into violence. After a drunken spree in Philadelphia, a male attendant assigned to watch an excited patient fell asleep at his post. The patient, attempting to arouse his keeper to get some medicine, became a little rough, and a general "fisticuff" ensued. Both parties gave and received blows, the doctor noted, but the attendant got the worst of it. He tendered his resignation, "which was immediately accepted."[103]

Quarrels among attendants and inmates commonly occurred in every nineteenth-century institution. But as Kirkbride well knew, such untoward events had particularly troublesome consequences for mental hospitals. A quarrel between two attendants, an unusually heavy amount of ward work, a moment's neglect – all could result in a patient's escape, suicide, or self-injury. Marks of abuse on a lunatic, who presumably could not control his own impulses, invariably had a more serious import than the same injuries on a sane patient. If publicized, attendant neglect or abuse could do irreparable harm to an asylum's reputation. And although he met infractions of discipline with heavy penalties – dismissal for attendants who quarreled repeatedly, struck a patient, or fell asleep on a watch – Kirkbride could not prevent lapses that detracted from the impression of constant kindness, watchfulness, and good order he projected for the asylum.

Several suicides occurring in the late 1860s illustrate the tragic consequences that even minor infractions might have. In the first case, a young woman known to be suicidal had been given the privilege of walking in the yard outside her ward, since the exercise seemed to calm her. The arrangement existed with the understanding that she was "never to be from under the eye of an attendant." But one morning while the attendant worked about the ward, the patient slipped through an improperly secured gate and drowned herself in the hospital pond. A similar incident took place within the year. An attendant, opening a door to sweep and dust, turned her back for a moment, and a patient slipped out unobserved and drowned herself. Unfortunately for the hospital, the first suicide received coverage in a "scurrilous sheet," as Kirkbride termed it, which printed an editorial containing "at least a dozen lies of the most unadulterated character" defaming the institution.[104]

Kirkbride did not dismiss the attendants involved in either case, since with this one exception, they had given able, conscientious service and could only be replaced by less experienced help. But the tragic results that seemingly insignificant errors produced reinforced his conviction that the most trivial aspects of asylum discipline had to be enforced in order to prevent suicide, a "great and never-ending source of anxiety" for him. As Kirkbride told the managers, "our regulations in regard to [suicide] have been so carefully matured, that if followed to the letter, such an accident could rarely occur. I say, *rarely*, because new modes of effecting this, never before thought of, seem to be constantly being devised. The immediate carrying out of rules, must necessarily be entrusted to others, and in both instances referred to, apparently very simple matters led to the fatal results."[105]

Even the most trivial lapses in the hospital's standard of care could have a devastating effect on the patrons' confidence in Kirkbride. Having convinced themselves (with the superintendent's eager assistance) that commitment represented a humane response to a relative's insanity, patrons felt betrayed when the asylum did not live up to the expectations Kirkbride had created for it. An indignant man, recalling the doctor's promises to keep his brother clean while in the hospital, could only conclude from the "considerable quantity of lice" on the patient's head that he had been "shamefully neglected by those whose duty it was to attend to such matters." Likewise, escapes contradicted the assumption of watchful care over the patients. After witnessing the hue and cry over an inmate's elopement while on a visit to the hospital, a woman wrote of her own relative, "I often feel unhappy fearing he may escape from the Asylum, as one did so while I was there." Patrons led to anticipate saintlike behavior from the staff understandably grew angry when they found "marks of maltreatment" on their relatives. Kirkbride usually managed to smooth over the ill feelings generated by asylum mishaps, but each one cost him time and effort and left the patrons' trust in him impaired.[106]

Herein lay the chief weakness of Kirkbride's asylum philosophy. However carefully he planned his hospital's building and administration, its operation eventually had to be entrusted to others. Kirkbride's own exertions, which were motivated by a compelling mixture of compassion and ambition, had to be supplemented by the efforts of less committed and less competent individuals. Thus, the superintendent's practice of asylum medicine inevitably became dependent upon the varied personalities who made up his staff. The assistant physician who could find nothing to do, the matron who gave ill-considered advice to patrons, the companion who lost her ability to brighten her charges, and the attendants who engaged in fisticuffs with the patients all created flaws in Kirkbride's great whole, flaws with the potential to damage the hospital's hard-won reputation.

Fortunately for his own sake, Thomas Story Kirkbride proved

to be adept at mending the cracks in his asylum's facade. By devoting considerable attention to the hospital's public relations, he kept the discrepancies between image and reality to manageable proportions. A superb diplomat as well as a principled humanitarian, Kirkbride seems to have had the ability to persuade those around him that despite its imperfections, his hospital was as faultless as it could possibly be. His efforts were greatly aided by his patrons' willingness to overlook the contradictions between Kirkbride's claims and the actual nature of hospital life. For ultimately, success in asylum practice depended less upon the realities of the institution's performance, than in its capacity to inspire the patrons' generous confidence in the physician's good intentions.

5

A new kind of existence

Thomas Story Kirkbride's therapeutic persuasion united the asylum doctor and the patient's family in a battle against insanity. As the first step, they defined the disease in common terms; its symptoms, as mutually agreed upon, consisted of intellectual impairment, irregular living habits, mood alterations, and delusions. To minimize the stigma attached to the patient's condition, doctor and patron equated the causes of insanity with morally neutral disturbances in the individual's recent past, such as physical illness or personal disappointments. But although desperately seeking to regard mental illness as an ordinary disease, the asylum's clientele accepted the necessity for a regimen of *institutional* treatment that was not imperative for other, purely physical disorders. Without a specially designed building and carefully chosen staff, the asylum doctor convinced them, the proper medical and moral measures for treating insanity could not be provided. The superintendent's special blend of moral authority and medical expertise, which his patrons hoped would modify the patient's aberrations dramatically, depended upon a totally controlled therapeutic environment for its exercise. By eliminating or curbing the individual's undesirable qualities, the hospital experience would exercise a restraining influence over insanity. The end result of their combined efforts, doctor and family concurred, was a humane, scientifically correct response to a frightening, perplexing human ailment.

The logic of this therapeutic persuasion was hardly so compelling to the patients, however. The very nature of their disorder made them unable or unwilling to accept the premises of asylum treatment. In the first place, those considered insane rarely viewed themselves as diseased or disordered in mind. What their relatives regarded as symptoms of insanity they often felt to be justifiable, even laudable, behavior. Consequently, their family's motivations in committing them struck many patients as highly suspect. Kirkbride, whom the family so obviously trusted, also became an immediate object of suspicion. In this frame of mind, patients naturally viewed every aspect of treatment as punitive and resisted Kirkbride's efforts to convince them otherwise. In short, the majority of the Pennsylvania Hospital for the Insane's inhabitants did not share in the therapeutic consensus upon which it had been so laboriously constructed.

Thus, asylum medicine involved a doctor–patient dynamic quite unlike that characterizing other forms of medical practice. With few exceptions, persons suffering from a physical disorder did not receive medical care against their wishes or find themselves involuntarily confined in a hospital. Although they might object to painful medical procedures, ordinary patients rarely had a vested interest in defying the physician's diagnosis or disputing his directions for treatment. In contrast, the asylum doctor worked with a perpetually hostile or unappreciative clientele. For all the superintendent's power within the institution, patients found ways to make their dissatisfactions felt: by escaping, committing suicide, starting a lawsuit, or simply complaining to their relatives. The superintendent ultimately had to respond to his charges' demands and expectations; for as a master had to heed his slaves or a prison guard conciliate his inmates, if the asylum's inhabitants grew too dissatisfied or troublesome, their behavior inevitably reflected poorly upon the chief physician and endangered public confidence in his abilities.[1] As a consequence, Kirkbride had a very important stake in gaining the patients' confidence, as well as that of their families. No understanding of mid-nineteenth-century asylum medicine can be complete, then, without considering the patients' experience of and influence upon their own treatment.

THE PATIENT POPULATION

The very diversity of the patients themselves enormously complicated the business of asylum medicine. The treatment of mental disorders, which by definition involved disturbances of the personality, necessarily had to take into account the social traits so crucial to character development, such as sex, age, marital status, ethnicity, and occupation. Moreover, both doctor and patron expected the hospital's accommodations and arrangements to preserve certain social relationships, particularly class and gender distinctions. Thus, every aspect of asylum medicine had to be carefully calibrated to harmonize with the patient's social condition. Without varying his methods in relation to these vital determinants of behavior, Kirkbride could hardly hope to meet either the patients' or patrons' expectations of hospital care.

A collective profile of the 8,852 individuals treated at the Pennsylvania Hospital for the Insane from 1841 to 1883 suggests the complexity of the patient population upon which Kirkbride practiced asylum medicine.[2] The sexes were about equally represented, with men making up 54 percent and women 46 percent of the total. Fifty-five percent had been married or widowed; the rest were single (see Table A.1). The majority of the patients were in the prime of adult life when committed to the asylum; only 6 percent were younger than twenty and 19 percent older than fifty (see Table A.2). Almost one-quarter (24 percent) had been born outside the United States, primarily in Ireland, Germany, and England (see Table A.3). Regardless of their origin, 81 percent of the patients resided in Pennsylvania at the time of admission; the rest came from all regions of the country, with the South contributing half of the out-of-state clientele (see Table A.4). Perhaps as a consequence, only a few black patients were admitted during the whole forty-three-year period.[3]

The occupational information Kirkbride kept on his patients provides some sense of their relative class positions. Of course, without additional information on the inmates' financial status, occupation gives only a crude approximation of their social standing. Categories such as "farmer" or "merchant," for example, blur the varying levels of wealth and prestige obtainable within the same general line of work. Still, a tally of the patients' occupations (or, in the case of women not employed outside the home, their male relatives' occupation) suggests the range of social groups represented in the hospital population. Of the men, 19 percent had professional or prestigious white-collar occupations (merchant, lawyer, physician, and the like); 35 percent were proprietors or held low-status white-collar jobs (e.g., clerk, grocer, manufacturer, farmer); 24 percent were skilled artisans (e.g., brickmaker, cooper, baker, wheelwright); and 7 percent were unskilled manual laborers. Fifteen percent of the men listed no occupation at all; this group included "gentlemen," that is, wealthy men who did not have to work for a living, as well as those who had lost their jobs. Of the women, 23 percent were related by birth or marriage to men in professional or prestigious white-collar occupations; 28 percent to proprietors or low-status white-collar workers; 16 percent to skilled artisans; and 9 percent to unskilled laborers. Twenty-four percent of the women had occupations of their own, the vast majority as domestics, seamstresses, or teachers.[4]

Asylum patients composed a heterogeneous group not only in terms of their social characteristics but also in the diversity of their mental disorders. The different diagnoses assigned to patients upon admission provide a good index of their variability. Based upon the family's case history, as well as his own initial observations, Kirkbride classified each individual as suffering from mania, monomania, melancholia, or dementia. This system of medical classification, which had been in use for centuries, depended upon symptomatic criteria to distinguish the types of insanity; the various forms of mental disease were not classified according to a distinctive etiological or developmental sequence (both of which remained obscure in the mid-nineteenth century), but rather by characteristic types of behavior.[5]

Of course, nineteenth-century physicians did distinguish between organic and functional disorders; the former clearly involved the physical deterioration, or "softening," of the brain, whereas the latter did not. But as was discussed in Chapter 2, physicians believed that all forms of insanity involved the physical derangement of the nervous system. The organic–functional distinction merely indicated a greater or lesser degree of certainty concerning the disease's physical origins. In any event, the suspected etiology of a disorder had no real bearing on its classification; physicians did not habitually refer to "organic mania" or "functional melancholia" in making a diagnosis. Nineteenth-century nosological conceptions also allowed little scope for systematically designating changes in the patients' behavior over time. Kirkbride recognized a periodic or intermittent insanity, in which spells of irrationality were followed by long periods of lucidity; similarly, some patients alternated between mania and melancholia. Maniacal or melancholic conditions, he observed, often degenerated into dementia. But the diagnostic framework itself did not incorporate developmental patterns in distinguishing the different forms of the disease.[6]

Although admittedly crude, Kirkbride's classificatory system enabled him to group his patients according to the features of their disorder that were most crucial to treatment; that is, their level of mental and physical activity. Mania designated the "high form" of madness, whose symptoms included, as Kirkbride recorded in a typical case, "general excitement, great loquacity, frequent declamation and gesticulation, with sleeplessness, a disposition to tear off his clothes, etc." Patients described by their relatives as suffering from "fits," "ebullitions of passion," or "paroxysms" would usually be diagnosed as maniacs. When suffering from monomania, patients manifested intellectual impairment and physical energy only in relation to certain subjects. For the most part, monomaniacs gave no striking evidence of derangement in their personal appearance or behavior, but if engaged on the subject of their delusions, the extent of their insanity became clear. "In general conversation and his behavior," Kirkbride noted of one such patient, "there is nothing noticed, indicating insanity" until the matter of politics came up; the gentleman believed he was to be the next president of the United States, and "other matters of the kind not more probable."[7]

Patients showing the opposite symptoms – listlessness, silence, passivity – would be diagnosed as suffering from melancholia or dementia. Individuals described by their families as despondent, sunk in "constant gloom and silence," and inclined to weep and moan were classed as melancholic. In this state, the patient "says little, never walks out without urging, thinks his friends avoid him, believes he is subject to scrofula, and there are plots against him," as Kirkbride noted in one case. The same man also showed less and less inclination to shave or change his linen, and was "much disposed to constipation." When the process of withdrawal from the world seemed complete, patients would be classed as demented. Those suffering from this, the most severe form of insanity, had become totally absorbed in their own thoughts and fancies and completely unaware of their surroundings. Occasionally, the demented patients became excited or violent, but in their usual state they remained "sitting in the same position during the whole day, without moving a limb or uttering a word." The most debilitated among them had to be cared for like infants.[8]

Clearly, the categories of mania, monomania, melancholia, and dementia encompassed a wide range of mental conditions; the physician's diagnosis only crudely classified an immensely variable disorder. Among the hospital's clientele, each form of insanity was well represented: Of the total number of patients treated at the Pennsylvania Hospital for the Insane between 1841 and 1883, 45 percent were diagnosed as suffering from mania, 13 percent from monomania, 28 percent from melancholia, and 14 percent from dementia (see Table A.5). Although the majority of patients admitted were diagnosed as suffering from mania and melancholia, these patients comprised only about a third of the resident hospital population at any given time, due to their relatively short lengths of stay; roughly 50 percent left within a year of admission. In comparison, the dementia patients, despite their small number in the total hospital population under treatment, made up approximately half, sometimes more, of the residents because of their tendency to stay for much longer periods of time. Between short-term, active treatment for violent or excited patients and long-term custodial care for the chronic insane, the asylum provided a variety of services. Simply to house and tend, much less provide medical treatment for, such a motley collection of aberrant individuals posed a herculean challenge to the asylum doctor.[9]

In structuring a therapeutic milieu, Kirkbride had to take into account both the social and mental diversity of his clients. He did so by devising a regimen that incorporated rather than sought to obliterate the patients' individual or social differences. Although a single standard of sanity may have dictated his concept of a cure, Kirkbride's methods for achieving his desired ends were not uniform for all patients.[10] Rather, moral treatment depended upon an elaborate incentive system that manipulated the patients' sense of class and mental differences so as to encourage their reformation. In retrospect, asylum life, as observed from the patients' perspective, appears to have been a curious mixture of regimentation and individualism quite unlike the total institution envisioned by modern-day observers.[11]

PATIENT TREATMENT

Psychotherapy as practiced at the Pennsylvania Hospital for the Insane attempted to eliminate or modify the patients' symptoms in varied ways. The most intrusive modes of treatment secured behavioral change by external, direct intervention. Although eminently useful in controlling the worst features of mental disorders, that is, violence and excitement, such measures had to be supplemented and eventually superseded by other, more inner-directed therapies. A carefully planned daily regimen, a system of rewards and punishments, and individual conversations between doctor and patient all provided the insane with incentives to behave in a rational fashion. Gradually, asylum treatment attempted to replace external forms of manipulation with more subtle measures that encouraged the patients to develop their own self-control. In this fashion, Kirkbride hoped that medical and moral means operating consecutively would break the "habits" of insanity, as he termed them, and slowly reacquaint the patients with the requisite standards of sanity.

Drug therapy

Perhaps the most reliable means Kirkbride possessed to secure a rapid change in his patients' mental and physical state was drug therapy, particularly the use of narcotics. Unlike the small number of therapeutic nihilists in his generation, Kirkbride never doubted the ability of medical measures to alter the course of insanity. Materia medica served the physician well, so he believed, by modifying violent, irrational behavior as well as removing the physical disorders underlying mental derangement. Although Kirkbride gave greater public emphasis to amusements and employments as the more innovative aspect of asylum treatment, he believed active medical treatment to be equally essential to the proper care of insanity. Furthermore, his ability to "exhibit" drugs, that is, to produce a demonstrable effect on the patient's physiology by administering a particular substance, considerably enhanced lay perceptions of Kirkbride's medical authority over mental disease.[12]

In the vast majority of cases, Kirkbride's drug of choice was morphine, an opium derivative capable of producing a sedative effect without the nausea or constipation frequently caused by continued opium use. Kirkbride usually combined morphine sulphate with antimony, a diaphoretic, or perspiration inducer, which helped to eliminate the red, dry tongue, contracted pupils, and dry skin occasionally caused by the narcotic. The mixture was dissolved in water or tea and then administered. Morphine appeared not only to control the excitement of mania and lift the depression of melancholia but also to weaken delusions. Kirkbride frequently noted in the casebooks, as in this entry, that morphine "exercises a decidedly evident influence in modifying her delusions and in calming her." Such was the power and reliability of morphine that Kirkbride prescribed it for 75–88 percent of the patients receiving medical treatment.[13]

When the patients had less violent symptoms, or when morphine disagreed with them, Kirkbride tried conium, a drug made from hemlock, which acted as a narcotic "without being decidedly stimulant or sedative." Conium supposedly worked as an "alterative," that is, a substance having the ability to modify, "in some inexplicable and insensible manner, certain morbid actions of the system." Given in combination with iron, a mixture that supposedly aided the digestion, it too could produce dramatic changes in behavior. A young man who "would neither eat, speak nor keep on clothes," was "filthy and appeared idiotic" underwent a dramatic transformation after taking conium. "Although he is not well," Kirkbride recorded, "the change has been most striking – his personal appearance, his general health, his habits and manners are totally changed."[14]

In cases of periodic insanity, in which regular intervals of madness and rationality alternated, Kirkbride used a mixture of quinine and iron. He reasoned that since the intermittent form of insanity resembled an intermittent fever, upon which quinine had a proven effect, the same drug might produce an antiperiodic effect if administered between paroxysms of madness. The quinine appeared to set in motion a "mysterious" action capable of overriding the "train of morbid actions... within the recesses of the nervous system." It also possessed "indirect" sedative properties, making it all the more useful for treating insanity.[15]

In addition to morphine, conium, and quinine, Kirkbride employed a variety of narcotics. For melancholic patients prone to constipation, he sometimes used succus hyocamus, or black henbane, as a substitute for opiates. "Moderately exhibited," according to Wood and Bache's pharmacopeia, hyocamus stimulated the pulse and led to "diminished sensibility and sometimes... such a general composure of the system as to induce sleep," while acting to "quiet irregular nervous action." Kirkbride found "Dover's Powders," a mixture of ipecacuanha, opium, and potassium sulphate, useful in producing a milder sedative effect. The potassium sulphate diluted the effect of the active ingredients and allowed for "division into minute doses," a property especially useful in women's cases. In the 1860s, Kirkbride also experimented with potassium bromide, a sedative with a supposedly powerful anti-aphrodisiac effect. When administered along with morphine, it seemed to work well on male patients suffering from venereal diseases.[16]

No drug seriously rivaled morphine, in Kirkbride's estimation, until the introduction of chloral hydrate in the 1870s. When first introduced, this derivative of chloroform excited considerable interest throughout the medical world. *The Dispensatory of the United States* published in 1878 stated that there was "probably no remedial agent more universally employed throughout the civilized world." As a sedative and soporific, chloral supposedly had no match but opium. But Kirkbride remained skeptical of claims concerning its superiority over morphine. Reporting on his experiments with the drug in 1870, he informed the AMSAII that in most cases, chloral induced sleep without side effects, yet occasionally produced a "kind of intoxication" or excitement. "Like the bromide of potassium," he concluded, "it is an adjunct to morphium, but in no way a substitute for it." In 1876, Kirkbride reported on several unexpected deaths among his patients taking chloral. "I confess I have become exceedingly cautious in its use," he told his fellow asylum superintendents, adding facetiously that he would prefer his medical friends not to administer it to him.[17]

To supplement the action of narcotics, Kirkbride used a variety of other medical remedies. For mania, he often ordered cups or blisters applied to the back of the patient's head or neck, warm baths with cold applications to the head, and mustard foot baths, all procedures thought to reduce local excitement. For the melancholic, he prescribed an opposite regimen designed to stimulate and open up the system, including cathartic pills, camphor rubs, and vigorous toweling after a bath. By far the largest number of nonnarcotic or nonsoporific prescriptions given to the patients aimed at regulating their bowels. To treat constipation, a chronic disorder among the insane, Kirkbride utilized a wide variety of preparations ranging from the mildest laxatives to very strong purges.[18]

Upon admission to the hospital, most patients began some combination of these medical prescriptions. Kirkbride omitted drug therapy only in cases of long-established, seemingly unresponsive forms of insanity. New patients continued to receive drugs for at least six months to a year; medication would be discontinued then only if a patient had shown no improvement. Once considered chronic, patients received only the medical care necessary to preserve their physical health, although narcotics might be used to control very noisy or destructive individuals. "For the purpose of producing quiet, [I] should not hesitate in chronic cases, to give opium," Kirkbride stated at an AMSAII meeting, on the grounds that it benefited the patient and "all around him." Various opium preparations served this purpose, including powder, tincture, "black drop," and paregoric. During his trial of chloral hydrate, Kirkbride noted its effectiveness in producing a quiet ward for the night "among a set of habitually noisy patients," but still rated it as less reliable than opium.[19]

Physical restraint

If, after being treated with narcotics, patients continued to behave in an extremely violent, life-threatening manner, Kirkbride felt impelled to confine them physically. Destructive inmates would be placed in a bare room, to see if their frenzy would pass off naturally. If the patients assaulted another person or attempted self-injury, they would be placed in some kind of restraining device: either the "sleeves," a form of partial straitjacket, holding the patient's arms immobile; the "mittens," confining only the hands; the "bed strap," a web of leather straps designed to keep the patient flat in bed; and the "canvas suit," which prevented destruction of clothing. The only patients kept confined were those who persistently attempted to mutilate themselves. The casebooks record, for example, a woman confined in mittens after she had picked at her face until it was covered with sores, and a man put in bed straps "to restrain and prevent further mutilation" after he seriously injured his eye with his finger.[20]

Similarly, the asylum physicians force-fed patients to prevent them from starving themselves to death. When a patient refused to eat, Kirkbride first had attendants with unusual "tact and patience" try to feed them. Only if this tactic failed and there existed "danger of serious prostration" did Kirkbride condone force. Usually, the attendants could "induce" patients to eat by pinching the nostrils shut, thereby forcing them to swallow, or by pouring "strongly nutritious liquids" down their throats. A nutritive enema might also be given. As a last resort, Kirkbride fed the patient beef extract with a stomach tube, a device he disliked intensely but regarded as an unavoidable necessity in the most stubborn cases. Often, the mere appearance of the tube convinced the recalcitrant to eat rather than suffer its use; "the sight of the stomach pump," the assistant reported in one case, caused a woman "to make an effort and eat the soup herself."[21]

No matter what the situation, Kirkbride appears to have used physical restraint very sparingly and carefully. An entry in the ward journal for 1871 suggests the painstaking nature of his methods. Dr. Bartles recorded a vigil over a male patient who had been placed in the bed straps "to prevent self-mutilation and injury to others." The man would sometimes remain quiet for a while just after awakening. "The straps are then removed from some of his limbs – until he again begins to move violently and distress himself," Bartles noted, and the straps would have to be replaced. If this degree of care was at all typical, the asylum staff did make a concerted effort to use physical restraint as little as possible.[22]

In public and private statements, Kirkbride frequently expressed his abhorrence of physical restraint. As he stated at the 1855 meeting of the AMSAII, he "never saw it in use without a feeling of mortification, nor without asking himself whether it was really necessary." At the same time, Kirkbride felt that restraint was justified to preserve the patient's life or prevent violence to others. This reservation put him at odds with his English colleagues, who wholeheartedly endorsed John Conolly's nonrestraint system. Regarding Kirkbride's practice as the closest American equivalent to their system, they could not comprehend and somewhat resented his refusal to endorse nonrestraint. After spending a week at the Pennsylvania Hospital for the Insane, the English alienist John Bucknill observed that Kirkbride practiced nonrestraint but simply chose not to call himself a "nonrestraint man," for reasons Bucknill did not understand. In all probability, Kirkbride's position on restraint stemmed from a deep-seated fear of patient violence, a fear that had its roots in his own personal experience, as we shall see later in the chapter.[23]

Daily regimen

Although narcotics and restraint were certainly the most direct methods Kirkbride possessed to modify the destructive impulses of insanity, neither measure had a lasting effect on the patients. No reformation produced by external or coercive means could be said to constitute a real cure. Thus, Kirkbride looked upon drug therapy and restraint only as preliminary measures designed to prepare the patients for moral or psychological forms of influence. To ensure a continued remission of mental disease, moral treatment had to stimulate and strengthen the patients' own powers of self-control. To this end, Kirkbride attempted to mold a "new kind of existence," a sane style of living for the patients, by careful regulation of the hospital milieu.[24]

Kirkbride believed that the "simple change in habits" forced by hospitalization did "more towards effecting cure than it commonly has credit for." From the patient's first day in the institution, a carefully planned routine began to counteract the irregularity in habits so closely associated with mental disease. Regular hours of sleep replaced those that tended "to break down the general health and excite the nervous system." Bad habits leading to "mental and physical enervation," such as inactivity and intemperance, had to be given up. "A life of indolence or morbid restlessness, is to be replaced by one of regulated and rational activity," Kirkbride declared. The hospital regimen, by mandating "system, active movements and variety of occupation," forced the insane to take the first step toward improvement.[25]

For patients at the Pennsylvania Hospital for the Insane, this new kind of existence began at 6:00 in the morning, when the attendants awakened them to dress for breakfast. The assistant physician distributed medications, and at 6:30 they went to breakfast in the ward dining rooms. After dining, usually on potatoes or mush with an occasional side dish of meat, the patients returned to the wards to await the physicians' visits. Kirkbride and his assistants made their rounds between 8:30 and 10:00 A.M., checking on each individual's mental and physical state. As soon as the medical visitation was over, the patients began their daily round of amusements. The morning's activities included at least one twenty-minute walk chaperoned by the attendants. In good weather, the patients might stay outside in the pleasure grounds near their wing as long as they wished. For indoor amusements, each ward had a library and a collection of games; the patients could also visit the billiard hall, calistheneum, or combination museum and reading room located on the hospital grounds. During the morning, the wing supervisor and teacher came through the wards with daily papers and magazines, trying to get everyone involved in some activity. At noon, medicine was again distributed, and at 12:30 the patients had their main meal of the day: soup, meat, vegetables, bread, and pie or pudding for dessert. Afternoon activities followed the same schedule as those of the morning, occasionally varied with the teacher's talks on amusing but improving topics. At 6:00 P.M. in the winter and 6:30 in the summer, the patients had a light evening meal, or "tea" as it was called, featuring bread, mush or chipped beef, and stewed fruit. After teatime, the medical officers made another round devoted to the "exercise of. . . personal influence" on the more promising patients. The regular daytime schedule varied only slightly on Sundays, to include morning and afternoon church services for convalescent patients and small Bible-reading classes for those left behind in the wards.[26]

During the winter, the evening entertainments began at 7:30. In the 1840s, the asylum program featured three lectures, accompanied by a magic lantern show and live music each week. Over the years, Kirkbride slowly expanded the nightly offerings to include a formal activity for the whole week. The Pennsylvania Hospital for the Insane justly became famous for its varied and extensive program of amusements. Some nights the patients saw magic lantern shows, based on the hospital's extensive collection of glass stereopticon slides; the patients particularly liked illustrations of foreign countries and cartoonlike "comic views" (see Figure 5). The ordinary fare of magic lantern shows was frequently enlivened by visiting speakers, who delivered lectures on improving topics such as "The History, Manufacture, and Uses of Illuminating Gas" and "The Early Domestic Habits of New England." Musicians from Philadelphia gave concerts, and theatrical groups performed plays with such racy titles as "A Kiss in the Dark" or "The Loan of a Lover." A Signor Blinz arrived several times a year to give exhibitions of singing canary birds and other trained animals, to the "especial gratification" of his audience. On nights when no special amusement was planned, the hospital officers and their wives often gave little parties for individual wards. On Sunday evenings, Kirkbride or his assistant led an hour-long service of Bible reading and singing. After the evening entertainment, the patients had gingerbread (if they had behaved well) and

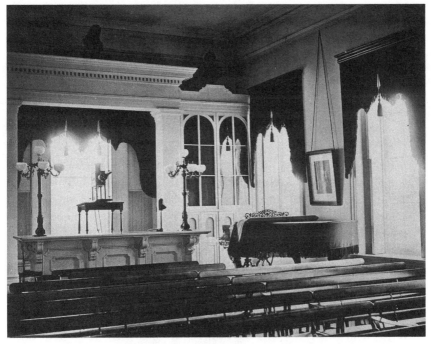

Figure 5. Auditorium, probably at the Female Department. Note the magic lantern projector on the table at the front. The benches had reversible backs, which could be switched from one side to the other to allow the patients to face the back or front of the auditorium. Photograph by A. Morse & Co., probably taken in the early 1870s. (Courtesy of the Historic Archives, Institute of the Pennsylvania Hospital.)

returned to their wards. If time remained before bed, they might sing hymns, play games, or enjoy other "diversions." Between 9:30 and 10:00, the assistant physicians distributed the last medication and everyone retired for the night except the night watchman, who made periodic rounds to make sure that all the patients were well.[27]

Although patients followed the same basic routine during the day, their surroundings and occupations varied according to their affluence. As Kirkbride made abundantly clear in his *Reports*, the asylum openly acknowledged the social distinctions among its clientele; he firmly believed that patients should be able to buy whatever conveniences they desired. "It is done in some respects as in a large hotel," he explained to a patron. "No man has a right to complain that his wealthy neighbor chooses to spend his money

in fine apartments and an abundance of servants." On this principle, patients could furnish their rooms with rugs, chairs, or
pictures they brought from home or had the steward purchase
especially for them. They wore their own clothes, supplemented
with whatever finery they possessed: gloves, hats, jewelry, and
the like. Patrons could leave money with the steward to buy little
delicacies or indulgences a patient might request, so long as the
doctors approved. The steward's expense book shows amounts
spent for food items, such as fruit, candy, and ice cream; amusements, including musical instruments, drawing paper, and chess
sets; and personal items, among them toilet soaps, hair brushes,
and even a spittoon (despite Kirkbride's pronounced aversion to
tobacco in any form). The same fund was used to advance inmates
small sums of pocket money. Relatives also sent packages from
home containing food, clothing, reading matter, and toilet articles.
A husband responded to his wife's requests by sending Kirkbride
a package, noting: "I send herewith as she desires, the woolen
thing for the head (as the maid supposes [this is] the one she asks
for), a bottle of Ring's ambrosia, and a jar of ginger which she is
fond of at dessert." The asylum regimen denied no patient such
expressions of individual taste, as long as the patrons paid for
them. Even with the poorer inmates, there were no concerted
attempts to impose uniformity in dress or to strip them of personal
effects; they were allowed any comforts they could afford to
purchase.[28]

As might be expected, patients of different social backgrounds
employed themselves in appropriate ways. Working-class male
patients were encouraged to work in the hospital garden and work-
shop; the women helped out in the kitchen, laundry, and ward
work. In return, Kirkbride reduced their board payments or recommended them for the free list; not infrequently, he offered hard-
working patients a job in the hospital employ once they recovered.
In contrast, the affluent inmates amused themselves during the day
by riding out in the hospital carriage and visiting the asylum's
recreational facilities. Although not ignoring her other charges,
the companion, as a higher grade of attendant, spent more time
with the gentlemen and ladies, encouraging the men to read newspapers or play at board games and the women to do fancy
needlework.[29]

In its accommodations and employments, then, the Pennsylvania Hospital for the Insane reflected a commitment to individuality, comfort, and class distinctions. Unlike other institutions of its era, such as the penitentiary or reform school, the corporate asylum did not seek to change its inmates through the imposition of a uniform, highly regimented discipline.[30] The patients did follow a regular schedule, but hardly a punitive or denying one. The hospital authorities sought to offer an appealing way of life, complete with homelike comforts, that would reconcile the patients to a prolonged stay. Since, in a noninstitutional setting, patients would have expected to see class distinctions in housing and employment, the asylum replicated those features of everyday life. It was indeed more like a hotel than a correctional institution. The difference in tone can be attributed partly to the hospital's voluntary status; it had no compulsory clientele, but rather had to attract patrons, especially affluent ones, in order to continue operating. But the principles of individuality and class distinctions incorporated into the daily regimen served a therapeutic function as well. The hospital's social hierarchy facilitated the operation of a system of rewards and punishments, which relied upon the patient's feelings of ambition and emulation to inspire good conduct. By making access to pleasant surroundings and attractive companions contingent upon sane behavior, Kirkbride tried to induce the insane to exercise more self-control.

The incentive system

The asylum's system of rewards and punishments depended primarily upon the manipulation of ward assignments (see Figure 6). As was outlined in Chapter 4, patients were placed on a ward according to two considerations: mental condition, as measured by the level of excitement and a propensity to violent or filthy habits (i.e., masturbation and incontinence); and social condition, as reflected in board rates. The best-behaved patients lived on the upper wards; excited but manageable individuals, along with quiet chronic patients, on the Third and Fourth wards; and violent and destructive ones in the lower divisions. The ward hierarchy was able to incorporate subtle differences in the patients' education and social rank. In the Female Department, for example, the South Wing was more genteel than the North; on the upper wards of the South Wing, the best-paying, best-behaved patients had the

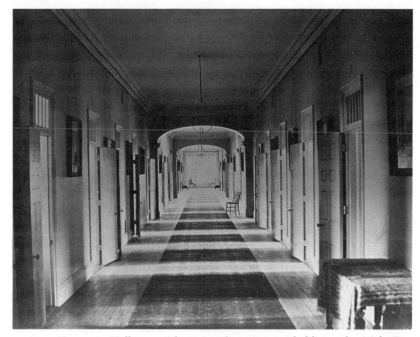

Figure 6. Hallway with patients' rooms, probably at the Male Department. At the far end, where the seated figure can be seen, was a small lounge area. Photograph probably taken in the early 1870s. (Courtesy of the Historic Archives, Institute of the Pennsylvania Hospital.)

Second Ward, the respectable but less refined ladies the First Ward. As the hospital's accommodations expanded and improved, so did the relative desirability of the various wards. For example, the Shields Wards, finished in 1880, superseded the First and Second South wards as the most exclusive accommodations in the women's division. The relative assessments might change, but the practice of ranking wards by the mental and social class of their inhabitants continued.[31]

This ward hierarchy was accepted not only by Kirkbride but also by the patients themselves, who quickly came to define their hospital status by ward number. They too regarded the First and Second wards as the most desirable and the lower wards as the most unpleasant. Thus, changing their ward assignments was an effective way for Kirkbride and his assistants to punish or reward patients. When an individual on the Third Ward became noisy or abusive, for example, the assistant would order him to spend the day on one of the lower wards, in the hope that a few hours among the asylum's least attractive inmates would frighten the malefactor into better deportment. If the undesirable behavior continued, the patient might remain on the lower ward all night. After a few days, if no improvement took place, the patient would be reassigned to the new ward indefinitely. Ward demotions were used primarily to punish noisiness, excitement, and violence. Removing a disruptive individual to a lower ward had the added benefit of setting an example for the other patients. A man who kept insisting loudly that "the doctors and attendants are hired to kill him" was moved to another ward, the assistant noted, "where his grumblings and denunciations will not disturb the calmer patients." Demotion also protected the better accommodations, for those who fouled their rooms or broke "considerable furniture" could be banished to a ward with fewer amenities.[32]

The hospital career of Miss R, as recorded in the supervisor's journal, illustrated the frequency with which patients might change wards as their mood and behavior fluctuated. Miss R started out on the Third Ward, occasionally taking tea with "the Ladies, Second Ward South," as a reward for good behavior. But she soon "got in the pond" and, in a "very excited" state, was sent to the Seventh Ward. Miss R remained "very distressed" the next day and was moved to the Eighth Ward. After ten days there, she gradually improved and slowly began to work her way back up the ward hierarchy. First, she spent the day and then slept over in the Fifth Ward. Finally, Miss R returned to the Second Ward, where she stayed for some time. In a grotesque parody of the rags-to-riches mythology of the time, a patient's progress could be measured by his or her social mobility within the ward hierarchy.[33]

On a more short-term basis, doctors and attendants regulated the patients' movements within the ward as a disciplinary measure. Patients who used obscenities or became violent would be denied the use of the hall and parlors, which formed the center of ward social life. The casebook noted a female patient whose "language is of such a character as renders it necessary she should remain in her room for a few days." A patient's isolation might be extended to mealtimes as well; noisy or violent individuals were made to sit at separate side tables in the dining room or eat alone in their rooms. As the worst punishment of all, the badly behaved inmates would not be allowed to attend the nightly entertainment. On a few occasions, a whole ward fell under such a ban due to collective misbehavior. The staff took a different tack with patients who manifested their peculiarities in private rather than in public. A gentleman able to behave perfectly well while "in company" nevertheless began laughing "immoderately" and "speaking or exhorting with much earnestness" as soon as he was left alone. To discourage his peculiarities, the attendants simply locked him out of his room. Similarly, patients prone to masturbation, excessive sleeping, or any other reclusive practices would be forced to remain in public view all day long as a deterrent to their insane habits.[34]

Another privilege of movement that the doctors could extend or revoke, depending upon the patient's behavior, was the "liberty of the grounds." As a mark of trust, Kirkbride allowed well-behaved patients to go anywhere on the hospital grounds they wished. If at any point they became excited or broke a hospital regulation, the privilege would be withdrawn. Similarly, convalescent patients could travel to Philadelphia, as long as they promised to come back at the appointed time; if they returned late, or in an excited or intoxicated state, the liberty of the grounds would be revoked.[35]

Such disciplinary measures reinforced the assumption implicit in every aspect of moral treatment: that the patients themselves must decide whether or not to act in a sane fashion. The hospital rules were clearly spelled out, so if an inmate chose to disregard them, Kirkbride could not help but view the act as conscious and deliberate in intent. "I very much regret," he wrote to a patron whose relative had been sent to a lower ward, "that your mother has compelled me to place her where she is, but her conduct and language left us no choice." Kirkbride justified removing a man to the lodge in similar terms: "in spite of repeated warnings, given in the kindest spirit and in the most respectful manner," the patient had forced the doctor "to show to others as well as to convince him that some order and discipline were to be observed in this institution, and that conduct of the most unbecoming kind could not be passed over, from week to week, without some notice." In Kirkbride's terms, every infraction represented a choice for insanity, and the process of discipline became a contest of wills between patient and doctor.[36]

Kirkbride sought to extend the therapeutic benefits of hospital

discipline by involving the patients more closely in its administration. Whenever possible, he recruited difficult but impression-
able inmates for special duty on the ward as a "doorkeeper" or
"health officer." By "working upon his ambition," Kirkbride wrote
of a patient whom he had appointed as doorkeeper, he hoped to
make the man identify with the hospital authorities and learn the
"necessity of order in such an establishment." To reinforce their
good intentions, patients who performed "little offices" about the
ward and cooperated with the attendants received little trinkets
and privileges. Kirkbride granted a chronic woman patient full
liberty of the house and grounds, noting that her behavior had
been "quiet and lady-like," and "frequently excited a very good
influence among other patients." At every opportunity, the superintendent went out of his way to praise inmates who helped
keep the wards in order. "Mr. W. is so pleasant and correct a man
in every respect," Kirkbride wrote to his family, "and his influence
among his fellow patients is always so decidedly for the good,
that we do not feel anxious to part with him." Commenting on
his patient "trustees," as he termed them in the *Report* for 1852,
Kirkbride stated that he had found it "exceedingly rare that a
patient selected for such a post disappoints us, or allows any one
to transgress the established regulations, while his own self-respect
and his confidence in those about him, are increased." A patient,
he concluded, often made the "most faithful and trustworthy
guardian" of his hospital peers.[37]

To a rather remarkable degree, the patients themselves appear
to have accepted Kirkbride's notion of peer guardianship, to the
point of preserving hospital discipline on their own initiative. The
following letter, written by a woman on behalf of the "Ladies of
the Second Ward," suggests the extent to which patients upheld
both class and behavioral standards on the wards.

The ladies of the 2nd ward are unanimous in the desire that Mrs. B. may
be kept in that part of the institution to which she belongs, until she is
prepared to behave in a manner more in accordance with the laws of
propriety and decorum. Their peace is much disturbed by her incessant
talking, and angry invectives, and they respectfully request that you will
give speedy attention to the state of things at present existing here. Much
dissatisfaction is also expressed that the feelings of the better class of
patients should be so often shocked by the gross vulgarity and profanity
of two of the patients who have their rooms on this floor. M.H. is a

disgrace and nuisance among us, and the other to whom I allude, Miss H. has acquired such a habit of swearing and scolding that we can no longer forbear a general complaint...we deem it unjust that ladies possessing any refinement of feeling, should be compelled to be listeners, or witnesses of such demoralizing conduct.[38]

Friendships on the ward had a therapeutic potential, quite apart from their disciplinary effect, which Kirkbride also tried to direct to his own ends. Patients performed a valuable service as confidants and counselors, and Kirkbride encouraged their relationships whenever he thought them conducive to either party's improvement. One woman tended another "as if she were her own sister and I think with benefit," Kirkbride noted approvingly. In another case, he felt that a patient's improvement could be "attributed to the care she has taken of a German lady for whom she acts as our interpreter, and in whose welfare she manifests the deepest interest." At the asylum parties, dinners, and entertainments, Kirkbride hoped that a similar spirit of good will would spring up between the patients and the hospital staff. Social occasions gave the superintendent an excellent opportunity to improve his public relations, especially with troublesome inmates. Kirkbride wrote of the weekly tea parties, first introduced in 1866, which he attended without fail, "Even those who are especially obtuse as to the relations and feelings of the officers toward the patients, very often express gratification, and acknowledge a new light dawning on them, when they so often find all the officers and their families giving up what ever private engagements may have been tendered them, in order to be present at these social gatherings."[39]

Hospital social activities apparently took on added excitement, from the patients' perspective, because they could extend their personal acquaintanceship with the hospital officers and their families. The instructor of the ladies' gymnasium class wrote of her charges' enthusiasm for their exercise hour: "In passing through the house, I often heard it said, 'Oh! I shall see the doctor in the hall [Kirkbride], for he is always at gymnastics,' and I do not hesitate to say that more petitions have been presented and their claims urged before the executive of this establishment, in this hall, than have been acted upon by the Congress of the United States within the same time" (see Figure 7). Patients also vied for the privilege of eating with a popular staff member; invitations to dine at the "matron's table," along with the teacher and wing

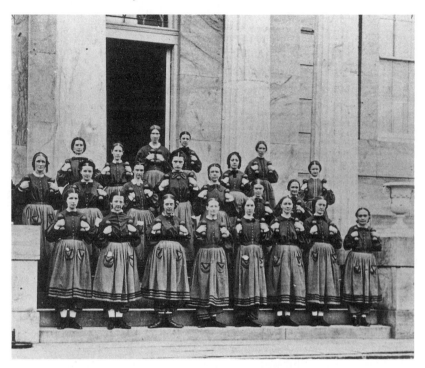

Figure 7. Women attendants with dumbbells, doing demonstration for the ladies' calisthenic class. Photograph taken in the early 1860s. (Courtesy of the Historic Archives, Pennsylvania Hospital for the Insane.)

supervisor, or, better yet, at the "family table" in Kirkbride's own home, were highly prized. Inmates, female and male alike, seemed especially pleased by attention from the hospital officers' female relatives. Women patients expressed "an extreme desire to be introduced" to Kirkbride's wife Eliza and considered attendance at her "reading circle" a great privilege. Similarly, the men enjoyed dinner parties given at the Male Department by Dr. Jones's wife.[40]

Sociability in the asylum not only functioned as an incentive for good behavior; it also fostered an attachment between patient and doctor that Kirkbride hoped to parlay into a more serious therapeutic relationship. If, after taking medication and participating in the hospital regimen, patients began to show signs of returning consciousness or rationality, Kirkbride and his assistants tried to engage them in a simple form of talk therapy. During their daily rounds, the doctors concentrated on those individuals who seemed "susceptible to influence," as Kirkbride put it, and sought to begin a dialogue on the nature, causes, and cure of the patients' insanity. Kirkbride had no formal theory or even term to define these efforts, referring only vaguely to his "advice," "opinions," or "personal influence" upon the insane. Yet, Kirkbride's conversations with his patients formed an important aspect of moral treatment, for it was in the course of these dialogues that he laid out the changes the insane would have to make in order to become cured. By giving his charges a "proper view" of their illness and convincing them of the wrongness of their former lives, Kirkbride hoped to enable patients to resist their insane impulses and control their own behavior. Only if he succeeded in this phase of treatment could Kirkbride truly claim to have cured the patient's mental disorder.[41]

The family role in therapy

Crucial to the success of Kirkbride's dialogues with the insane was the wholehearted cooperation of the patients' families. In order for treatment to proceed, they had to be convinced to leave their relatives in Kirkbride's hands, no matter how much the patients complained of asylum life. A considerable portion of his work as a superintendent involved the maintenance of a good working relationship with the patients' families. Not only did Kirkbride have to meet with patrons when they visited the asylum; he also had to keep up an extensive correspondence, answering their queries concerning the patients' progress.[42] These conversations and letters served Kirkbride as a more personal medium for driving home the general truths he outlined in the *Reports*. In the course of describing the patient's health, adjustment to hospital life, and prognosis, Kirkbride lost no opportunity to encourage his patron's generous confidence in the asylum and its chief physician. Thus, Kirkbride turned psychotherapy at the Pennsylvania Hospital for the Insane into a three-sided interaction involving doctor, patient, and family.

In the first place, Kirkbride was quick to reassure family members that the decision to commit a relative was a wise one, by emphasizing the special effort needed to control the patient even in the hospital. "I fear that you would have great difficulty in controlling your wife at home," he informed one patron, "without resorting to means, that would be a constant source of pain and mortification to yourself and family." Kirkbride concluded, "there is no little difficulty in controlling Mrs. M by mild means even here, and at home the difficulties must necessarily be greater."[43]

Kirkbride's reports on the patients' physical condition allowed him to reinforce the notion that insanity was a very serious disease. He felt compelled to mention a trifling matter such as a sore throat, as he wrote in one letter, for "occasionally in patients like Mr. G, small acute ailments sometimes terminate more seriously than we would have any right to expect among sane persons." Then if the patient died in the hospital, the family would not be quite so surprised or guilt-stricken. Kirkbride consoled the family of an aged relative who died in the asylum by offering a medical explanation for his insanity (as well as his death): "His brain was much diseased, but the starting point was probably in the stomach, added to his continued labors when his advanced age and failing health demanded repose of both mind and body."[44]

In dispensing his medical opinions, Kirkbride aimed at gaining the patrons' cooperation in a general sense, rather than drawing them into every aspect of the patient's medical treatment. When relatives got too involved in the details of a case, the superintendent found that they tended to become meddlesome. To avoid such overinvolvement, Kirkbride described the regimen he pursued with a patient only in very general terms, such as a "mild tonic treatment" or a trial of "active medicines." Ordinarily, the superintendent confined himself to statements of this sort: "We have commenced the course of treatment which I suggested to you – and I can assure you everything shall be done which seems to offer even a small chance of alleviating your son's malady." Kirkbride's remarks rarely went beyond reassuring generalities unless the patron repeatedly requested a more detailed account of the medical treatment being pursued. However meddlesome patrons might be, Kirkbride politely acknowledged their suggestions concerning medical treatment, replying that such requests, coming as they did from "one so deeply concerned," would be "allowed all proper weight in deciding upon the mode of treatment." Rather than dismissing the family's suggestions out of hand, Kirkbride preferred instead to accede to them whenever possible, so as to strengthen their resolve to leave the patient in his hands. At the same time, his patience with patrons did have its limits. He refused the frequent requests from relatives who wanted private doctors to attend the patient in the asylum. Although willing to consult with family doctors concerning the course of treatment, Kirkbride nonetheless felt that it was "entirely impracticable" to let outside physicians practice within his asylum. Such a course, he believed, could only undermine his authority over the patients.[45]

Kirkbride's opinions on the patients' prognosis had to be couched in careful terms. He needed to secure his patrons' willingness to give asylum treatment a fair trial – which took at least a year, according to Kirkbride – without raising false expectations concerning a cure. When a patient appeared to improve, Kirkbride's course with the family was comparatively easy; he could detail the signs of progress and express "entire confidence in the patient's recovery." "There is encouragement for a long trial of her present remedies," he concluded in a hopeful case, thereby associating the cure with continuance of his remedies. But when an individual's case appeared discouraging, Kirkbride could offer no such reasons for continuing treatment. Instead, the superintendent argued that the prognosis was by no means fixed. "The prospect for the future, judging from his present symptoms, is not very promising," Kirkbride wrote in one instance, "and yet, I should not think of giving up his case as an entirely hopeless one." In this manner, Kirkbride continued to counsel hospital care even when the patient seemed to gain little benefit from it.[46]

To offset the family's eagerness to have a relative come home, whether better or not, Kirkbride emphasized the positive aspects of the patient's hospital experience. Although sparing of details about medical treatment in his letters, the superintendent willingly supplied information about the inmates' everyday activities in the asylum, such as the type of exercise they took, the activities they participated in, and the friends they had made on the ward. Kirkbride informed one family that their relative had an "excellent man" for a private attendant, and that the two got along very well. As with their suggestions regarding medical remedies, Kirkbride reassured his patrons that he heeded their advice about the patient's moral treatment. As he wrote to a man concerned about a reclusive female relative, "I fully agree with you that it is important that she should be out of her room and particularly out of her bed as much as possible." Kirkbride acknowledged the innumerable little favors patrons asked to be done for an inmate. "We take pains to consult about any little matters that may contribute in any way to his comfort," he assured an anxious relative. Whenever possible, Kirkbride sought to place the most favorable construction on the patient's experience of hospital life. Commenting on a young man's first month at the asylum, Kirkbride wrote to his parents that "everyone about the place is much interested in him, and his pleasant disposition and courteous manners make him a general favorite."[47]

But when patients were newly admitted and highly dissatisfied, Kirkbride's efforts to make hospitalization seem both urgent and attractive were often less than persuasive. To prevent a "premature removal," the superintendent had to assure the family that the patient's misery was only temporary. One patron admitted that although he meant to give the hospital treatment a fair trial, his wife's appeals to be taken home were "very trying...but if she is not rational long enough to feel deep and lasting the emotions which dictate them it will be a palliation to me." Kirkbride responded soothingly in such cases by claiming that the patient's desire to go home resulted "almost entirely because she thinks nothing can be done for her – if we succeed in convincing her that she may be benefited I have no doubt she would be very glad to remain some time with us." He warned families that unless they stood firm in the beginning, the patient would never be persuaded to cooperate in the treatment. He wrote to a man concerned about his son, "I need hardly express to you the importance of his understanding that his friends are determined to give a full trial to a proper course of treatment, and that his removal from the hospital will depend upon their judgment and not his own." His son's willingness to get well depended on this, Kirkbride claimed. "Whenever he ceases to look forward to an early return home, or to visits from members of his family or acquaintances, whom he believes he could persuade to remove him, I have every reason to believe we shall be able to make his time pass pleasantly and profitably."[48]

The curative process

Having reaffirmed the family's compliance with the terms of treatment, Kirkbride then turned his attention to the patient. As the first objective in treatment, Kirkbride tried to induce the insane person to take the proper attitude toward the hospital itself. Often

during their first weeks in the institution patients refused to acknowledge the necessity for their commitment, and expressed
great anger or misery at being left there by their families. Many
insisted that their minds were not affected, that their detention in
the asylum was at best a mistake or at worst a conspiracy necessitating prompt legal action. One gentleman, who claimed that
the physicians attesting to his insanity were "in error or attended
him only to get their fees," thought that the hospital was in fact
a prison. Another young man, "believing that little is the matter
with him, thinks it strange that he is in a hospital," Kirkbride
reported. Not convinced of their own insanity, such patients naturally suspected their relatives of "some sinister motive" in committing them. A woman, brooding over the "supposed harshness
of her treatment," said that "she was deceived and...her sister
did it to get possession of her clothes." Kirkbride noted in another
case that a young man "does not yet exactly comprehend what
his situation has been and as a consequence has some idea that he
had been suffering neglect."[49]

To overcome the patients' resistance to treatment, as well as
soothe the patrons' guilt, Kirkbride tried to get the insane to acknowledge that their families had acted wisely in committing them.
He held long conversations with a young man, trying to convince
him "that his family felt the deepest and most anxious interest in
his welfare." To another patient, anxious to return home to his
family and business, Kirkbride stated over and over "that his friends
have nothing in view but his own good and that whenever they
felt satisfied that he was perfectly restored and not liable to an
early relapse, they would be glad to have him among them." At
this point in the treatment, Kirkbride often solicited letters from
the family to underscore his efforts with the patient. He requested
a man to write to his despondent father and tell him "that in your
neighborhood, it is universally understood that from loss of physical health or other causes, his mind has become affected, and that
as soon as that is restored, everybody will be glad to welcome
him home...but that until his health is restored, he had better
make up his mind to remain contentedly where he is." Following
Kirkbride's advice, a man wrote to his wife, "we should advise
you to be attentive to your Physician and to obey the regulations
of the Hospital," adding that she should "cheer up and not let
your hopes droop." Some patrons sought to gain the patient's coop-

eration with a bribe, as did a husband who promised his wife that "if she would take her medicine regularly" as the doctor prescribed it, he would take her into the city for a day.[50]

Once the patients' misery over their confinement began to lessen, Kirkbride encouraged them to participate in the asylum activities. If they showed the least inclination to read or converse, their activities were "carefully encouraged." "I shall use all my influence," Kirkbride assured a patron, to induce his son to "adopt a more active and varied course of exercise, and to associate more with some of the very intelligent gentlemen who are in the same ward with him, which I am convinced cannot fail to be beneficial to him." The doctor sometimes overcame a patient's reluctance to follow the hospital regimen by promising that compliance would eventually lead to discharge. "I have taken considerable pains to induce her to take more interest in things," Kirkbride wrote of a woman patient, "by the assurance that if she did so," her husband would be "glad to gratify her in her wish" to return home.[51]

When inmates began to respond to fellow patients and pay more attention to their appearance, Kirkbride felt that they had taken another major step toward a cure. He described a patient as "greatly improved" because "she now begins to speak more pleasantly with the ladies who are around her and occasionally indulges in lively remarks and to enter into general conversation." He continued, "She begins, too, to take more interest in her dress and has had some small purchases made for her." Kirkbride recorded great jubilation at getting a patient who had kept his eyes closed since admission to put on a pair of spectacles and begin reading. "So far as I can estimate," he wrote to the man's wife, "this is the first time he has ever opened his eyes since he entered this institution and the event has created quite a sensation among his fellow patients – and certainly gives us grounds for stronger hopes respecting his case than we have before been able to indulge."[52]

Once patients began to participate more freely in asylum life, Kirkbride tried to talk more pointedly with them about their disordered thoughts and feelings. Sometimes the patients' initial anger at being hospitalized included the doctor as well, and they had to be persuaded to trust him. He wrote to a patient's husband that although she accepted the remedies provided for her, "towards myself she does not express any very good feeling, mainly I believe from an idea, that you would take her home at once, if I did not interpose some objection." Kirkbride wrote resignedly of another patient that he found it "exceedingly difficult to induce [him] to converse with me or even to answer questions of any kind." For that reason, he concluded, "we are very much at a loss to know his feelings or wishes." This resistance had to be overcome, for without access to the patients' inner thoughts, the doctor could have no hope of influencing their behavior. A willingness to talk with Kirkbride thus became an important precursor of a cure.[53]

If he could gain some knowledge of the patients' thoughts and emotions, Kirkbride then focused attention on the particular symptoms of insanity the family had complained about or that he himself had observed. When the patient suffered from delusions, the doctor tried straightforward denial of the irrational beliefs. "I have stated to him that they were delusions and that no one could consider him well while he entertained them," Kirkbride reported to a patron. If the patients wavered in the least, Kirkbride worked to increase their doubt. "On one or two occasions," he noted of a gentleman who erroneously believed himself to be a defaulter, "he has appeared to me to have some doubts whether his suppositions were true – but generally he will not listen to a doubt on the subject." Sometimes these direct denials had no effect on the patients' delusions; as Kirkbride wrote of one man, "I find it quite impossible to satisfy him that he is wrong in any of these particulars." In the more stubborn cases, the doctor might try marshaling evidence to contradict the delusion. When a patient kept insisting that he had a recipe "by which four times the usual amount of grain can be raised," Kirkbride kept asking to see it, in the hope that the patient's inability to produce the document would shake his faith in his "extravagant plans." Kirkbride also solicited help from the family in confronting the patient's delusions. Kirkbride advised the husband of a woman patient, who believed that her family doctor remained near the hospital waiting to take her home, "it might not be amiss for the doctor to write her a short letter and enlighten her on this point." A man reported to Kirkbride that, as the doctor had requested, he had written to his wife that very day, "earnestly entreating her to abandon her strange notions about conspiracies and poisoning, etc." Kirkbride once asked President Zachary Taylor to write a letter reassuring a former army surgeon, who believed himself wanted for desertion, that no such charge was being held against him. "He attaches so much importance to such a letter from yourself that I have believed it of great importance in removing his delusion," Kirkbride wrote to Taylor.[54]

Since many insane delusions consisted primarily of a settled dislike or lack of interest in relatives, Kirkbride devoted considerable effort to restoring the patients' supposedly "natural feelings" of love, respect, and obedience toward their kin. As long as they responded to mentions of the family with "symptoms of anger or excitement," Kirkbride believed the patients' disease to be in full force. To weaken this type of delusion, the physician tried "to fix [their minds] on friends" at home and get them "to express a proper interest" in the family. He recorded a "very favorable" change in a woman patient who "last evening for the first time...spoke of her infant with some approach to the natural affection of a mother." While the woman was insane, he observed, "she appeared to have little or no feeling of interest in it." A young man's improvement could be clearly seen, Kirkbride assured a patron, in a letter the youth had written to his family, giving "evidence that many of his feelings are perfectly natural." When it seemed beneficial, the asylum superintendent encouraged relatives to write, hoping that, as one patron said, "it would keep up an interest in home and so incite self-exertions to get well" and return there.[55]

When patients first acknowledged that they had been unjustly hostile to their family and doctor, or that a cherished belief was in fact a delusion, they often felt ashamed and revolted by their insane behavior. Kirkbride believed this sensation of guilt to be a sign of returning rationality and encouraged its expression. As long as the patient remained, as Kirkbride put it, "totally unconscious of the character of his actions or conversation," there could be no real improvement; in order to be cured, the insane had to admit that their former actions and attitudes had been wrong. Kirkbride complained of a patient, "she cannot be made to believe that her conduct at home, was ever improper...which goes to show conclusively that she is far from well." In contrast, he noted approvingly that a woman who had physically and verbally abused the physicians for several days, had become "much depressed, and regrets exceedingly what has passed – the recollection of which is mortifying to her." Another patient manifested his return to sanity by admitting that his "conduct at home was wrong, and that he shall have to answer hereafter for doing wrong knowingly but that he might have stopped if he had chosen to do so." A convalescent woman expressed her "repentence" and "resolution" to do right: "Hitherto I have acted from impulse, in the future I shall be guided by thoughts and principle."[56]

Kirkbride tried to use the shame and guilt that individuals came to feel about their past behavior to increase their determination to resist or overcome their insane impulses. Once aware that their behavior was wrong, patients could more easily be helped to prevent the recurrence of their symptoms. In essence, Kirkbride presented the return to sanity as a moral choice. He explained what the patient had to do in order to be considered cured and then tried to induce the necessary emotions, whether shame, desire to return to a normal life, or admiration for himself, to enable them to make the choice and abide by it. He told a convalescent patient, "There is no one anywhere, who will dream of your being insane after you leave here, unless you force that opinion upon them, by excitement of manner, striking peculiarity of conduct, or opinions." He advised a man whose sanity had returned, "You have it almost entirely in your power to continue to enjoy these blessings. You must be thoroughly convinced of the importance in every point, of some regular employment, and of resisting fancies that may sometimes enter your mind, but which if harbored there can only give you uneasiness and lead you into difficulty."[57]

For patients who had once experienced delusions, Kirkbride counseled distraction from and repression of the troublesome material. They should avoid conversing about topics on which they had formerly shown "unsoundness." The doctor viewed a patient's ability to resist talking about a delusion, whether it had disappeared entirely or not, as a desirable improvement. To a man bothered by sexual obsessions, Kirkbride explained "that a great deal of danger is to be apprehended from allowing the mind to dwell upon the matter." The patient agreed, writing, "I shall endeavor as much as possible to direct my thoughts in other channels." Kirkbride told a youth to avoid talking about his "unnatural feelings" toward his father: "Whatever may be your own views about these matters...say little about them...introduce the subject rarely if ever." The doctor concluded, "Their expression can do good to no one and may do you much harm, in the estimation of nearly everyone."[58]

Kirkbride also gave patients special counsel about the habits of intemperance and irregularity that he felt aggravated mental disease. He wrote of a convalescent patient, whose clandestine use of tobacco made him excitable on occasion, "could he give up this to him very pernicious habit," he could return to his family. Kirkbride often sought patients' pledges to give up their vices. "I have conversed with him freely on the subject" of masturbation, he assured a father regarding his son, and the youth had promised "that he would take my advice." With the intemperate, "the only safety is water," Kirkbride warned. "I shall lose no opportunity to impress upon Charles, the immense important of his avoiding everything that can intoxicate – it is the only safety for him, mentally or physically," he wrote to a relative. With another intemperate young man, the physician stressed "the importance. . .of avoiding all sources of great excitement, the immense advantage of regularity in your habits, and above all, the deep interest you have in adhering to the pledge, which you have now so faithfully kept for the best part of a year."[59]

To be pronounced cured, patients not only had to be free of all symptoms of insanity and able to resist undesirable impulses; they also had to believe in their own reformation and state their determination to lead, as one man put it, "a totally different course of life, from that which he led previous to coming to the Hospital." Kirkbride could not consider the inmate well who, despite his improved behavior, said that "he still feels a despondency about him, which he does not believe treatment can ever relieve." The truly convalescent patient wished to tell her family "that she feels much better and now believes that she will get entirely well." Kirkbride happily reported such signs of progress to the family, as in this letter: "Mr. D. says that his feelings toward his wife are now different from what they have previously been, and he has a firmer determination than he ever had before, to avoid the causes which have before led to his separation from his family." A patient who once denied his family's existence now felt "confident he shall never again have any uneasiness on the subject, that he feels perfectly able and so very anxious to return to the office and to engage in active occupation." Kirkbride added, "he appears to me serious in these sentiments and if so, of course must be nearly, if not quite well."[60]

Patients showing strong signs of improvement entered a period of convalescence that usually lasted for several months. They received additional privileges to come and go about the hospital as they liked and take short trips into town. Throughout this period, Kirkbride watched the convalescents carefully, trying to ascertain whether their improvements were indeed permanent. He suspected in some cases that the patients merely appeared to accede to his wishes and opinions, although their actual feelings or delusions remained unchanged. "The fear of returning to the hospital," he wrote of an inmate, "may possibly induce her to conduct with greater propriety but I fear that in reality, there is little improvement in her feelings toward her family." Kirkbride frequently asked the family's cooperation in testing a recovery by asking them to write letters calculated to provoke the patient to "break out" on any remaining delusions. In the case just mentioned, the superintendent suggested that the woman's husband inform her of her family's health and request an "early answer." "In that answer," Kirkbride wrote, "I have little doubt she will show the true state of her feelings much better than in her conversations with myself." In another instance, a man appeared much better, except for "a degree of absence and of restlessness about him." Kirkbride wrote to his parents, "if you asked for an answer filled with details, you would probably be better able to judge of his strength of mind and powers of observation."[61]

Kirkbride also judged convalescent patients by their reaction to family visits or news from home. A woman who formerly had shown much hostility and excitement toward her family when they visited now "conducted herself with entire propriety" during their calls, a sure sign of improvement. In another case, Kirkbride noted, "The permanency of his improvement has been tested by his hearing of the sudden death of his only remaining child and the continued illness of his wife." Although the man spoke "feelingly of the loss he has sustained," he showed no symptoms of derangement, whereas formerly, "any great mental anxiety caused this patient to become excited and incoherent."[62]

If, after several months, an individual continued well, wrote rational and pleasant letters home, and responded calmly to visits, Kirkbride began to prepare him or her for discharge. First, he reduced any medication the patient might still be taking to make sure that no symptoms recurred. Then doctor and patient began to discuss the latter's postdischarge plans. Kirkbride directed special attention to the young male patient's choice of an appropriate employment. Usually, the doctor did not advise against engaging in any particular employment, but rather stressed the individual's determination "to resolve upon a perfectly temperate and regular course of life and to join with his mental labor, a very decided amount of physical exercise." He then sent the patient off with some final advice and directions for a healthy regimen. A "memorandum" prepared for a patient in 1843 included the receipts for the "pills he has been taking for some time," the "fluid he has found to exercise such a soothing effect," and an "anoydyne enema" for his diarrhea. Kirkbride added in a postscript that the patient should take special care of his diet – "errors in quantity are as bad as those of quality" – and take frequent exercise. In a lengthy letter to a recently recovered gentleman, Kirkbride spelled out the elements of a prudent daily regimen:

I would suggest to you a trial of your present plan of early rising – to sponge your body with cold water, and immediately after drying it, to rub the whole surface with a "salted towel" [a towel dipped in a saturated solution of salt and dried] until a decided glow is produced, to eat in moderation of what you find to agree with you, to keep your bowels regular – if possible by diet and exercise and regular visits to the temple of Cloacina – if not, by mild laxatives, say a little rhubarb chewed; – if you use tobacco at all, the less the better; to take exercise in the open air, on foot or on horseback, if possible with company – every day, unless the weather is decidedly stormy; to wear flannel next to your skin and to retire early at night, after using the salted towel as recommended for the morning. A moderately stimulating plaster, of good size, over the loins might be serviceable, and a mild tonic, like the cold camomile tea, could be of no disadvantage to you. Use your mind, of course, but do not work it to excess and remember that most sound minds cannot be worked much without injury, unless their muscles have a fair share of labor.[63]

Thus, by influence and persuasion, Kirkbride guided receptive patients through a personal transformation somewhat like a religious conversion. Although not strictly spiritual in content, the sequence of self-criticism that the asylum doctor sought to produce in his patients had definite religious overtones. The recognition of wrongdoing in insane actions; the repentence and willingness to reform that was necessary for amendment; the emphasis on choosing to be sane; the personal conviction of "salvation," or freedom from insanity; the public profession of an altered state of mind; and the commitment to a new post-hospital existence – each step toward recovery involved concepts and terms strongly charged with religious values.

In a sense, then, early asylum therapy might be regarded as a secularized version of the conversion experience. Despite their reservation about revivalism, nineteenth-century physicians such as Kirkbride essentially had only a religious model of personality change to draw upon; moreover, the very conception of the moral faculties to which their measures appealed fused emotional and religious sensibilities. Thus, it was perhaps inevitable that the psychological aspects of moral treatment took on religious overtones. Significantly, Kirkbride referred to his Sunday morning visits to the wards, which he set aside especially for the influence of receptive patients, as "going to...his Meeting." By invoking his spiritual qualities as a Christian and physician, he invested the older religious rituals with the scientific authority of medicine. The result was a therapeutic technique apparently capable of inducing lasting personality transformations.[64]

PATIENT RESPONSE

Not surprisingly, only a portion of Kirkbride's patients, an average of 47 percent during his career, completed this demanding process of change. Another 26 percent made some improvement while under his care, 13.5 percent remained unchanged, and 13.5 percent died[65] (see Tables A.6 and A.7). One might argue that those patients who improved would have improved anyway, regardless of the treatment they received at the Pennsylvania Hospital for the Insane. Modern therapies produce very similar rates of outcome, suggesting that the prognosis is determined by some underlying dynamic of mental disorder rather than by a specific form of treatment. Yet, contemporary studies also have shown that the patients' confidence in the therapist does seem to affect their ability to recover. Certainly, Kirkbride's cured patients attributed their changed outlook and behavior to him and him alone. Whether correct in their assumptions or not, the patients' declaration of gratitude toward and respect for the asylum doctor strongly reinforced Kirkbride's reputation as a healer.[66]

The compliant patient

The many letters written to Kirkbride by grateful patients, both during and after their hospital stay, provide some insight into the attitudes conducive to a cure. Patients invariably expressed an intense attachment to their physician, prefacing their notes with "my dear friend" or "my kind and patient doctor." Kirkbride's "kind and consoling" manner, grateful patients recalled, had encouraged them to share their anxieties with him. As a male patient wrote, "I would unburthen my overloaded heart in confidence to you, feeling sure it would be a relief." The doctor's reassurance inspired the patient's confidence in himself or herself, as well as in the future. A woman testified that "Dr. Kirkbride...always had the power of imparting a ray of hope when others failed." Once the patient began to trust him, Kirkbride's very presence became a source of reassurance and security. Inmates described a "peculiar feeling of restfulness and help in the mere knowledge of his being near," so much so that his absences brought a "strange sense of loss" for them.[67]

Kirkbride's sympathetic demeanor proved all the more compelling to his charges because he possessed such authority in their eyes. In part, his influence was associated with his medical knowledge; cured patients often expressed admiration for Kirkbride's "scientific and strictly correct course of treatment," as one former inmate remembered it. But the doctor's authority went beyond mere scientific knowledge to encompass spiritual guidance as well; the "presence of goodness and kind wisdom" informed his medical authority over the patients. This combination of scientific and spiritual qualities gave the asylum doctor his unique "healing, strengthening power"; as a cured patient wrote, it was Kirkbride's "skillful kind attention, united with heavenly aid," that had changed her from "a comparative state of misery and despair to Light, Love and Happiness."[68]

Acceptance of Kirkbride's authority, in turn, led patients to adopt his interpretation of their disease. Under the doctor's guidance, they gradually came to regard their insanity as a weakness or indulgence that might be controlled by their own willpower. "I have great instability of nerves and temper to contend with," a woman admitted to Kirkbride, "but knowing the necessity of self-control I try always to exercise it." Another announced that she had resolved to stay at home "and see what strength of will may do. . .that is of course strength of will for the right." Cured patients often referred to their efforts to overcome the "bad habits" of insanity. A young man, professing to follow all of Kirkbride's advice, declared, "I hope gradually to conquer any bad habit that threatens me such as sleeping too much, sedentary habits and other slight faults which indulged in engender others."[69]

A letter written to Kirkbride by a newly recovered young woman nicely conveys the manner in which cured patients conflated personal morality with disease. "*I see now clearly that it was disease* which led me to pursue the course of conduct I did," she wrote. "Now my feelings of integrity have returned and though my affliction has humbled me yet I trust it has been for my own good." Recalling her delusions, she commented, "How in the wide world I ever believed in them so firmly as I did I cannot now imagine. . .owing to your constant and unvarying kindness. . .I was first led seriously to reflect, to reason with myself about it. . .It is my earnest and fervent prayer that I may never be led into such error again."[70]

Devotion to and respect for their "beloved physician" inspired compliant patients with a desire to abide by Kirkbride's guidance. To win his approval, they pledged with "earnestness and solemnity" to avoid any untoward behavior that might cause the doctor "to withdraw your usual attention and kindness," as one man put it. A woman announced, "I am determined to manifest my respect for you by complying on all occasions with the regulation by which you govern the institution." At home, convalescent patients followed the routines begun in the asylum almost as if they constituted a magical defense against insanity, eagerly assuring Kirkbride that they observed his directions for medication and regimen to the letter. "I have made every exertion to keep up my spirits," wrote a woman, as "well as to do many other things for the improvement of my health. . .I hope I shall be rewarded for it." A reformed drunkard, referring to his "splendid champagne firestone water," affirmed, "I. . .never expected to be sick again with my entire temperate habits."[71]

Cured patients often felt an intense devotion to Kirkbride long after leaving the hospital. In fact, the persistence of their sanity appeared to depend in large part upon how successfully they managed to internalize the "love and sympathizing care" they associated with him. Former inmates sustained their connection with Kirkbride in a variety of ways. Many asked for photographs of the doctor and hospital, which they displayed in a shrinelike manner at home. "My attention is frequently drawn to your admirable likeness," a woman reported to Kirkbride. Dr. Smith, the assistant physician, had suggested that she mount it on black paper; and so fixed, it now hung "prettily framed and suspended in my own room." In this fashion, the woman declared, she had made Kirkbride a "close prisoner" and could recall his face at any moment, with a "calm and benign expression, in just such a happy mood as you were wont to be on Sunday morning when giving a round of the various wards to say a kind word to each and all." Many patients wrote to Kirkbride, especially in the first year after discharge, asking advice about personal matters from pursuing an education to choosing a new cookstove. They also recounted memories of hospital life and sent messages to friends still under Kirkbride's care. Not infrequently, patients included small gifts such as books, handmade items, and poems with their letters. A schoolgirl ended her missive to the doctor with a bit of affectionate doggerel: "My pen is bad, my ink is pale, but my love for you will never fail."[72]

These fervent expressions of devotion evidently strengthened the patients' resolve to stay well. They often begged for a few "encouraging words" from the doctor to help them in their trials. "If you only knew how much it would strengthen and console me," confided a woman, "you would not hesitate to write me." Sometimes simply summoning up Kirkbride's memory caused fears and doubts to recede. "When I sometimes tremble for the *future* there arises a strong feeling of confidence in looking towards you," wrote one patient. Another one recalled, "It was only the other night I woke in great fright; I was too frightened to call, but I suddenly thought of Dr. Kirkbride, and, as I thought, it seemed to me, that I could see him distinctly though the room was dark, and immediately I felt that peace and freedom from danger that Dr. Kirkbride always inspired."[73]

The patients' memories of the asylum played a similar, if less intense, function in strengthening their determination to stay well. Some took comfort in the fact that, if their troubles became too great, they could return to their "sweet quiet home" in the asylum. Other former patients liked to recall the friends they had made there. "The truth is I never in my life met with such congenial people as yourself and some others in the Pennsylvania Hospital," wrote one. The compliant patients thought of their hospital stay not as an ordeal but as a "green spot" in their past. As one man declared, the asylum was "the finest place in the world to get well." A more poetic gentleman declared that he "cherished" his memories of the asylum "as among the purest, the brightest and the most beautiful gems set in the sky of my heart's sorrow."[74]

In their letters to Kirkbride, men and women alike expressed the peculiar combination of affection and respect for him that contributed so much to a successful asylum stay. But the greatest intensity of affect was definitely reserved for the female patients. The gender differential in attachment might be explained in several ways. First, after the opening of the Male Department in 1859, Kirkbride concentrated his therapeutic efforts on the women, leaving S. Preston Jones to attend more closely to the men. This division of labor alone could account for the women's greater attachment to the superintendent. In addition, one would expect women to express more fervent declarations of affection for their doctor simply because they had fewer cultural constraints on emotional display. It also seems likely that women made better patients than men. The mixture of love and deference called for in the therapeutic process perhaps came easier to them, because they could easily place Kirkbride in the place of a father, brother, or even lover. For men, this brand of paternal authority may have aroused more ambivalence, thereby making Kirkbride's direction harder to accept. Even if men did respond less positively to Kirkbride's therapeutic authority, it made little difference in the cure rates, for before 1859, Kirkbride had roughly the same rate of success for both sexes. But one might still suspect that Kirkbride found women patients more rewarding to treat. His decision to remain at the Female Department in 1859, rather than take possession of the new hospital that represented the fulfillment of his architectural ideals, lends some credence to such a supposition.[75]

Patient profile: Eliza Butler

The complexities of the male doctor–female patient interaction can nowhere better be observed than in Kirkbride's relationship with Eliza Butler, a young woman he treated in 1858 and married in

1866, several years after his wife Ann's death. Eliza Butler's accounts of her illness provide a sensitive look at the patient's experience of insanity. Although by no means a typical occurrence in asylum practice, the Butler–Kirkbride relationship does allow insight into the dynamics of the therapeutic relationship.

Eliza Odgen Butler came from precisely the sort of affluent, cultured family that made up most of the Pennsylvania Hospital for the Insane's clientele. Her father, Benjamin Franklin Butler (not to be confused with the Civil War general of the same name), was a prominent New York lawyer and politician who served as attorney general during the Jackson and Van Buren administrations. Eliza grew up in Washington, D.C., and New York City in a household structured around her father's busy political and social schedule. Her upbringing stressed the cardinal virtues of the mid-Victorian urban middle class: sociability, piety, scholarship, and devotion to family. The girls as well as the boys were encouraged to be "hard scholars"; Eliza attended private school and took additional lessons in French and music. Her mother, Harriet Allen Butler, took an exacting interest in her children's religious training, making particularly sure to see that they never suffered from the sin of spiritual complacency.[76]

In Eliza's case, the self-critical religious consciousness fostered by her mother eventually took on a destructive force. Her mental distress began to manifest itself after Harriet Butler's death in 1853, which left the eighteen-year-old Eliza in charge of the household. The older Butler children, having all married and begun families of their own, evidently expected Eliza and her younger sister, Lydia, to take care of their aging father. Besides keeping house for him, Eliza filled her days with household chores, volunteer work, and cultural improvement; she taught Sunday school at the juvenile asylum, took German lessons, attended weekly lectures and read extensively. But all her occupations apparently failed to satisfy her and her physical health became more precarious, her mood despondent. "Religious gloom," as her father termed it, was a prominent feature of Eliza's depression. It was probably an overwhelming conviction of her own sinfulness that led her to attempt suicide sometime in late 1857 or early 1858.[77]

Thinking back over his daughter's mental decline, Benjamin Franklin Butler was inclined to attribute it to overwork. "I now see that she was entirely overtaxed," he wrote to Kirkbride in

1858. Yet, from a modern perspective, it seems just as likely that Eliza's unhappiness, along with the host of nervous diseases suffered by nineteenth-century middle-class women, resulted from too little rather than too much challenging work. A well-educated young woman, condemned to years of household drudgery on behalf of an aging parent rather than her own family, certainly had legitimate cause for despair.[78]

On January 13, 1858, Eliza Ogden Butler became a patient at the Pennsylvania Hospital for the Insane. The course of her illness can be only sketchily reconstructed. The hospital medical register listed Eliza Butler's disorder as melancholia of two months' duration, caused by "impaired health and mental anxiety." From her father's correspondence, it seems apparent that an attempted suicide had prompted her commitment. Eliza's case records no longer exist, but Butler's letters to Kirkbride supply some information concerning her hospital stay. Upon admission, Kirkbride had her placed under special watch and attempted to overcome her reluctance to eat. "Untiring vigilance and a decided, though kindly control," in Butler's words, brought about some improvement by March; he thought that Eliza looked better but was "yet the victim of the great delusion," presumably the necessity of destroying herself. Like most new patients, she hated the asylum at first and wrote to her father begging him to secure her release; when he refused, she stopped writing to him for a time. But by the spring, Eliza professed a willingness to stay, although never abandoning her "first preference for 'home.'" Despite her improvement, Butler feared that his daughter wanted to get home only so that she might try to kill herself again. She must have considered suicide again, for in May her father referred to a "very recent" incident that showed her "yet considerably under the influence of the terrible monomania by which she has been possessed the last five months." Butler also expressed distress over her lack of affection for himself and the rest of her family.[79]

In the meantime, Kirkbride began to have some success in his conversations with Eliza. The superintendent felt a special interest in her case, not only because Benjamin Franklin Butler was a prominent man but also because he was a friend of Kirkbride's sister-in-law and her husband, Hannah and Stacy Collins of New York City. Moreover, Eliza had a relatively mild and tractable form of insanity. For her part, Eliza found herself much affected by Kirkbride's influence. Years later, in a letter to Dorothea Dix, she recalled his habit of "sitting down by the patients and talking to them in the calm way, which I know from my personal experience, carries help and light to helpless, clouded minds." Besides, she wrote on another occasion, "How could anyone resist craving the sympathy of those tender eyes?" Having won Eliza's trust, Kirkbride extracted a promise from her that she would not harm herself, and she began to improve more rapidly. By June, the assistant physician, Edward Smith, could congratulate Kirkbride on "Miss Butler's progress in your confidence."[80]

Kirkbride's confidence worked so effectively with Eliza Butler that by August, barely seven months after her admission, she seemed ready for a trial at home. On the 24th of that month, Benjamin Franklin Butler arrived at the hospital to take his daughter back to New York. Butler thanked the physician for his "many special endeavors to promote the happiness and consequently, the entire restoration of my dear daughter." A few days after her release, he reported that Eliza seemed to continue in good health; she took long walks, slept more soundly, and had a return of her menses. "Insensibly to herself, probably, she begins to use terms of endearment towards her family." Other signs of improvement included attendance at family worship and the absence of any disposition to avoid her old acquaintances. Her sister Lydia reported that when alone with her, Eliza had shown some "impatience, and spoken morbidly of her condition," but generally she seemed quite well.[81]

In September 1858, Butler took his two youngest daughters on a European tour to seal Eliza's return to health. After a few weeks of traveling, Butler himself began to succumb to Bright's disease, a kidney disorder from which he had suffered for several years. Attended by his daughters and several family friends, Benjamin Franklin Butler died in Paris on November 8. In the following days, Eliza showed herself to be truly cured by her calm, rational response to her father's unexpected demise. An observer described her as a "stouthearted, glorious minded woman" who "controlled herself like a heroine." Eliza wrote her sister a long account of Butler's death, describing it as a supremely religious, "heavenly" experience. As for Lydia and herself, Eliza concluded, "it is very strange to feel ourselves alone; to decide for ourselves and on our own responsibility what it is right and best for us to do."[82]

After her father's death, Eliza returned to New York, to an existence not unlike the one she had known before her hospitalization. At first, she and Lydia kept house and pursued the usual round of religious and cultural activities. Sometime in 1861, Eliza took charge of her sister Margaret's large family. In November of that year, Margaret Butler Crosby, fifteen years Eliza's senior, had been admitted to the Pennsylvania Hospital for the Insane for "melancholia due to ill health." Unlike Eliza, Margaret made a slow recovery, remaining at the Pennsylvania Hospital and then at the Bloomingdale hospital for several years. While her sister was in the asylum, Eliza devoted her energies to caring for Margaret's large family.[83]

Once again finding herself in a demanding but ultimately unfulfilling family situation, Eliza Butler continually had to resist her "evil tendencies," as she thought of them, toward mental disease. The prayers for heavenly assistance transcribed in her devotional diary frequently mentioned the psychological problems she faced. On a good day, Eliza could thank God that "I have been kept almost entirely from my enemy (speaking crossly or being in a nervous state of irritability)." When her enemy possessed her, Eliza felt a deep sense of sinfulness; she wrote on one occasion, "I have again to repent a wicked nervousness...I must strive, God helping me, to restrain my evil temper." In discussing her mental state, Eliza invariably employed moral or religious language. Her sins were "fits of ill temper," crossness, and disrespectful comments. She felt that her inability to control these sins represented a willful turning away from God; since she knew the correct way to act, only her sinful nature kept her from right behavior. Eliza's equation of her mental distress with sin comes across clearly in the entry for November 6, 1863. "Again I must take up an old confession of old sin...This evening as we were walking up to Teachers Meeting, I gave myself up to a fit of hysterics...And I did this notwithstanding all the answers to my prayers, notwithstanding all thy Mercy oh Lord." When Eliza managed to control her evil tendencies, she still felt far from comfortable. Her sister Margaret's prolonged illness could have added little to her confidence. In addition, the same scrupulous religious sense that made her mental sins seem so enormous also acted to limit her sense of self-worth. Echoing her mother's concern about philistines, Eliza prayed to be kept "from forgetfulness of my past Insanity and recovery, from selfishness and self-seeking." Her achievements had to be balanced by remembrance of her former sins, especially her insanity. "Keep me from being puffed up and thinking too highly of myself," she concluded a prayer.[84]

Eliza Butler's diaries for the early 1860s suggest the mental dilemmas of a young woman leading a life little to her liking. Unable to forget her past insanity, yet seemingly powerless to resolve her personal dilemmas, Eliza envied her married sisters with their families but hardly expected to emulate their domestic state. An episode of mental illness, however favorably terminated, no doubt made her hopes of marriage quite remote. Besides, Eliza felt herself to have few graces with the opposite sex; thus, she seemed destined for the life of a spinster aunt caring for other people's families rather than her own. Fighting desperately to accept this reality without slipping back into insanity, Eliza prayed for resignation: "Keep me from wanting to have God's will otherwise concerning my lot in life," she wrote in 1863. "I pray that I may learn how to grow old, not to feel painfully that I am growing old, but to feel about it just as I ought to."[85]

As it happened, Eliza Butler's lot in life turned out to be quite unlike her anticipations. In September 1862, Ann West Kirkbride died at the age of forty-nine after a long, debilitating illness. Since the 1840s, she had been invalided by a "protracted and serious disease," most likely tuberculosis. After the birth of a daughter in 1840 and a son in 1842, Ann Kirkbride had borne no more children. Her illness eventually curtailed her ability to travel and even work about her own house. "Although greatly afflicted for many years," Kirkbride wrote of Ann, she had "so many admirable traits of character, and bore all her sorrows, with such perfect Christian resignation, that her whole life has been a living sermon to all around her." Ann's death left an emotional void in Kirkbride's life, which he eventually determined to fill. As Eliza observed of him years later, "neither sons nor daughters can count with the men who are lost without a nearer companionship."[86]

Kirkbride had kept in more or less constant contact with Eliza Butler after her discharge in 1858. While at the Pennsylvania Hospital for the Insane, Eliza had become friends with Kirkbride's daughter Annie, and after Eliza's departure, the girls continued to exchange visits. Eliza wrote occasionally to her former doctor and visited the hospital periodically. When in New York City, Kirkbride usually paid a call at the Butler house. Margaret Crosby's illness fostered the exchange of messages and visits. Sometime in 1860, Kirkbride enlisted Eliza's help on an asylum-related project. "Before there was the least thought of my being his wife," as Eliza explained to her sister-in-law years later, "Dr. Kirkbride asked me to look up 'the promises' in the Bible, as he wanted to have them printed for use of his patients, who were only too apt to pick out the most inappropriate passages for their peace of mind." The resulting volume, entitled *Comforting Promises*, appeared in 1861 in "quite a large edition," as Eliza recalled. An entry in her diary for October 1863 indicates that her feeling for Kirkbride had already deepened beyond mere admiration. His visit left her "full of old foolish fancies," she noted, and launched into a furiously penitent prayer: "free me from folly, make me pure and holy, forgive my sins and make me very penitent." For days after this entry, Eliza's diary referred to an ongoing battle against the "temptation of weak, wicked thoughts."[87]

Eliza Butler stopped keeping her diary early in 1864, and so left unrecorded the courtship that eventually led to her union with the object of her "foolish fancies." Thomas Story Kirkbride and Eliza Odgen Butler were married in New York at the Mercer Avenue Presbyterian Church on May 17, 1866. Kirkbride's union with a woman twenty-seven years his junior, and a former patient as well, must have provoked some comment among his professional acquaintances, yet their correspondence (at least that preserved) made few references to Kirkbride's remarriage. Writing to Pliny Earle in 1872, Isaac Ray referred in passing to his friend's new family, describing Kirkbride as "very happy both in his professional duties and his domestic joys." In their letters to Kirkbride, his close friends always mentioned Eliza in a cordial fashion. But it is difficult to believe that the brethren did not remark further on the unusual circumstances of Kirkbride's remarriage, given the interest they showed in a similar union undertaken by another superintendent, William H. Prince. "Did you know," wrote D. T. Brown to Kirkbride in 1861, that "Prince of Northhampton has married one of his patients, causing great surprise in the village and intense horror among its marriageable ladies?" Several years later, Brown wrote to Pliny Earle in a more somber tone that Prince's wife had had a relapse and been taken to the Hartford Retreat. As their letters make obvious, the superintendents generally kept up on the details of one another's personal lives, so the fact of Dr. Kirkbride's having married a former patient cannot have escaped public notice. A passing reference to Eliza Butler's case by a man far removed from Kirkbride's personal circle of friends confirms this supposition. In a letter to Pliny Earle, Charles Folsom, a Massachusetts physician active in the State Board of Charities, recommended as a mental hygiene measure "what seems sensible to me, judicious marriages among those predisposed to mental disease – in fact among those who have been 'cured' of one attack – a principle which Dr. Kirkbride advocates and has put in practice in his own case."[88]

In all likelihood, Kirkbride's associates regarded Eliza Butler Kirkbride's past history not as a source of embarrassment but rather as a testimonial to asylum treatment. Certainly, Eliza saw herself in this light, as her correspondence with Dorothea Dix reveals. She once told Dix that she was "able in her own experience to measure what hospital treatment has already done for the Insane." Eliza's example did indeed bear eloquent witness to the productive lives that cured patients could live, if allowed to return to society without permanent stigma. By all accounts, her marriage to Thomas Story Kirkbride was an extremely happy one. Between 1867 and 1874, Eliza bore two sons and two daughters, all of whom went on to have distinguished careers of their own. During Kirkbride's lifetime, Eliza took an active role in asylum work, running a Bible class for the women patients and holding small social gatherings for their benefit. Throughout the controversies that plagued the specialty in her husband's last years, Eliza remained a staunch advocate of asylum medicine. Her memorial to him, published in the hospital's 1883 *Report*, provided not only a moving tribute to Kirkbride but also a resounding defense of the whole concept of moral treatment. After Kirkbride's death, Eliza turned to other areas of reform and remained active in Philadelphia philanthropy, especially the support of public education, until her death in 1919.[89]

Possibly one of the greatest achievements of nineteenth-century asylum medicine was its creation of an institutional process by which individuals such as Eliza Odgen Butler could recover from a mental disturbance and return to a reasonably normal life. Although prejudice against the formerly insane still remained, hospital treatment undoubtedly facilitated their acceptance back into society. Rather than become a permanent member of a deviant population, the insane patient might choose to accept the sick role and be cured. The lives of patients such as Eliza Butler who made this choice lent impressive weight to the basic premises of moral treatment. As Kirkbride argued in his 1842 *Report*, insanity was a terrible affliction in large part because society reacted to it with such horror: "More than half of these horrors will be destroyed, and the chances of recovery increased," he wrote, "whenever the whole community can look upon the insane as upon other sick, suffering under a disease...and can believe that when restored, an individual who has been thus afflicted, is as worthy of confidence and respect, and as capable of resuming his position in the world, as though he had recovered from a fever or other affection, in which the manifestations of his mind had been temporarily deranged." At best, then, the concept of insanity as a curable disease provided a new method for reclaiming those who suffered a temporary mental disturbance.[90]

The fact that only half of Kirkbride's patients ever recovered and resumed their positions in the world did not necessarily diminish the perception of medicine's success in treating insanity. Critics could argue, as many did, that the mental hospital did not cure *enough* patients, but they could not deny that it appeared to benefit some. The testimony of recovered patients such as Eliza Butler, who believed themselves healed by Kirkbride, offered convincing proof of medicine's power over insanity. For even a few to be helped by treatment, and thereby overcome a terrifying condition, remained an impressive achievement, especially to the individuals involved. The gratitude patrons and patients felt toward Kirkbride and his hospital formed a constant source of support for moral treatment, support that could withstand the most determined assault upon asylum medicine.

The noncompliant patient

But to present a truly complete picture of asylum treatment, this favorable testimony of cured patients and their families must be set alongside the experience of those who never accepted Kirkbride's persuasion: the inmates who refused or were unable to accept the physician's authority, adopt the sick role, and recover. The sizable pockets of indifference and resistance these patients formed within the institution shaped Kirkbride's medical practice as much as did his relations with the more compliant. The dissatisfied patients' perceptions of asylum care too frequently contradicted the superintendent's therapeutic vision of the asylum to be ignored. When magnified by legal action, patient complaints led to public controversies that plagued Kirkbride during the last two decades of his career.

Forms of patient resistance

At the most elemental level, the asylum's chronic patients provided mute testimony against moral treatment's effectiveness simply by remaining insane. Whether they intended it or not, their presence on the wards mocked Kirkbride's therapeutic persuasion. Over the years, that presence became more and more noticeable as chronic patients gradually accumulated on the wards. In part, the rising population of chronic patients reflected certain changes in Kirkbride's administrative policies. After completing the Male Department in 1859, Kirkbride found that he had overestimated the need for additional hospital accommodations and had trouble filling its beds. To utilize it more fully, he evidently accepted more chronic patients, for from 1860 to 1870, there was a dramatic increase in the proportion of dementia patients admitted, from 13 to 24 percent. In comparison, the female dementia admissions remained at 9 percent. Above and beyond this policy change, the proportion of chronic patients naturally tended to grow because these individuals stayed for such long periods of time (see Table A.8).

Chronic patients not only failed to respond to treatment; they also tended to be troublesome patients who expressed their dislike of the hospital in destructive and disruptive ways. Although Kirkbride vehemently denied the existence of "hospital-made" patients, as critics termed individuals made insane by institutionalization itself, it seems evident that some patients used their symptoms to express hostility toward both the doctor and the hospital. Their disruptive behavior may not have been originally provoked by the hospital; clearly, many patients had been noisy or destructive long before commitment. Still, once they were confined in the asylum, the continuation of those behaviors did not occur solely as a response to inner compulsions having no relation to the hospital experience. Whether acting consciously or unconsciously to resist treatment, troublesome patients posed an unavoidable and significant problem in Kirkbride's asylum practice. Their noncompliant behavior served as an ever-present reminder to the physician, as well as the other patients, that his authority was indeed limited.[91]

Refusing to eat represented one of the most frequent means used by patients, particularly women, to express their hostility toward the hospital. From the patient's perspective, self-starvation served two purposes. First, this behavior attracted constant attention from the staff and caused the doctor "a vast deal of trouble and uneasiness," as Kirkbride put it. Forced feeding was an unpleasant, dangerous procedure that at best barely kept the patient alive; in a weakened condition, the undernourished easily succumbed to other diseases. Thus, the refusal to eat placed Kirkbride in the painful position of watching a patient slowly starve to death without being able to prevent it. In addition, the tactic had a dramatic effect on the patient's family. New inmates who wanted desperately to leave the hospital often refused to eat as a ploy to get relatives to remove them. Only when a disgruntled newcomer finally gave up the "determination to try and get home by starving," as William Moon once described it, could the doctors relax. Self-starvation also served to punish relatives for leaving the patient in the hospital. Moon noted in one case that a woman had to be force-fed for a week after her husband reneged on a promise to take her home.[92]

The destruction of hospital property was another frequent outlet for patient dissatisfaction. In the chronic and excited wards, furniture and glass breaking, shredding of clothes or bedding, and "filthy habits" such as masturbation, incontinence, and feces smearing were all common. In some cases, the patients who went on destructive rampages expressly related their misbehavior to anger at a hospital officer or policy. A woman patient, for example, explained that a glass-breaking spree had been prompted by the attendants' "ridicule" of her. Even when inmates gave no explanation for their actions, Kirkbride seemed to perceive their destructiveness as a deliberate attempt to annoy him. His characterization of patients who repeatedly dirtied themselves or destroyed their clothes as "troublesome," "careless in their habits," or "lost to all sense of shame" attributed a conscious defiance to their actions. The superintendent's annoyance came across clearly in an account of an "extremely troublesome" male patient, who waited purposely to have his bowel movements at night and then used "every means in his power to daub his room in nearly every part," in spite of the staff's efforts to prevent him.[93]

Self-mutilation, like self-starvation, figured among the most troublesome inmate behaviors, having very serious consequences for both the patients and their families, yet proving difficult to prevent. In one case, Kirkbride noted that a young man's "fixed and determined" desire to injure himself necessitated "incessant watching." While in the asylum, the young man was observed "day and night, and no other patients in the house gave so much anxiety or required such an amount of vigilance," he wrote. Despite these efforts, the man succeeded in a mutilation that understandably horrified his family and put Kirkbride in a very difficult position. The superintendent apologetically wrote to the family's doctor, "you may assure Mr. B's father, the utmost vigilance was used and the manner in which he effected the removal of his testicle is one of the most surprising things of the kind I ever knew."[94]

Although Kirkbride regarded certain patients as deliberately aggravating, he forgave their misbehavior as long as they appeared sufficiently unable to control it or unconscious of its effect. Much more vexing were cases in which insanity seemed to border on simple and deliberate "wickedness." One such patient, a merchant's widow, spent nine months in the hospital, continually "profane, obscene and lost to shame" as well as abusive to all about her. Kirkbride wrote, "she has been excessively noisy, profane and indecent in her language and habits, has been guilty of the most filthy acts to annoy those about her and has had the deepest hostility to all who have the direction of the institution." Even the attendants recognized – and resented – the deliberate quality of the woman's defiant misbehavior. Kirkbride observed, "With all her noise, *etc.* she declares it is not insanity but *simple passion* and her disease is one of that moral kind in which it is exceedingly difficult for me to convince the attendants that she does not judge correctly about her case." Undoubtedly, the attendants' willingness to tolerate abusive individuals depended in part on their conviction that the patients were indeed insane and thus not responsible for their actions.[95]

Some patients opted for a less equivocal rejection of hospital

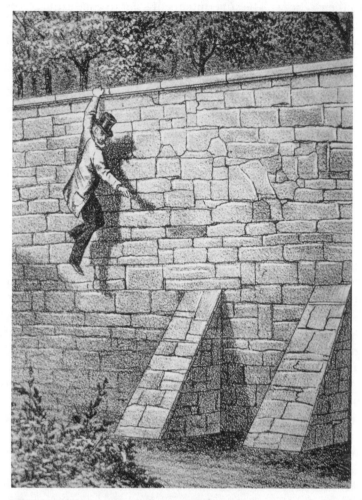

Figure 8. "Ebenezer Haskell escaping from the Pennsylvania Hospital for the Insane...Sept. 9th, 1868." Illustration from Ebenezer Haskell, *The Trial of Ebenezer Haskell* (Philadelphia, 1869), between pp. 8 and 9. Haskell broke his leg in this fall.

treatment: escape. "Elopements," as the staff referred to them, often involved great ingenuity on the patients' part; they loosened iron bars, crawled through culverts, made ropes out of torn sheets, and scaled tall fences in their quest for freedom (see Figure 8). Besides allowing them to remove themselves from an unpleasant environment, escape provided patients the added satisfaction of causing great disturbance in the asylum. A search party had to be formed to try to catch the patient while he or she was still in the neighborhood; anxious letters had to be dispatched to warn relatives that they might soon have an unexpected, perhaps unwanted visitor; and the staff behavior had to be examined to account for the breach of discipline. So all in all, elopements were a gratifying way for a patient to pay his "respects" to his "jailers," as one expressed it. This man, who escaped after ingeniously cutting away his door lock, left a message chalked on his mirror: "Patient Skill vs. Mercenary Stupidity."[96]

Surprisingly, many male patients escaped from the asylum only to return after a brief absence. A ward journal for the Male Department often included entries such as this one: "Frank B. gets over the wall, comes home drunk, runs away again, and goes home." On another occasion, two patients escaped together and "started on a spree"; one ended up at the stationhouse, and the other came back "gloriously drunk." For some patients, eloping served only as a short-term release during which they eluded supervision and tasted forbidden pleasures (chiefly liquor), with every intention of returning to the asylum's security. Thus, escape did not necessarily involve a wholehearted rejection of the hospital. Kirkbride received a letter from one patron whose son had escaped, explaining that the boy had been "very well pleased with his treatment" and that he was "very sorry" he had gone. The "instant he was over the wall, he would not have left could he have gotten back without going through the gate." The frequency of such incidents suggests that the nineteenth-century mental hospital did not provide the complete isolation or confinement of its inmates that it promised both the patrons and the general public. However stringent the institution's rules, the boundary between the hospital and the community could not be made impermeable.[97]

For the patient determined to defy the hospital's authorities, physical violence was another dramatic form of resistance. As letters, case records, and ward journals make evident, inmate attacks on doctors, attendants, and other patients were a commonplace aspect of ward life. Although comparatively more frequent and severe among the men, attacks occurred on the women's wards as well. Ordinarily, the fighting involved little more than a scuffle, in which some incident of communal life prompted an unpremeditated bout of punching, kicking, or biting. Since patients suspected of violent tendencies had limited access to items that might be used as weapons, ordinarily they could do only limited damage and were subdued quickly. But asylum violence sometimes assumed more threatening dimensions, especially when more than one inmate became involved. In a journal kept during his first year of asylum practice, Kirkbride tersely described a "very unpleasant scene" in a male ward that suggests the explosive potential of patient violence. During the superintendent's morning visit to the ward, a patient named Mr. T. became very excited and raised a chair to strike Kirkbride. As the ward attendants hastened to secure him, another patient named Jasper tried to interfere. "Upon my requesting him to desist," Kirkbride wrote, Jasper hit him in the face, and then attacked the assistant physician and attendants. Had not staff members from an adjacent ward heard the noise and come to assist them, Kirkbride remarked, "we should have been very unpleasantly situated." Jasper, the superintendent concluded, had "shown himself one of the most treacherous men in the house," and claimed that he could not think of three other inmates who would have acted in the same malevolent fashion.[98]

Kirkbride correctly understood that the treacherous patient who was rational enough to plot deliberate violence, but too diseased to realize the immorality of his actions, represented a grave threat to the asylum order. In contrast, unpremeditated outbursts of an excited inmate could be easily handled by the rational deployment of hospital resources. Collective violence, however frightening in theory, posed no real threat; as Kirkbride well knew, the insane, unlike prisoners or slaves, could not cooperate with each other long enough to foment an organized rebellion against the hospital authorities. But the planned violence of an individual such as Jasper could not be so easily guarded against; the most violent experience of Kirkbride's career was a premeditated assault by just such a "treacherous" former patient.

Patient profile: Wiley Williams

In February 1848, Kirkbride admitted a twenty-two-year-old Georgian named Wiley Williams, who was diagnosed as a monomaniac. In a letter to the superintendent, Wiley's brother described him as an eccentric individual whose peculiarities had lately taken a sinister turn. The family had been unwilling to think him insane, however, until the previous summer, when the youth had become unable to care for himself and "unconscious of all." Wiley had recovered somewhat since then, but the family still thought him "not safe at times to their persons and property."[99]

From his first day at the Pennsylvania Hospital for the Insane, Wiley Williams proved to be an uncooperative patient. Although calm most of the time, he evinced a "bad feeling" toward Kirkbride and refused to speak to him. He had his ward assignment demoted "for making a noise." Because the youth constantly expressed his desire to leave the asylum, Kirkbride kept a "strict watch" on him. Nonetheless, Wiley managed to escape, only to have his relatives return him to Philadelphia. Then in November 1848, Wiley escaped again, using a clever ruse: He arranged a roll of his clothing, complete with a night cap, to look like his body in the bed, hid in the water closet, and escaped as soon as the watchman made his round. This time his family decided not to return Wiley to the hospital, so as to "see if he can take care of himself and conduct with the propriety of a man in his senses."[100]

Although he had regained his freedom, Wiley Williams did not forget his grievances against Kirkbride and the Pennsylvania Hospital. In April 1849, almost six months after his successful escape, Wiley wrote a letter to Kirkbride, threatening to kill the superintendent before the year was out. He wanted his revenge, so Wiley wrote, because Kirkbride had mistreated him. "I remember how closely I was watched, whilst to others many liberties were given," he complained; other patients came and went, but he, Wiley, had to remain. In this manner, the doctor had "robbed me of friends, money, happiness itself, all in pay for which I will rob thee of life." Describing himself as Kirkbride's "judge and executioner," Wiley concluded, "thy death warrant is sealed."[101]

Upon receiving Wiley's letter, Kirkbride showed it to a few friends at the hospital, and soon forgot about it. Then in October 1849, while walking from his home to the hospital at 7:30 in the morning, the superintendent met his young son Joseph, who informed him that someone was up in a nearby tree. Assuming the tree climber to be a patient, Kirkbride sent the boy to get the gatekeeper and went over to see who it was. As soon as the man in the tree spoke, the doctor realized that Wiley Williams had returned and probably meant to shoot him; he turned to run away, whereupon Wiley shot him in the back of the head. Kirkbride's hat evidently deflected the shot, for the ball penetrated only the scalp and scraped along the skull. The gatekeeper soon appeared and captured Wiley, who was taken off to jail. Kirkbride's wound proved not to be serious; after spending two weeks in bed, he returned to work without feeling any lasting ill effects from the injury. In December 1849, Wiley stood trial for assault and battery with intent to kill and received a life sentence. He spent the remainder of his life at the Eastern State Penitentiary, classified as an "insane criminal."[102]

At the trial, Wiley claimed that he had shot Kirkbride to "get him out of the way." In recounting his motivation, he seemed particularly aggrieved that the superintendent had been so "slow" in deciding whether or not he was insane. But in 1850, Wiley wrote to Kirkbride from prison, saying that he had never meant to murder him at all. According to Wiley, the gun had been purposely loaded with small shot and fired over the doctor's head; the young man professed himself "very mortified when I heard that even one shot had took effect." Referring to himself as one of Kirkbride's "warmest friends," Wiley concluded, "I have ever cherished the most kindly feelings from the time I became acquainted with you."[103]

Notwithstanding these kindly sentiments, Kirkbride clearly believed, at least for an instant, that he would die at the hands of his former patient. As he later wrote to Wiley's family, "under all the circumstances my escape was certainly a surprising one, and one which no one situated as I was at the time could reasonably expect." Yet Kirkbride expressed no malice toward his assailant. "I can assure you in all sincerity," he wrote to Wiley's father, "that I should be as glad as ever to do anything that could be of service to him." Kirkbride expressed no desire for vengeance at the trial, but rather stated his belief that Williams was insane and therefore not responsible for his violent act. In later life, Kirkbride made no public references to the incident, although it was clearly spoken of in the family; his son Franklin Butler, born in 1867, recalled the "thrill" he had as a child in being allowed to feel the bullet that still remained under his father's scalp. Despite Kirkbride's silence on the subject, one cannot help but speculate that this incident affected certain of his professional views, such as his conviction that the nonrestraint system could not be instituted in American asylums. Perhaps it even affected his decision to let another doctor have immediate charge of the male patients after the new hospital opened. At the very least, this violent experience gave Thomas Story Kirkbride a sobering view of the dangers involved in asylum work.[104]

Patient complaints

On a day-to-day basis, Kirkbride found his asylum practice profoundly affected by a gentler, less dramatic form of patient resistance: the act of complaining itself. Violence produced an immediate reaction, yet inevitably discredited the perpetrator and turned the victim into a martyr. In contrast, a well-formulated reproach brought attention to the inmate's grievances at the same time that it discomfited the doctor. When addressed to the guilt-stricken relatives responsible for the commitment, patient complaints prompted speedy inquiries and expressions of concern. Realizing the advantages of this form of resistance, Kirkbride's disgruntled charges sought redress by complaining constantly. Their accusations are especially useful to the historian, insomuch as such complaints give voice to the noncompliant patients' perception of the asylum – suggesting the emotions that may have motivated less articulate or more disabled inmates to tear their clothes or daub their rooms with feces.

The disgruntled patients' attitude toward asylum treatment, like the perceptions of their more satisfied peers, can be documented from their numerous letters to the superintendent. In addition to such firsthand accounts, the patients' families frequently relayed their relatives' complaints about the institution. Unfortunately, the actual circumstances referred to in many cases are almost impossible to document. In particular, patients detailed incidents of neglect and abuse that simply cannot be verified from available records. Kirkbride dismissed most of the accusations he received, portraying the inmates' unfavorable perceptions of asylum life as the products of disordered minds. Yet, he cannot be regarded as an impartial observer, since he had an obvious interest in denying hostile accounts. The letters themselves suggest varying degrees of reliability. When a patient's note expressed an undying hatred for Kirkbride, it stands as a straightforward expression of feeling; one is not inclined to doubt that the individual felt that dislike at least at the time of writing the message. But when a patient claimed to be confined in "mittens covered with sharp iron spikes," as one lady did, the statement seems more suspect. The hospital officers did indeed use mittens as a restraining device, but none conforming to such a description; one is inclined to believe that the patient endowed the plain canvas mittens with spikes of her own imagining. Obviously, many individuals ended up in the asylum precisely because their perceptions of reality were disordered. Thus, it is impossible to endow their statements with any more credibility than those of the hospital authorities. Still, patient complaints deserve careful consideration, for even the most blatant delusions reveal the features of hospital care that the inmates disliked most. By highlighting the therapeutic claims that the patients found hardest to accept, complaints draw attention to the weakest aspects of Kirkbride's asylum regimen.[105]

The most frequent complaints lodged by the patients concerned the attendants, whom they repeatedly accused of being insensitive, "bullying," and violent. In a typical letter, a patron relayed an escaped patient's observation on asylum life: "he speaks very highly of your institution, and seems grateful for your attention, but complains very much of [a] certain...attendant M., who he says used unnecessary violence, choked him and then confined him in a room where he had to sleep on the floor, without bed or bedstead." The young man in question apparently accepted the attendant's violence as a given, for he expressed himself "quite willing to return" if only he did not have to sleep on the floor again, making no mention of the abusive Mr. M. A patient writing directly to Kirkbride adopted a more indignant tone: "I have been most shamefully abused by the attendant William," who he claimed "threw me on the floor and jumped on my breast with both knees." Other patients felt strongly about ridicule or rebuke from the attendants. A woman explained to the assistant physician that she had been driven to a destructive rampage "because the attendants had laughed at her." Their ridicule, the doctor concluded, had hurt her far more than all the other "indignities" she felt she had to suffer. In a more genteel fashion, a young lady "seemed to be suffering intensely," her mother reported, because the wing supervisor had intimated that the girl lied about some ward matter. Not surprisingly, patients resented the staff's intrusive surveillance of their activities. A woman refused to have a private attendant, "as she had the idea that the attendant was a spy upon her." Not a few inmates believed that the attendants used their free access to the patients' quarters to steal money and clothing.[106]

Next to their attendants, patients had the fewest kind words to say about their wardmates. Belying Kirkbride's contentions about the benefits of patient friendships, they complained bitterly "of being surrounded by crazy people," as one woman wrote. More specifically, they disliked noisy, aggravating ward companions. A patron wrote of his relative's situation, "He is compelled during his whole time *whether sick or well* to stay confined to a ward wherein both from his own statements and my personal observations there is more than one obstreperous patient, whose continued noises very seriously affect him." Another distressed relative reported a man's complaint "of being greatly annoyed by the inmates near his rooms, who were constantly using profane language." Outbursts of violence had an even more upsetting effect. After an excited wardmate broke a woman patient's cup and saucer at dinner, she felt considerable agitation: "these things excite her very much and make her nervous and uncomfortable," her daughter reported. The more timid individuals quickly grew frightened of other patients. As a young girl told her aunt, "I am afraid of every inmate I meet and shudder with horror when I come in contact with them." Some desperately troubled patients found the companionship of other "unhappy and miserable" souls intolerable. "I ought not to be with such people," insisted one woman. "It affects me very much. You cannot begin to know the amount of harm being among such people as are here has done me."[107]

Not only did some patients resent their ward companions, they also found the hospital environment itself far from homelike. Their letters home complained about every aspect of institutional existence, from the quality of the food to the lack of privacy. A girl trying to get her mother to bring her home described the hospital as "icy cold, not a particle of fire or heat" in it, and claimed that she had gotten a bad cold as a result. Lack of privacy was another common grievance. Patients complained that their wardmates and attendants wore their clothes and read their mail. One patron reported that his brother "has discontinued using his toothbrush, having taken up the opinion that some of the inmates of the hospital make use of it." Although in some cases they involved only imaginary invasions of privacy, such frequently voiced suspicions suggest a strongly felt aversion to collective living.[108]

For all of Kirkbride's efforts to provide entertainment, the carefully structured hospital regimen left many patients bored. Men in particular voiced a dislike for the passive "invalid" life they were forced to lead in the asylum. Even the size of the building itself militated against the asylum's appeal; the very features that Kirkbride hoped would inspire patients' confidence became intimidating to them. "How shall I get up those steps again and pass thru those long entries," worried a despondent young woman. Another patient who escaped from the Pennsylvania Hospital for the Insane and took up residence at the Friends Asylum wrote to Kirkbride, "We have a much smaller establishment here for which reason it seems more like home."[109]

The amenities allowed wealthy residents in the asylum sometimes exacerbated the resentment patients felt toward their institutional surroundings. Some patients and patrons interpreted the superintendents' argument that the rich had the right to purchase luxury in the asylum to mean that the poorer charges would be slighted. The fear of being treated like a charity case emerged in numerous letters. One old gentleman refused to have his weekly board lowered from $8 to $5 because he did not want "to be looked upon as a pauper and maintained accordingly." A woman patient feared that her attendant knew her to be "under the care of the county" and neglected her as a result. Special signs of favor from Kirkbride brewed discontent among the inmates. Several patients complained, for example, that they had never been asked to dine at the family table in the superintendent's home, a privilege they assumed the lucky ones had purchased. Resentments over special privileges at times united a whole ward. After an oil painting was hung in the Second Ward of the Woman's Division, Kirkbride reported to the managers that the ladies in the First Ward felt that some "favoritism" had been at work, and urged the managers to buy another painting as soon as possible.[110]

The discontented patients' resistance to asylum life often included a marked hostility to the chief physician. Many patients distrusted Kirkbride because he so openly sided with their relatives over questions of treatment. As one young man put it, the superintendent was his relatives' "cat's paw," always working against his, the patient's, best interest. A former inmate who felt some affection for Kirkbride still expressed a common reservation: "I must say, a great deal more weight was given, by you particularly, to statements made by real and professed friends (some of whom were bitter and astute enemies) than your own observation of the actual condition I was in justified." Kirkbride's well-wisher concluded by cautioning his former doctor, "it is well not to rely too entirely on the statements of others although made in due form." As subsequent court cases would show, this man pointed to a fundamental flaw in Kirkbride's relationship with his patients. What patrons and admirers praised as the doctor's diplomacy, disgruntled patients often perceived as deceit. When the superintendent appeared to be sympathetic but failed to accede to some heartfelt request, patients were left all the more outraged. As a male patient wrote, Kirkbride's reluctance to release him had been all the more painful because "having gained my friendship, you play upon my feelings almost as you please, under the restraint of unyielding rules."[11]

To the extent that some patients found it hard to trust Kirkbride, they also found it difficult to share his therapeutic vision of the hospital. Not understanding or accepting the basic premises of medical treatment – that insanity was a disease best cured in a hospital, and that they themselves were insane – patients could not help but comprehend commitment as a form of punishment. Repeatedly, inmates referred to the asylum as a prison rather than a hospital. Some, believing themselves to be terrible "sinners" or "criminals," viewed their imprisonment as justified. One such patient comprehended his commitment in these terms: "his friends was [sic] tired of him and wanted to get him out of the way and did not like to kill him themselves, so they took him to the hospital to get the doctors to do it." Accepting this sentence, the man simply spent his days at the asylum waiting to be hung, the style of execution he believed the doctors to prefer. Other patients accepted their fate far less passively, insisting that they had been wrongly confined by malicious relatives. Vigorously protesting their imprisonment, they spoke as one woman did: "I say with Patrick Henry, 'Give me liberty or give me death!' " Inmates of this persuasion wrote indignant letters, harassed the staff, and eventually hired lawyers to contest their commitment. One of the assistant physicians described a resourceful fellow who lay in wait for visitors to the ward; when they appeared, "he would harangue them in what he meant for an oratorical style, about the great injury and wrong done him in locking him up in an asylum."

Underlying both the resigned and defiant stances was the same lack of agreement with the hospital's therapeutic purpose; without sharing its assumptions, patients could only regard the institution with fear or indignation.[112]

The most articulate of the defiant patients described asylum treatment in terms quite unlike those employed by Eliza Butler Kirkbride. In their tirades against the "Quaker inquisition and French Bastille," as one patient termed the hospital, one can in fact behold a mirror image, an inverted reflection of the persuasive institution Kirkbride claimed to oversee. An angry letter from a former patient named William eloquently expressed the defiant inmates' countervision of the asylum. William had been compelled to write, he explained to Kirkbride, because in a letter to his parents, the doctor had expressed confidence that his former patient felt no ill will toward the hospital or its head. So strongly did William take issue with this statement that he felt he had to disabuse Kirkbride of his comfortable assumptions. "I have not a very high opinion of your medical skill [or] your regard for principle or home," began William. He had no doubt that a properly run hospital might aid the insane; but as Kirkbride conducted the asylum, it did not heal the sick, but rather "robbed [them] of their rights – to the detriment of their health, reputation and fortunes." By "neglect and temporizing treatment," William claimed, "you take more reason from your patients than you give." The physician's only motivation in running the hospital had to be profit, for he showed no concern for its inmates. Until he himself had been in the asylum, William concluded, he would never have believed that "so hateful a system of oppression" could exist in America. With Kirkbride at its head, the Pennsylvania Hospital for the Insane, "which we were led to believe was the pride and glory of our state, . . . is used for no other purpose than as a vast charnel house to bury souls in."[113]

Although only a few patients expressed this kind of rage, many sought aggressively to redress their grievances against Kirkbride and his hospital. Despite the obvious disadvantages the insane faced in confronting the asylum authorities, they persisted resourcefully in their efforts to be heard. Consequently, in the course of an average working day, Kirkbride had to respond to a wide range of inmate protests. Even what little record remains of their resistance suggests that the asylum milieu did not much resemble that of a total institution.

To translate complaints into redress, some patients used the hospital rulebook. When indignant about abusive attendants, inmates often showed a shrewd knowledge of the standards Kirkbride set for his staff. The man who claimed that the attendant William had "shamefully abused him" concluded his letter by stating, "I believe the regulations governing the attendants state that they are not to get in a passion, not to inflict more punishment than is necessary." Patients relied not only on the published rules to make their point but also on the verbal orders they heard the physicians give. The ladies in the Second Ward, who wrote to Kirkbride complaining about their unrefined neighbors, had attempted to enforce Kirkbride's orders in his absence. Knowing the unpopular Mrs. B had been forbidden by "the Doctor" to visit their ward until her manners improved, the ladies wrote indignantly to the superintendent, "we were somewhat surprised to hear her voice in angry abuse in the hall, and upon repairing to the attendants to inquire why they did not discharge their duty by taking her downstairs, heard them express their unwillingness to do so, as it was not their place." The ladies disagreed, replying "that it was the duty of the attendants to preserve order in the ward, and that as they understood the Doctor's order, they [the attendants] had disregarded the rules and neglected to fulfill their duty."[14]

In trying to turn the superintendent's regulations to their own advantage, patients displayed considerable faith in the doctor's good will. They often stated the assumption that Kirkbride need only be made aware of the unjustices they suffered in order to set matters right. One trusting patient, complaining of "most awful rough" handling at the hands of his "tenders," stated his conviction that the abuse occurred behind Kirkbride's back, "contrary to the rules of this fine institution." He gave a very believable account of how this irregularity took place without the superintendent's knowledge: "I had often taken notice when the time came that you came to visit the patients they put on a very smooth face and [are] very friendly and the moment you were gone they were savage." Out of terror, the patient claimed, he had done the attendants' work for them and never told anyone of their brutality, "for fear they would get to hear it again and be more severe on me." Believing in Kirkbride's kindliness, he had written secretly to ask for help. Kirkbride's papers make no mention of whether or not he investigated these charges; an attendant named in the account was still on the payroll a year later.[115]

Patients who lost (or never possessed) any faith in the doctor's good intentions often turned to their families for assistance. Because Kirkbride made such an effort to enlist the family in a patient's therapy, his disgruntled charges had a ready-made channel of communication. When relatives wrote to a patient pleading for cooperation with the doctor, he or she could respond with long lists of the grievances that kept them from improvement. Many a patron received in answer to inquiries about hospital life, as one informed Kirkbride, "long letters complaining grievously of bad treatment and bitterly denouncing [his] keepers."[116]

In most cases, Kirkbride could effectively counter the patient's claims by simply reminding patrons that the dissatisfied parties were in fact insane and characterizing their complaints as delusions. To perturbed relatives, the superintendent frequently repeated an observation published in his 1854 *Report:* "In my experience, patients who are thoroughly cured rarely leave an institution with other than the most kindly feelings toward it, and with a disposition to cultivate the most friendly relations with those who have been engaged in their care." In other words, only those patients who still had a "morbid condition of their minds" spoke badly of the hospital. "Too often," Kirkbride explained, their insanity caused them "to interpret erroneously what has passed under their observation, even if there is not a willful perversion of truth."[117]

The majority of patrons apparently accepted Kirkbride's logic and dismissed the patients' negative perceptions of the asylum as symptoms of mental disease. "His mind is so injured," wrote one man after receiving a scathing letter from his father, "that he is ready to imagine anything no difference how foolish." When forced to choose between two conflicting interpretations of hospital events, most families accepted the doctor's version as the more authoritative. Still, few patrons turned an entirely deaf ear to complaints, and particularly plausible accounts of injury prompted concerned inquiries from them. In a somewhat apologetic tone, a patron explained to Kirkbride that the family knew the patient to be insane but felt that there might be some truth in his charges of abuse, "for although his mind wanders very much, he has a good memory, tells a connected and plausible story and has always been in the habit of telling the truth." To assuage the patrons' guilt and concern, Kirkbride had to investigate, if only nominally, the circumstances surrounding the complaint, so as to satisfy their inquiries. In the process, the patients got some audience, if not complete redress, for their grievances.[118]

Kirkbride's attention to patient complaints, a sensitivity amply demonstrated in his correspondence, points up an important factor in his asylum practice. A private institution such as the Pennsylvania Hospital for the Insane depended heavily on the good will of its patrons. The patrons' satisfaction with the institution, in turn, hinged on the patient's level of contentment; feeling immense guilt and anxiety over the commitment, families often reacted strongly to a patient's claims of neglect or abuse. As a result, Kirkbride had a vested interest in eliminating as many sources of patient dissatisfaction as he could. His hospital regimen could not be too exacting nor his attendants too abusive, or else his patrons might take their relatives elsewhere. Thus, although on paper the asylum appeared to be a total institution in which no checks existed on the physician's control, in practice the patronage factor softened its rigidity and gave the patients some scope for expression.

Patients' legal action

Even inmates whose families would not intervene on their behalf found a way to limit and influence the exercise of Kirkbride's authority: by appealing to Pennsylvania's courts. Threats of legal action were in fact a commonplace gesture on the part of disgruntled patients. Some began letters to their lawyers as soon as they arrived at the asylum. Others quickly learned that the mere threat of legal measures served effectively to punish the parties responsible for the commitment. Kirkbride often received hysterical letters from patrons fearful of courtroom disclosure of their private affairs. One woman wrote agitatedly that her daughter meant to take her case to the Supreme Court and thereby give her mother "the pleasure of seeing her name in all the papers from the *New York Herald* to the *New Orleans Picayune*." Advice and encouragement from like-minded patients often amplified such threats. One litigious individual in a ward could easily start other discontented patients thinking of legal recourse. Kirkbride described a particular gentleman as "a little troublesome to us, from his volunteer opinions and the legal counsel which he is constantly giving to patients who are not entirely satisfied." After this patient had convinced a wardmate to threaten a lawsuit, Kirkbride wrote apologetically to the family concerned, "The Mr. M. who has volunteered his assistance in getting your uncle released, I need hardly tell you, is like himself a patient, and the intimacy which has recently sprung up between them has been of no advantage to Mr. S."[119]

Until the passage of the Pennsylvania commitment law in 1869, the superintendent had no obligation to facilitate patients' demands for court hearings and could exercise his discretion even in allowing them counsel. Although Kirkbride strongly discouraged any form of legal action, he still felt bound to allow individuals to contact a lawyer. As he explained to a patron in 1845, "In cases of the kind where a patient insists upon having legal advice, I do not generally feel at liberty to refuse forwarding a letter to his counsel." At the same time, Kirkbride felt an equal responsibility to protect the patron's interests: "I always inform the friends of the patient of the fact," he continued in the same letter, "and give them every opportunity to prevent unnecessary trouble." The 1869 law eliminated the asylum superintendent's scope for discretion by guaranteeing all patients the right to secure legal counsel and procure a court hearing on their insanity through application for a writ of habeas corpus.[120]

The vast majority of disgruntled patients never actually availed themselves of their legal opportunities for redress. During Kirkbride's superintendency, no more than sixteen inmates out of the more than 8,000 admitted to the Pennsylvania Hospital for the Insane brought suits alleging wrongful confinement. Yet, this small minority of court cases had a damaging effect far out of proportion to their number. Not only did they place a tremendous strain on the superintendent and his officers by forcing them to make frequent, wearying court appearances; they also created unfavorable newspaper publicity for the hospital, which undercut the therapeutic image Kirkbride had labored so long to establish.[121]

The habeas corpus cases all had certain common features. The inmates in question usually had difficult to define forms of insanity. Of the sixteen, at least four had alcohol-related problems; when intoxicated, they might be violent and dangerous, but as sober men, they could appear quite sane, even by the doctors' standards. Of one intemperate man seeking legal redress, Kirkbride admitted, "there is little doubt that he would be released by any judge before whom he might be taken." Other cases involved eccentric or peculiar patients whose disorder manifested itself in harmless compulsions or violent dislike of family members. Again, such eccentric individuals might easily go among strangers and appear sane. Thus, by and large, legal controversy centered on borderline patients brought into the asylum by a broadening definition of insanity and a heightened concern for family discipline, as discussed in Chapter 3.[122]

Patient profile: Ebenezer Haskell

The case of Ebenezer Haskell, Kirkbride's most successful patient adversary, well illustrates the social and legal issues involved in mid-nineteenth-century commitment controversies. Haskell, a carriage maker and mechanic by trade, had been committed to the Pennsylvania Hospital in 1866 by his wife and sons, who claimed that he threatened them with a knife, ran through the streets in his nightdress, and wasted their money on extravagant business schemes. Haskell asserted that he had been committed only because he wished to get a rightful settlement from a financial deal with his wife's family. Insisting that he had been unjustly committed, Haskell escaped from the asylum four times between 1866 and 1868. Finally, in November 1868, he obtained a jury trial before Judge Carrol Brewster.[123]

Haskell's trial centered on two issues: the determination of his insanity and the legality of his commitment. The debate over his insanity hinged on the proof that there had been a sudden change in his feelings toward his family. The prosecution insisted that his attitude toward his in-laws was perfectly justifiable; his own lawyer admitted that Haskell had always been peculiar, but argued that he was eccentric rather than insane. The defense counsel countered by claiming that Haskell's "enmity toward family" and "aversion to relatives" constituted sufficient proof of his derangement. But the most important evidence in the case centered not on Haskell's mental condition but rather on the legality of the commitment papers. The original certificate of insanity had been signed by a physician who admitted that he did not know Haskell and had based his judgment on the sons' account of their father's behavior. At the conclusion of testimony, Brewster charged the jury, "If such proceedings can be tolerated, our constitution and laws professing to guard human liberty are all waste paper." At the same time, the judge disclaimed any intention of "reflecting upon the excellent physicians in charge of the hospital," whom he believed "deservedly in high repute here and elsewhere" and guilty of no crime. Instead, Brewster couched his remarks as a plea for a sound commitment law. The jury found in Haskell's favor; whether they were in sympathy with Brewster's constitutional argument or believed in Haskell's sanity is unknown.[124]

In the other habeas corpus decisions, the court by and large echoed Brewster's divided sentiments. On the one hand, the judges' opinions all praised the Pennsylvania Hospital for the Insane as a model institution and expressed admiration for its superintendent. In almost half of the cases, the court upheld Kirkbride's decision to admit the patients in question and returned them to his care. Judges also displayed tolerance toward irregular commitment procedures prompted by emergencies. For example, in an 1870 case, a patient had been left at the asylum by a relative, who then went off to Europe and neglected to supply the requisite doctors' certificates for eight months. Although this was a clear violation of the 1869 law, the judge reviewing the case agreed that the patient was insane and understood why the asylum officials had refused to release him "to run at large at the risk of doing injury to himself, possibly others." The court ordered the man released and readmitted with proper papers. In other instances, judges denounced the parties bringing the legal action as irresponsible. In Amelia Mintzer's case, the presiding officer declared that the lawsuit involved a family disagreement, not a case of disputed insanity, and asked for dismissal: "This court cannot regulate all the domestic affairs of our citizens," he concluded. At Sarah Livesay's trial, the judge rebuked her counsel for bringing the writ without the patient's knowledge or approval. (Ebenezer Haskell had in fact persuaded the lawyer to act on her behalf.) Clearly, the judges presiding over the commitment controversies did not take a hostile stance toward the asylum. On the other hand, they did not hesitate to criticize its admission policies, as did Brewster, when they seemed to deny the patient due process of law. In half of the cases reviewed, the patient gained release not necessarily on the grounds that he was not insane, but because the papers attesting to his condition had not been properly sworn. In particular, the courts refused to accept certificates of insanity signed by physicians who knew little of a patient's past history or recent behavior. Although acknowledging Kirkbride's expertise, the legal authorities still asked for better safeguards against wrongful confinement.[125]

The controversial habeas corpus trials that beset the Pennsylvania Hospital for the Insane during the 1860s and 1870s inaugurated a new era of legal involvement in the asylum's internal affairs. Perhaps inevitably, the informality of the hospital's traditional commitment procedures led to greater judicial intervention. Within the expanding legal community of mid-century Philadelphia, hospital patients easily found advocates for their challenges to the process. Isaac Ray wrote scornfully, "the scrub lawyers in this village seem to think they have found a big Bonanza in Kirkbride's place, for they have kept up a running fire of habeas corpuses all winter." As a result, the courts gradually came to play a larger role not only in the commitment process but also in asylum policy as a whole. Judge Brewster, perhaps as a result of his widely publicized role in Haskell's trial, found himself receiving letters from asylum patients alleging abuse from attendants; he naturally called upon Kirkbride to account for the complaints, stating, "I know how trying must be the situation of an attendant under such circumstances but at the same time you are aware how seriously the Law would regard any attack upon the person of a patient." In another instance, a local judge got involved in the question of denying visiting rights to certain relatives. Whereas previously Kirkbride had been allowed to handle such matters more or less by himself, he now had a legal "conscience" to whom he had to answer. Slowly but surely, the court had become a third party, although not necessarily a hostile one, in the commitment and treatment of the insane.[126]

Kirkbride by no means rejoiced at the court's increased interest in his institutional affairs. The trials and visits to the judge's chambers added nothing but a wearying, aggravating burden to his already overloaded asylum practice. Yet on the whole, Kirkbride probably would have accepted this new legal relationship without perturbation, had its consequences been limited primarily to the courtroom. His legal brethren, especially those on the bench, were a fairly sympathetic group who respected the physician's claims to professional expertise. Although Kirkbride himself felt that further safeguards on the commitment process were unnecessary, he did not strenuously oppose the principle his legal adversaries upheld, that is, the necessity to show sufficient cause for voluntary confinement. Had the impact of the habeas corpus trials remained at the level of judicial review, requiring only that Kirkbride observe more circumspection in admitting borderline patients, the superintendent might have survived his legal appearances without grave distress. Kirkbride's real anguish came not from the lawyers, but from the journalists who parlayed the commitment controversies into a full-scale assault on the asylum. It was the public outcry rather than the court decisions themselves that had the more serious consequences for Kirkbride's asylum practice.

PUBLIC CONTROVERSY CONCERNING THE
ASYLUM

Once again, Ebenezer Haskell played a central role in mobilizing the press's hostility toward the asylum. Soon after his release, Haskell published a harrowing tale of his incarceration in the Pennsylvania Hospital for the Insane (refer to Figure 8). Although his disjointed, confused narrative does little to dispel doubts about Haskell's sanity, his book does present a crude but compelling view of asylum treatment as seen from the noncompliant patient's perspective. Haskell introduced his readers to the horrors of the dreaded Seventh Ward, where the "yelling and howling" of the other patients continually upset him. The attendants choked their charges into submission or tortured them with the "douche" (a bucket of cold water thrown into the face) and the "saddle" (Haskell's term for the bedstraps). The nurses threatened Haskell with the saddle, he claimed, "if I kept on talking or tried to escape." When finally promoted to the Second Ward, he found matters no better. There he met a bookkeeper whom the doctors had fed with a stomach pump, despite the fact that the poor man's stomach passages were inflamed with disease. "He had such a dread of the pumping," wrote Haskell, that "he told me death was preferable to life." The bookkeeper finally committed suicide by jumping off the hospital portico, according to Haskell. As for Kirkbride and the managers, they were worthy of nothing but scorn. The asylum superintendent cared only for his emoluments, and his managers were easily bought off with a good dinner.[127]

Ebenezer Haskell's exposé wove together into a dramatic narrative all the complaints uncooperative patients had been making about the asylum for years. But this former patient did not rest content with publishing his unflattering vision of the hospital; he became a one-man crusade against the institution. Throughout the late 1860s and early 1870s, Haskell occupied himself with a variety of anti-asylum stratagems. He lobbied in Harrisburg for the 1869 law requiring two doctors' certificates of insanity; encouraged the habeas corpus trials of other patients, particularly Amelia Minzer and Sarah Livesay; and published letters and editorials in the local papers about asylum abuses. Like Wiley Williams, Haskell claimed to have no particular malice toward Kirkbride or the Pennsylvania Hospital for the Insane. In a letter to Kirkbride written in 1871, he expressed his belief that the hospital was "a good and useful Institution" that "outside parties," meaning conniving relatives, used "to carry out their wicked designs." The issue in Haskell's mind was not the propriety of hospital treatment but the method of selecting its subjects. As Haskell wrote to the *Evening Star* in 1873 concerning the Minzer trial, "There is a principle involved in this case of importance to me and the public, to know who is safe to walk in the streets of Philadelphia, without being kidnapped and ushered into a madhouse, without being heard before a judge of one of these courts."[128]

Haskell's crusade, joined with the drama inherent in commitment controversies, made the Pennsylvania Hospital for the Insane the focus of increasing publicity in the late 1860s and 1870s. In the competitive environment of post-Civil War journalism, the local newspapers quickly realized that insanity trials made newsworthy items and closely followed Haskell's case, as well as the subsequent suits involving "Kirkbride's," as they often referred to the Pennsylvania Hospital for the Insane. Coverage of the trials did not necessarily bring with it editorial censure, however. Philadelphia's biggest and best-established dailies, the *Public Ledger, Evening Bulletin*, and *Philadelphia Inquirer*, all defended Kirkbride and the asylum in their editorial columns. Only the newer, more aggressive practitioners of yellow journalism among the city's newspapers, particularly the *North American* and *The Times and Dispatch*, attacked the local institution. By far the most scathing journalistic assaults came from outside the state altogether, from two well-established sources: the *Atlantic Monthly* and the *New York Tribune*.[129]

In May 1868, the *Atlantic Monthly*, a New York City-based magazine, published an anonymous article, attributed by Kirkbride to L. Clarke Davis, entitled a "Modern 'Lettre de Cachet.' " Comparing the certificate of insanity committing a patient to the hospital with "that old 'lettre' of France which with like silence and secrecy, consigned its victim to the Bastille," the author presented a thorough critique of asylum management. The Pennsylvania Hospital for the Insane, along with several other institutions, came in for some pointed observations. Although praising Kirkbride as "a gentleman noble and good as he is wise" (a disclaimer his critics seem compelled to offer), the author nevertheless took issue with the Philadelphia superintendent's philosophy of asylum management. Kirkbride's insistence on the chief physician's authority over every aspect of the hospital's operations struck him as an ill-conceived notion. "We cannot fail to see the capacity for evil with which he is clothed, since every officer of the institution, from the physician to the scullery maid, depends upon his favor to maintain position under him," Davis wrote of Kirkbride. Given the fact that abuses had occurred even in the Pennsylvania Hospital for the Insane, admittedly the "oldest, if not the ablest and most useful of its class" – here the article referred to Haskell's case, not yet come to trial but already publicized – such a doctrine became even more dangerous in the hands of unscrupulous doctors running private madhouses. More importantly, Kirkbride's opposition to nonrestraint made the asylum no better than a prison; any attempt to make it appear less oppressive, whether by using handsome lawns or "ornamental cast-iron screens," was doomed to fail. The abuses occurring behind its "frowning stone edifice" went unnoticed, due to the "immense influence yielded by the Pennsylvania Hospital in Philadelphia, which, lifting up its heavy granite front to intimidate legislature, judge and citizen alike, sternly questions if anything so solid, so eminently respectable as it is, can be suspected of wrong, ignorance or lack of care."[130]

Not surprisingly, the *Atlantic Monthly* piece infuriated Kirkbride, who quickly persuaded his friend Isaac Ray, recently retired from the Butler Hospital, to write a reply, which appeared in the August 1868 number of the monthly. But neither Ray's rebuttal nor any of Kirkbride's subsequent attempts to defend his philosophy of asylum management could stem the growing public debate over the mental hospital. Within two years came another powerful attack, this time from an influential New York City newspaper.[131]

The *New York Tribune* turned its attention to the Pennsylvania Hospital for the Insane during the same period that it published a relentless series of exposés on the New York Hospital's Bloomingdale Asylum. Perhaps not wanting to appear uncivic-minded by its attacks on a local institution, the well-respected, conservative daily began to search other cities for asylum abuses. In the wake of Ebenezer Haskell's trial, the *Tribune* found a convenient target in nearby Philadelphia. Referring scornfully to the cowardice of the local press, which was so "ominously silent when required to mention anything that may cast obloquy upon a powerful local institution," in contrast to itself, the New York newspaper sent its own correspondent to investigate Kirkbride's asylum. The superintendent, no doubt hoping to convert the reporter's distrust into approval, spent an afternoon showing him the institution, only to be rewarded with an unflattering feature about the great "suburban palace–prison" of Philadelphia.[132]

For all its invective, this 1869 *Tribune* article, like the *Atlantic* piece, rather shrewdly addressed the obvious weaknesses in Kirkbride's philosophy of hospital management. The reporter acknowledged the efforts the superintendent had made to create a pleasant institutional environment: "The floors well-scrubbed, the parlors richly furnished, the stairs carpeted, the bedrooms cleanly, the curtains expensive, the grounds extensive, the ventilation good and the supper excellent." But instead of applauding these outward signs of a well-run hospital, the reporter characterized them as "the cheap bids which the Superintendent offers to an easily satisfied public." Like a whited sepulcher, an attractive exterior covered all sorts of spiritual horrors: the kidnapping of patients, their confinement in "holes not fit for a dog," and other hideous atrocities. No amount of "improvements" could counteract the injustices detailed by former patients such as Ebenezer Haskell, the author of the article concluded. To him, Kirkbride's concern for the asylum's image seemed so much "bribery."[133]

The criticisms of the Pennsylvania Hospital for the Insane, first appearing in relatively respectable publications such as the *Tribune* and the *Atlantic Monthly*, soon became a staple of the penny press. In far less measured tones, the popular papers picked up the same themes and exaggerated them. According to the penny press, the asylum was used primarily by wicked relatives to defraud innocent souls of their money. Kirkbride, always the bland but scheming showman in these caricatures, cooperated with the family's schemes because the asylum provided him with a fine house, carriage, and salary. Since the medical definition of insanity was so imprecise, the doctor could declare anyone insane just by magnifying some harmless peculiarity. As one paper commented scornfully in a case in which a patient's lack of truthfulness had been alleged as a symptom, "If lying is to be made a test of insanity, the entire area of West Philadelphia will not be large enough for a building with capacity to contain the insane portion of the community." In similar fashion, the so-called tests of insanity furnished skeptical journalists with endless material with which to ridicule the asylum doctors. Although the whole system of commitment was "bosh," as the same article termed it, Kirkbride and his fellow superintendents opposed needed reform for pecuniary reasons.[134]

Of course, the Pennsylvania Hospital had its journalistic supporters as well. The pro-asylum press engaged the anti-Kirkbride faction in frequent editorial combat. The superintendent's defenders upheld the physician's ability to diagnose so subtle a disease as insanity, maintained that abuses rarely happened "outside works of fiction," and questioned the sanity of the asylum's detractors. The local medical weekly proclaimed that the "vulgar notion of sane people being shut up in hospitals for the sake of their money (or something worse) is nothing better than a bugaboo story for frightening children that have got their growth." According to the conservative local papers, the whole asylum controversy was the work of a few half-sane patients and unscrupulous lawyers who had taken advantage of an ignorant, sentimental public. As a result, a noble charity and a fine doctor had suffered "a piece of wholly gratuitous hardship and injustice."[135]

Despite his passionate defenders, Kirkbride was wounded by the public attacks on himself and his institution. Although he rarely mentioned his difficulties in public, those around Kirkbride observed that the controversy distressed him. His friend and protégé John Curwen observed that "like all genuinely conscientious natures," Kirkbride could not help but be "very sensitive to...and harassed by the malicious attacks of designing persons." To many,

Kirkbride's fate seemed indicative of the vicissitudes of asylum work; "you will labor on for years, and then, like Dr. Kirkbride, lose a well-earned reputation by the clamor of uncured lunatics," wrote J. A. Reed of the Western Pennsylvania Hospital for the Insane. In fact, his reputation was hardly so fragile; in spite of the negative publicity, the Pennsylvania Hospital for the Insane continued to function, with no noticeable decline in admissions or contributions.[136]

Yet without a doubt, the increasing level of public controversy signaled a new, more hostile era in the asylum's existence. Despite the very personal form that the "clamor" of former patients took, Kirkbride's experience reflected not so much a censure of his individual practice as an indictment of the whole asylum movement. As will be shown in the next chapter, hardly a superintendent of Kirkbride's generation escaped without being the object of a newspaper attack or a former patient's diatribe. From the 1860s on, asylum exposés became a nationwide, indeed international, phenomenon. As the Philadelphia situation suggests, the factors producing a more antagonistic stance toward the asylum were many and complex. Certainly, the expansionist mood of both the legal profession and the popular press encouraged the critical mood; lawyers looking for clients and editors searching for newsworthy stories both found what they wanted in the dissatisfied mental patient. The attacks on the mental hospital also constituted part of a larger questioning of urban institutions and political authorities. Decades before the Progressive-era muckrakers began to investigate corporate abuses, the large city papers had already found a ready audience for stories of municipal corruption. Investigations of local institutions such as the asylum served a variety of political ends. If the institution was a public venture, exposure of abuses embarrassed the party in power. If a private concern such as the Pennsylvania Hospital was involved, the asylum became a convenient symbol of the city's social and economic elite, who sat on its board and sent relatives to its best wards. In a broader sense, asylum exposés can be seen as part of an ongoing tradition of anxiety about centralized power and its abuses, which predates the American Revolution. As Eliza Butler Kirkbride wrote of the asylum's critics, they spoke in the "prevailing spirits of the moment": a "general distrust of private motives, and of the good faith of corporations."[137]

Although these external political considerations were important factors precipitating criticism, the ferment concerning the late-nineteenth-century asylum also reflected dramatic changes in its internal organization. The public might have been less anxious about the institution's structure and function had they not changed so radically since the eighteenth century. The medical superintendent's position within the new mental hospital represented an unprecedented concentration of institutional power, a trend that might easily be seen as contrary to the democratic ethos of the times. Furthermore, the asylum had increased the number of mental disorders considered suitable for treatment, thereby multiplying the number of borderline or less severe cases among its patients. The increasing utilization of asylum treatment for drug- and alcohol-related mental problems created a whole new category of troublesome patients with whom Kirkbride had to deal. The morally insane, that is, individuals whose insanity manifested itself solely on moral or emotional issues, constituted another difficult new set of inmates. Although the actual mental condition of defiant former patients such as Ebenezer Haskell will always be a matter of conjecture, they obviously had sufficient reason and stability to persuade juries, legislators, and many other sane parties that their claim of wrongful commitment had some merit. In all probability, given the limited institutional resources of the eighteenth century, such individuals would not have been in a hospital before the early nineteenth century.

The new alliance that the physician forged between the family and the asylum also played a role in precipitating the mid-nineteenth-century debate over commitment. The theme of family conflict appears in the asylum exposés with predictable regularity. Fear of relatives' schemes to deny the individual "money, liberty and personal happiness" loomed even larger than the distrust of institutional power in the debate over commitment. Obviously, family conflict did not constitute a new development in the mid-nineteenth century. But the link between the family's interests and the asylum had grown much stronger over the preceding century. The increasing intensity and exactitude of notions concerning domestic life may very well have heightened suspicions and tensions among family members. To the extent that families came to look upon institutionalization as a solution to their internal disruption, the asylum inevitably became the focus of familial conflicts. Since the asylum existed to preserve the family order, those individuals who challenged that order had to indict the doctor and the institution as well.

Finally, commitment controversies can be traced to an inherent flaw in moral treatment itself. As Kirkbride envisioned it, the hospital's rationale depended upon a therapeutic persuasion, an agreed upon set of beliefs about mental disorders and their treatment. But however well executed this program was – and the Pennsylvania Hospital for the Insane represented the best of its type – asylum medicine rested upon an untenable premise: that the patient, as well as the patron, accepted the necessity for treatment. In truth, the vast majority of patients were confined and forced to submit to asylum care without their consent. Not surprisingly, many refused to believe the convenient fictions about hospital life – that attendants never behaved harshly, that their fellow patients were pleasant, reasonable companions – so gratefully accepted by their families. To patients who did not believe in their own insanity, the hospital did indeed seem like a prison. Out of this disparity in perceptions grew the endless allegations of abuse.

So, the Pennsylvania Hospital for the Insane, viewed from the perspective of its patients, resembled neither the benignly therapeutic institution imagined by its admirers nor the endless trial envisioned by its critics. Some patients came to accept its fundamental principles and responded to the advice and consolation offered by the physicians. Others resisted treatment, despite all the means used to control their behavior, and expressed hostility toward the institution in a variety of ways. For all patients, whether compliant or not, the hospital milieu never assumed the regularity or regimentation Kirkbride might have wished. Boundaries between the asylum and the community, and within the institution itself, were neither rigid nor impenetrable. And the patients' experiences with each other never corresponded to the relationships Kirkbride projected for them. Thus, in describing this nineteenth-century mental hospital, the balance must be struck between the spheres of compliance and rebellion among the patients and the ideal and reality of asylum life.

6

The perils of asylum practice

As the preceding chapters make evident, Thomas Story Kirkbride faced no easy task as an asylum superintendent. His daily practice represented nothing less than a continual struggle to counteract or deny fundamental characteristics of the asylum environment. Only by ceaseless planning and vigilance could he keep the inevitable disparity between therapeutic ideal and hospital reality to an acceptable minimum. If Kirkbride allowed that disparity to become too obvious, he risked losing the generous confidence of the managers and patrons, whose good will was essential to his enterprise. Thus, in a fundamental way, his success as an asylum doctor depended upon "keeping his house in good order," to use his phrase.

For various reasons, Kirkbride proved especially adept at the delicate legerdemain involved in asylum management. In an era when moral and scientific knowledge were seen as mutually reinforcing, his reputation as both a Christian and physician gave him a commanding personal authority. Sharing the same social background as his managers and most of his patrons, he could exercise his influence with comparatively little effort. This common bond with his patrons contributed to Kirkbride's special sensitivity to their fears and anxieties about insanity, an empathy that enabled him to anticipate their expectations of asylum treatment. In addition, the Pennsylvania Hospital's ample financial resources allowed Kirkbride the opportunity to translate the patrons' desires into an impressive array of improvements. Given all these assets, he managed to overcome the problems of asylum practice and to maintain a large measure of public confidence in his institution. Although the habeas corpus trials of the 1860s and 1870s undoubtedly damaged the hospital's public image, they did not destroy its superintendent's reputation for either integrity or expertise.

Perhaps more than any other asylum doctor of his generation, Kirkbride succeeded in making the principles of moral treatment into an institutional reality.

The particular era of asylum medicine in which Kirkbride came to maturity gave his success in hospital practice a significance beyond the walls of his own institution. His prominence within the specialty coincided with a period of rapid institution building. Between 1840 and 1880, the number of mental hospitals increased from 18 to 139. Particularly dramatic was the development of state-funded institutions, which increased almost tenfold in less than four decades. The Association of Superintendents of the American Institutions for the Insane grew rapidly from its original thirteen members to an organization of more than fifty members. During this period of rapid growth, Kirkbride's personal charisma and practical wisdom made him a natural leader within the new specialty. In the unfamiliar business of hospital construction, he provided general guidelines and concrete suggestions through his professional writings and correspondence. Younger superintendents found in him an accessible and discreet confidant. Perhaps most importantly, Kirkbride's reputation for unfailing honesty and kindness made him an excellent spokesman in the specialty's campaign to win the public's trust.[1]

Not only did Kirkbride play an important leadership role in early asylum medicine; his approach to hospital management profoundly influenced a whole generation of American asylum doctors. In the form of twenty-six propositions on hospital construction and management, which Kirkbride wrote and the AMSAII ratified in 1851 and 1853, his viewpoints became the specialty's official stance on institutional standards. The "propositions," as they were familiarly known, essentially codified Kirkbride's structural prerequisites for the successful practice of moral treatment: that mental hospitals have no more than 250 patients; that the hospital building be carefully planned and constructed; that the institution be organized and administered so as to accommodate a mixed clientele, that is, curable and chronic, paying and charity patients together in the same hospital; and that the medical superintendent have complete control over every facet of the hospital's management. These principles, which Kirkbride drew from his own asylum practice and from observation of his peers' experience, remained the specialty's official policy on hospital design for almost forty years. Such was the power of Kirkbride's asylum philosophy that even in the late 1880s, when his viewpoints no longer commanded widespread support, the AMSAII chose to make the propositions nonbinding, rather than reject them outright.

The status of Kirkbride's propositions reflected the larger fate of moral treatment as the dominant therapeutic rationale of nineteenth-century asylum medicine. In the 1850s and 1860s, when moral treatment reigned supreme, Kirkbride's asylum philosophy expressed the aspirations, if not the actual experience, of most asylum superintendents. Kirkbride's professional writings articulated a wide range of concerns shared by all the brethren, whether they served in state or corporate hospitals. But as conditions in the state institutions rapidly deteriorated in the 1860s and 1870s, the professional consensus underlying the propositions began to erode. Critics, both from within and without the AMSAII, called for larger, less expensive state hospitals that would more effectively serve the insane pauper and segregate recent from chronic patients. By the late 1870s, the mid-nineteenth-century vision of the small, multiclass, multipurpose asylum was being widely contested by both physicians and welfare officials. So, before his death in 1883, Kirkbride saw his asylum design, along with the fundamental premises of moral treatment it embodied, attacked on both scientific and humanitarian grounds.

To assess fully the significance of Kirkbride's asylum practice and philosophy, then, we must go beyond the walls of the Pennsylvania Hospital for the Insane, which up to this point has been the main focus of concern, and examine Kirkbride's influence in a wider purview: the professional politics of mid-nineteenth-century asylum medicine. This final chapter places his career within a broader context, first by examining the common perils of asylum practice experienced by Kirkbride's fellow superintendents, to demonstrate how well his formulations on asylum design addressed their common needs and concerns. Then the chapter discusses the changing institutional circumstances, particularly the deterioration of the older state hospitals, that led to increasing controversy over the propositions. The final section uses the career of Kirkbride's protégé, John Curwen, at the Pennsylvania State Lunatic Asylum to link the state hospital's problems with the asylum superintendents' decline as a political force in Pennsylvania politics. Thus, this chapter traces the rise and fall of Kirkbride's political influence from the AMSAII's adoption of the propositions in the 1850s to the foundation of the Pennsylvania State Lunacy Commission in 1883.

MID-NINETEENTH-CENTURY ASYLUM
PRACTICE

Kirkbride's standing within the field of asylum medicine reflected not only his personal concerns but also the centrality of institutional issues to the early American specialty. That asylum matters dominated its professional agenda during Kirkbride's heyday has long been recognized by historians.[2] The proceedings of the AMSAII's annual meetings, the papers published in the *American Journal of Insanity*, and the superintendents' correspondence with one another all attest to their preoccupation with hospital management. In the specialty's hierarchy of professional concerns, the subjects Kirkbride took as his life's work had very high priority.

Asylum design and professional aspiration

The "brethren," as the inner circle of superintendents frequently referred to themselves, had a lively interest in hospital planning. Although Kirkbride was widely regarded as the foremost authority on the subject, his prominence did not dampen other asylum doctors' exploration of design issues. His contemporaries, Isaac Ray and Luther Bell, for example, established their own reputations for expertise in the area. Bell, who headed the prestigious McLean Hospital in the 1840s, Pliny Earle, another physician interested in hospital design, and Ray had more varied intellectual interests than did Kirkbride, yet none of them characterized problems of asylum construction and management as of secondary importance. Likewise, the younger men entering the field in the 1850s and 1860s pursued the study of hospital planning as a recognized avenue to professional prominence. An ambitious young superintendent such as Charles Nichols, for example, tried to enhance his budding professional reputation by improving upon Kirkbride's linear plan.[3]

The superintendents not only associated the art of asylum design with successful advancement in the specialty, they also equated their personal prestige with the desirability of their particular hospital's building and administrative arrangements. To have charge of a poorly planned or unimproved institution lowered a physician's self-regard, as well as his estimation among his fellow asylum doctors. The superintendency of an asylum such as the Bloomingdale Hospital, long known for its managers' illiberality and its practice of divided responsibility between steward and chief physician, represented a professional cul-de-sac. James McDonald, Pliny Earle, and Charles Nichols all left Bloomingdale's employ because its management deviated so widely from the practices prevailing at other hospitals. D. Tilden Brown, who remained there from 1857 to 1877, appears to have suffered from feelings of professional inferiority, despite his seemingly dispassionate references to the hospital's flaws. As he wrote to Dorothea Dix in 1857, "Few men *enjoy* an inferior position in their profession, however philosophic they may talk and *write in reports*."[4]

Not surprisingly, the superintendents' definition of institutional desirability mirrored the standards set in the affluent corporate asylums such as the Pennsylvania Hospital for the Insane and the McLean Hospital. The closer a superintendent's institution approximated the external elegance and internal harmony prevailing in the leading institutions, the more prestige he enjoyed. Even a doctor with limited financial resources might aspire to emulate some aspect of Kirkbride's ideal asylum, if only by acquiring a bowling alley, a reading room, or a magic lantern. S. S. Schulz of the Danville Asylum in Pennsylvania bragged to Dorothea Dix in 1878 of his new greenhouse, taking pride in the observation that "If Dr. Kirkbride's Green House lasted 30 years, I am quite confident this will last fifty." In a similar vein, Horace Buttolph of the New Jersey State Asylum wrote that although his institution could not compare to Kirkbride's "noble Hospital," he hoped to make it "a very pleasant and comfortable establishment." To approximate in any degree the features of the best asylums constituted the mark of a successful asylum doctor.[5]

A spirit of emulation inspired the heads of public asylums no less than their counterparts in the private sphere. In part, their outlook stemmed from the perhaps inevitable tendency to equate the most elite hospitals with the epitome of professional achievement. The standards of asylum success also reflected the relatively confused sense of public and private spheres characteristic of mid-nineteenth-century America. Before the Civil War, the sharp differences in clientele, quality of care, and efficacy later to be associated with the private–state distinction did not yet exist. By attempting to replicate the practices typical of the corporate asylums, the early state superintendents had no a priori sense that they aspired to an inappropriate or unrealizable goal. That disillusionment came later.[6]

In addition, the need to establish legitimacy through asylum design necessarily concerned the superintendents of state as well as corporate institutions. The state superintendents faced problems of procuring public support similar in kind if not degree to those encountered by their counterparts in private institutions. Until the 1870s, many public asylums took in a percentage of paying patients, in a few cases as much as one-half the total, whose board rates made a crucial difference to the institution's financial stability.[7] In addition, paying patients were often of a class and mental condition that made them desirable inmates in the superintendents' estimation. To secure attractive patients and patrons, state asylums had to have the same persuasive assets as private institutions. Even more importantly, heads of public hospitals had to win the financial support of local officials and state legislators, who judged the asylum by its appearance and good order. With the almshouse and jail as inexpensive alternatives, the state hospital had to project a strong therapeutic image to obtain needed appropriations. Thus, the problem of legitimacy affected both state and corporate hospital superintendents, albeit in somewhat different ways.

Much of Kirkbride's authority within the mid-century profession can be attributed to his ability to articulate the shared problems of asylum practice and to propose practical measures for their solution. As Kirkbride rightly understood, asylum superintendents judged and were judged by others according to their administrative ability. Furthermore, building and management details often had a far-reaching influence on a physician's ability to treat insanity. The points Kirkbride made in his prescriptive literature concerning the necessity for a well-planned building, harmonious staff, and supportive board of managers were evident truths to his colleagues. For all his privileged position in an affluent corporate hospital, he spoke directly and eloquently to the whole specialty's daily experience of asylum practice.

Thus, the superintendents' accounts of their successes and failures in asylum practice, especially the more revealing admissions they made in their private correspondence, provide a useful commentary on the professional culture that accorded Kirkbride's achievements such high respect. The superintendents' perceptions of asylum work suggest the profound dilemma they faced, having sought and in large part won absolute authority in the asylum. For despite the unusual degree of power physicians managed to obtain within the new asylum, the exercise of their authority proved to be difficult. Having claimed to be building experts, farm managers, hospital administrators, fund raisers, family counselors, and clinicians, asylum superintendents found the multiple demands of their institutions hard to meet. Few men had the requisite energy, versatility, and good health necessary to perform well in all these roles. As a result, the profession soon had firsthand knowledge of the difficulties a superintendent faced when he failed to keep his house in order as Kirkbride advised.

"Living over a volcano"

In chronicling the perils of asylum practice, the superintendents naturally thought first of the problems caused by flawed hospital plans and construction. Examples of exceptionally bad hospital architecture were common points of reference among them, frequently invoked as proof that asylum doctors must have the dominant role in designing hospitals. Without a physician's guidance, ignorant building committees put up "gross enormities of construction," to use Isaac Ray's phrase, such as the Taunton, Massachusetts, State Hospital: an asylum located far from any roads, on such a "waste of sand" that its farms could never be productive; whose patients' rooms had expensive wallpaper, but were so badly ventilated that the beds might as well have stood in a foul-air flue, according to Ray. Understandably, no doctor could speak well of hospitals having heating systems so faulty that the patients stood in danger of freezing to death; with tubs installed without plumbing, requiring water to be ladled in and out each time a patient bathed; or, worse yet, so deficient a water supply as to allow no baths at all; yet errors such as these were commonplaces of mid-nineteenth-century hospital construction.[8]

From the asylum doctor's standpoint, flaws of this order resulted in tremendous hardship for both doctor and patient. The superintendents' correspondence frequently attested to the destructive impact that seemingly inconsequential building details could have on the quality of asylum practice. John Curwen, writing to Kirkbride to get a new pattern for window guards, explained that with his old ones, "I have had so many escapes by men breaking them and women creeping under them that I have had no comfort." Henry Stabb encountered "great difficulties," as he confided to Dorothea Dix, because his building plan forced him to place male and female patients on different floors of the same structure, rather than in separate wings; when one sex went outdoors for exercise, the other overlooked them from the windows, which inevitably created a disturbance. For the physician spending twenty-four hours a day in an institution and responsible for a volatile class of patients, such building flaws caused more than a slight inconvenience. Unfortunately, undoing the work of an incompetent building committee could take years, and in some instances, the problems could never really be rectified.[9]

In determining the superintendent's working conditions, the asylum's internal arrangements played as important a part as its architectural features. The problems with attendants, stewards, matrons, and assistant physicians, so frequently discussed in the doctors' correspondence, suggest that personnel issues concerned them only a little less than hospital construction. Kirkbride's directions concerning the asylum hierarchy, particularly his insistence upon the superintendent's right to hire and fire all hospital workers, reflected the difficulties that asylum doctors felt they had suffered at the hands of incompetent or insubordinate employees.

Incompetence seemed to be the special scourge of the asylum superintendents. Whether from ingrained laziness or momentary inattention, dereliction of duty greatly multiplied the probability of suicide, fire, or other untoward events capable of undermining public confidence in the institution. The average attendant had little sense of responsibility, less intelligence, and no sympathy with patients, according to the doctors' private estimation. (This was in marked contrast to their statements in annual reports.) To explain the attendants' poor performance, most doctors (although not Kirkbride) pointed to the predominance of the Irish among hospital workers. When it came to other hospital officers, the superintendents cited political patronage, rather than ethnic origin, as the source of rampant incompetence. State superintendents in particular complained bitterly of the "outside interests," usually meaning trustees or legislators, who saddled them with useless staff members. Richard Patterson, the superintendent of the Indianapolis Hospital for the Insane, informed Kirkbride in 1852 that he had just been given a new steward and assistant physician, "both young and neither of them any better suited to their places than they should be." On the steward, Patterson commented further, "He has not the remotest qualification for the place he occupies, except perhaps his honesty, and that may result from the fact he don't know enough to steal. However he is a *relative* of one of the Commissioners, and a warm family friend of another, and a *good Democrat* and that will do."[10]

Although the physicians bemoaned the problems caused by unqualified underlings, the tone of their remarks suggests that they viewed such failings as inevitable, especially among the attendant class. The superintendents could well afford to be charitable, inasmuch as the staff's lapses often provided a convenient excuse for accidents or oversights in patient care. Insubordination was another matter entirely. Employees who directly defied the superintendent represented a grave threat to his authority. Not only could one disgruntled individual disrupt a whole institution by galvanizing dissatisfied patients or employees into rebellion, he or she might also gain the ear of trustees and legislators, and make even worse trouble for the chief physician. The superintendents' letters to one another were filled with tales of "outrages" committed by disgruntled employees. By far the worst perfidies involved assistant physicians who, in an attempt to win a better position, betrayed their chief. Upon hearing that John P. Gray, an assistant at the Utica Asylum, was rumored to have aided in the downfall of his superior, N. D. Benedict, Edward Fisher, a young southern doctor, wrote indignantly to Kirkbride: "If it be true that Dr. Gray in any manner or form lent himself to the perpetration of so shameful an act after the kindness so lavishly bestowed upon him by Dr. Benedict, I really hardly know how to express my detestation of such ingratitude."[11]

In coping with the perils of asylum practice, whether treacherous employees or construction problems, superintendents often felt that they received little support from the asylum's governing board. In fact, many a chief physician, especially those in public institutions, found their trustees to be more of a hindrance than a help

in managing the asylum. Sometimes the board's retrogressive nature stemmed from an unwieldy structure; extremes in size, whether
the twenty-six-man board at the Bloomingdale Asylum or the sole
governor of the Trenton State Hospital, entailed inherent problems. More often, the superintendents felt that their difficulties
originated in the managers' character. Charles Nichols's tenure at
Bloomingdale convinced him that even a new organization would
not transform the uncooperative governors; "the best of them have
been too long under bad training," he wrote, and "the worst I
won't speak of." The superintendents agreed that politically motivated men made particularly bad trustees. Isaac Ray wrote dis-
gustedly of the board appointed in 1859 to oversee the Philadelphia
General Hospital's new insane department, "the only idea they
have is to take counsel from nobody who has ever been connected
with hospitals. So far their movements have been governed by a
spirit of ringism, having in it a large mixture of general cussed-
ness." Lacking any real understanding of asylum medicine, trustees could cause endless trouble for the superintendent by opposing
needed improvements, demanding jobs for unqualified protégés,
or interfering in the asylum routine. All too frequently, financial
success rather than medical ability determined a board's estimation
of their chief physician. They seemed to regard any large outlay
of money, however justifiable, as a black mark against a superintendent's performance.[12]

Whether stemming from personnel problems or financial difficulties, internal discord within the asylum could rapidly bring
about a doctor's downfall. Kirkbride and his brethren all were
familiar with instances such as Mark Ranney's dismissal from the
Wisconsin State Hospital. Since Ranney was not a particularly
well-liked or well-respected superintendent, his difficulties did not
touch his colleagues' sympathies very deeply. Still, his experience
well illustrated the chaos that could result when a superintendent
lost the respect and obedience of his staff and governors. In a long
letter to Isaac Ray, Ranney detailed the escalating tensions that led
to his firing. From the first, he claimed, the assistant physicians
had not only neglected their duties but also were determined to
resist him and spread "disaffection" to other employees. At the
same time, Ranney's attempts to tighten asylum discipline generated resentment among the attendants; they opposed losing privileges such as skimming the patients' milk to make their own

butter, having undisputed possession of ward keys, running about the house "at all hours for some trifling reasons," and holding "disorderly and noisy gatherings" in their quarters every night. Finding common cause, the assistant physicians and attendants banded together to defy the superintendent openly. Matters came "to such a pitch of boldness," as Ranney put it, that the staff held a secret masquerade party during which both the superintendent and his wife were "grossly caricatured." When the trustees became aware of the contretemps, they did little to aid Ranney. Their attempts to lessen tension by granting more authority to neutral parties such as the steward, the matron, and their own executive committee only further undermined the superintendent's position. "I need not say to you, of course," Ranney wrote to Ray, "that anything of the kind may have a widespread demoralizing effect in and about a Hospital for the Insane." The superintendent's efforts to reassert his sole authority resulted only in charges that he was "tyrannical" and "aristocratic." After almost two years of controversy, the trustees finally fired all the medical officers and the steward.[13]

Patient-related disputes also contributed to the problems of asylum practice. Harassment by legal writ, which so plagued Thomas Story Kirkbride in the 1860s and 1870s, affected most superintendents at one time or another; they all had their "Ebenezer Haskell," as a manager at the Government Hospital nicknamed one of his litigious former patients.[14] Although annoying and time-consuming, such disputes did not necessarily cause an asylum doctor serious trouble, because their patients' testimony tended to carry little weight with managers. Unless accompanied by other gross administrative failures, no board would fire its chief physician over an inmate's complaint. But whenever patient grievances became highly publicized, the potential for more serious complications increased.

Andrew McFarland's experience at the Illinois State Hospital gave Kirkbride and the brethren dramatic proof of this unpleasant reality. McFarland's nemesis was a former patient named Elizabeth Packard, who in persuasiveness and industriousness outstripped even Ebenezer Haskell. Packard was committed to the Jacksonville asylum in 1860 by her clergyman husband, who claimed that she had become a danger to himself and their children. Throughout her three years of confinement, Packard insisted otherwise: that her husband, who disagreed with her unorthodox religious beliefs, which tended toward spiritualism rather than congregationalism, had locked her up only to punish her and save his ministerial reputation. While in the asylum, Packard began to write about the injustices of her confinement, particularly the Illinois law that allowed a husband to commit his wife without the usual formalities. Although initially impressed by McFarland's ability, Packard soon came to believe that he abused his patients and cooperated with evildoers such as her husband who wished to lock up sane relatives. Theophilus Packard removed his wife from the asylum in 1863, whereupon she sued him for imprisoning her in her own home; after a five-day trial, a jury pronounced her sane. Packard then left her husband to pursue a career of writing and lecturing against asylum abuse that took her across the country. Specifically, she sought to reform court laws so as to provide patients, particularly married women, with safeguards against wrongful confinement, including jury commitment trials and postal rights. As the result of her lobbying, "Packard laws," as they came to be known, were introduced in many state legislatures during the 1860s and 1870s.[15]

In 1866, Elizabeth Packard used her considerable lobbying skills to seek retribution against Andrew McFarland. Not only did she convince the Illinois state legislature to adopt a new commitment law guaranteeing jury trials for all patients committed to the state asylum; she also persuaded them to set up a committee to investigate McFarland's asylum practice. For six months, the five-member panel heard testimony, including Packard's evidence, for and against the superintendent. The results were widely, indeed sensationally publicized, and the Illinois State Hospital gained considerable notoriety as an "American bastille," which specialized in incarcerating and torturing sane people. The committee's final reports, although absolving McFarland of any intentional patient abuse or financial irregularities, charged him with illegal commitment practices and recommended that he be dismissed.[16]

The managers of the Illinois State Hospital refused to fire McFarland, however, and he remained in the post until 1870, when he left to start a private mental hospital in Jacksonville. McFarland insisted throughout the investigation (and the other superintendents supported his view) that Packard was morally insane, and railed against the credence given her statements by the legislators.

"You are supposing from some years of the management of an important public trust, that you have some reputation for science, humanity, skill in your profession, etc., etc., throughout a state," he wrote to Edward Jarvis. "Yet here comes a crazy woman, whose influence, compared with yours, you, at first sight, think as nothing." But then, he concluded, "The whole legislative body is at the feet of a crazy woman, and you are nowhere. I have drunk at the very deepest wells of humiliation and am humiliated."[17]

State hospital superintendents were particularly at risk in "insane asylum warfare," as McFarland once termed it, because of their liability to legislative intervention. State representatives, as "guardians of the public interest," were especially sensitive to charges that a superintendent abused either state monies or patients. Even when a state hospital's trustees had investigated and dismissed charges against an asylum doctor, legislators did not hesitate to conduct their own inquiries. Being "unskilled in logrolling and subsoiling with legislators," Richard Patterson decided to leave his post at the Indiana state asylum and go into private practice. He wrote to Kirkbride in 1852, "These state institutions are horrible establishments, and no sensitive man – none but one who has the skin of a *rhinocerus* has any business in one of them." Horace Buttolph expressed similar complaints: "I have become so tired of making explanations and requests to members of the legislature that they do not heed, that I am resolved to avoid it in the future and only procure what can be had in other ways," he wrote to Kirkbride in 1859. "I really have too much important work to do, to afford to waste mind and voice upon a class of men who are so ready to sacrifice the public to political pique and interest."[18]

The legislative investigations of Charles Nichols, an influential superintendent respected by his colleagues (and a particular friend of Kirkbride's), were even more inimical to the specialty's self-image than the travails of less popular men such as Ranney and McFarland. When Nichols won appointment to the prestigious Government Hospital (now known as St. Elizabeths) in 1855, his elders in the specialty considered him among the most promising men of his generation. Dorothea Dix, as well as Kirkbride and Earle, showed him special favor. Nichols enjoyed the involvement in the capital's political and social life that came with his post, yet he eventually paid the price of this visibility.[19]

Even though Nichols developed a relatively cordial relationship with his trustees at the Government Hospital, he still found himself the target of frequent congressional scrutiny. During his twenty-year tenure at the Washington, D.C., hospital, Nichols underwent two major investigations, in 1869 and 1876, as well as numerous informal inquisitions. He was accused of a variety of crimes, from Confederate sympathies to theft of public funds. Although Nichols survived the inquiries with his professional reputation intact, the recurring controversies took a heavy toll on him personally. In 1869, waiting while the secretary of the interior reviewed his accounts, Nichols complained bitterly to Dix of the ingratitude shown toward him. The secretary would find errors in the accounts, he admitted, because the war had unsettled his administration of the asylum. "Since the war and the death of my wife," he continued, "I have had some irresistible, or not wholly resisted, propensities to delay and not to do certain things until I was absolutely compelled to, that may have occasioned some mistakes – mistakes I ought to have apprehended but did not." After six months of investigation, in a "broken and depressed condition," Nichols described himself as "struggling to surmount" his "terrible trials" and regain his confidence. He confessed to Dix, "I realize that I must not allow myself to go down any lower and if my brain does not give way I will certainly rise." Nichols finally left the Government Hospital for the Bloomingdale Asylum in 1878, after a second round of investigation, hoping to escape the intense scrutiny focused on the national asylum.[20]

Assaults on the better-liked and respected doctors reinforced the superintendents' tendency to see asylum work as a special form of martyrdom. "The good tree in the orchard of superintendents," proclaimed J. A. Reed to the long-suffering Nichols, "will be known by the number of stones and clubs found about it." After enduring his own investigation, which was sparked by a disgruntled matron, Reed wrote to Kirkbride, "the question very often comes into my mind, does it pay to give all one's time and energies in the cause of humanity, and be abused by those we serve until our characters are not worth much." Nichols perhaps best captured the profession's sense of vulnerability when he wrote to Dix: "I feel as if I was living over a volcano all the time, and cannot command the security necessary either to happiness or the highest usefulness."[21]

The pressures of mid-nineteenth-century asylum practice certainly reinforced the profession's attention to institutional detail. "Living over a volcano," as Nichols so aptly phrased it, hardly disposed a superintendent toward a bold approach to asylum medicine. To turn his mind from innovation, an imaginative asylum doctor need only be reminded of N. D. Benedict, who lost his post at the Utica Asylum because his managers viewed his medical experiments as too costly. The uncertain political climate also left little time for intellectual growth. John Curwen, struggling to produce his paper for the AMSAII's annual meeting, complained to Edward Jarvis, "My time is really so much broken up that I can scarce sit down uninterrupted an hour at a time and to write as I would like is almost an impossibility in such a state of mind." For a young doctor anxious to get ahead, Kirkbride's best advice was not to study or reflect on the nature of insanity; rather, "let him always keep his whole house and affairs in such order that the more they are *investigated* the better they will appear." Increasingly, the measure of a successful asylum practice became the ability to avoid public controversy. T. M. Franklin of the New York City Lunatic Asylum wrote to Pliny Earle in 1881, "We have been much favored...during the year in keeping out of the newspapers – for which I have been repeatedly congratulated – it being a new experience for this Institution for some few years."[22]

The superintendents perceived their job not only as politically perilous but also as personally threatening. That the strains of asylum work took a heavy toll on the superintendents' physical and mental health seemed evident from their personal histories. In fact, the brethren took a grim satisfaction in recounting the illnesses that plagued them. Samuel Woodward and Amariah Brigham were both considered victims of their zealous, self-denying labors. A number of superintendents, among them Luther Bell and Isaac Ray, retired early from asylum work for health reasons. Bell, returning to manage the McLean Hospital for a short time after his successor's health failed, confided to Pliny Earle, "no human inducement could tempt me to re-engage permanently in duties so onerous. I am amazed to think I ever stood them for twenty years. I do not allude to the physical labor, for I do not feel *that*, but the sense of responsibility and anxiety."[23]

An additional threat to physical well-being was patient violence. After being shot by Wiley Williams, Kirkbride received letters from other asylum doctors recounting their own exposure to physical danger. "Twice within four years my life has been in jeopardy from deadly weapons in the hands of infuriated madmen," James Bates of the Maine Asylum claimed. In subsequent years, several well-known doctors, including George Cook and John Gray, were killed in the line of duty. Referring to the violence against asylum doctors, D. T. Brown found it appropriate to extend Nichols's volcano metaphor: "Truly we live among assassins, as well as on volcanoes," he wrote to Kirkbride in 1858.[24]

Sadly, in a few cases, superintendents fell victim to the very mental disorders they sought to cure. In the mid-1860s, Merrick Bemis, superintendent of the Worcester Hospital, became so debilitated by depression that he could no longer work. Considering Kirkbride to be one of "his few really true friends," he asked to be admitted to the Pennsylvania Hospital for the Insane. "Now that he is suffering he feels that you will have a sort of fatherly care over him and that you can help him if anybody can," Bemis's wife wrote to Kirkbride. Edward Jarvis, a trustee of the Worcester Hospital, wrote several months later, "You are right in charging his failure of health to overwork. . . . We imposed too great a burden on him." Eventually, Bemis recovered and returned to work. In less fortunate circumstances, Andrew McFarland and D. T. Brown committed suicide after resigning their superintendent posts. Although their reasons for suicides were undoubtedly complex, the brethren, not unnaturally, saw the pressures of asylum practice as the major cause. Brown's death had particularly tragic overtones. After a decade of anxiety over newspaper exposés and family illnesses, Brown resigned from the Bloomingdale Asylum in 1877, stating that his own health had become impaired. After seeking treatment in several institutions, including the Royal Edinburgh Asylum, Brown retired to a farm in Illinois. In August 1889, a reporter for the *New York World* learned of the former superintendent's whereabouts and published a remarkably insensitive account of Brown's mental breakdown. Less than two weeks later, he hung himself.[25]

One cannot help but see the tragedies of mid-nineteenth-century asylum practice as the inevitable price the superintendents paid for their own ambitions. Granted, theirs was a very demanding job, even allowing for the superintendents' natural tendency to exaggerate their tribulations so as to reinforce their claims to an altruism unsullied by professional self-interest. But in subjecting themselves to such an ordeal, asylum doctors surely got no more than they asked for. Having sought unlimited institutional power, they paid for their gains in the currency of overwork, ill health, and political harassment. Not unlike the southern slaveholder's regime, asylum paternalism depended upon an absolute authority impossible to maintain in practice.[26]

Yet, the superintendents' concept of asylum paternalism had strong reinforcement from a very influential source: their patrons. Although attendants and legislators might characterize the asylum doctor's power as tyrannical, the patients' families more often than not regarded his assumption of authority as providential. As their letters to Kirkbride reveal, the patrons' expectations of hospital treatment revolved around the belief that the superintendent would exercise a degree of control over the insane that the family had failed to provide at home. The aspects of asylum care that patrons prized most – the moderation of symptoms, the preservation of privacy, the quality of surveillance – seemed directly dependent upon the chief physician's control over the asylum milieu. If he appeared to be a weak figure, unable to shape the building and staff in his own image, the patrons' confidence in him might well have been shaken.

With their patrons in mind, superintendents advanced their claim to one-man rule without believing that they acted out of a narrow professional self-interest. For them, the autonomy issue became fused with the needs of the patients and their families. To meet the patrons' expectations, so the doctors argued, the superintendent had to have complete control over the asylum, so as to make it a persuasive institution. Kirkbride's peculiar facility with this line of argument no doubt greatly contributed to his durability as a professional leader. More eloquently than any of his peers, Kirkbride rationalized the superintendent's institutional power in terms of the family's interests: In so many words, he professed to show that what was good for the asylum doctor was good for the asylum patron.

Although in public forums Kirkbride and his associates stressed the humanitarian impulse of their professional agenda, they were hardly oblivious to its personal benefits. In a very emotional way, the brethren came to look upon institutional autonomy as the only just reward for living on top of the volcano. If good men were to enter and remain in the specialty, they had to be assured certain prerequisites essential to professional esteem, chief among them an impressive, well-organized hospital and a manageable number of patients who were varied in both social and mental condition. Few doctors could serve well, the brethren argued, when forced to work in decrepit hospitals filled with only paupers and the incurable insane. Unless a superintendent could identify with both his institution and his clientele, he would never withstand the stress of asylum practice. Thus, the maintenance of favorable working conditions depended almost entirely upon the chief physician's ability to control such matters as asylum expenditures, staffing, and admission policies.

THE DEBATE OVER HOSPITAL DESIGN

Thus, from their shared asylum experience grew the AMSAII's resolute insistence upon a unitary plan of hospital construction and management. Kirkbride's propositions constituted not a set of architectural fixations (as their critics often maintained) but rather a manifesto of hospital efficacy and physician autonomy. The limits set on the asylum's size, the stipulation that both curable and chronic patients be treated in the same institution, the insistence upon the superintendent's undivided authority – these were measures the brethren viewed as essential to their successful execution of asylum practice. In other words, the propositions were the best defense the superintendents could muster in the "insane asylum warfare" that plagued them.[27]

But increasingly, state hospital superintendents found it difficult to maintain the AMSAII's standards of asylum practice. Kirkbride had formulated the propositions in an era when conditions in corporate and state hospitals were not radically different. But in the next two decades, a marked disparity between private and state care began to develop. The accumulation of the chronic pauper insane in almshouses and jails, as well as state mental hospitals, combined with rising costs of operation to force asylum doctors in private and state institutions to pursue very different strategies of survival. Corporate hospitals such as the Pennsylvania Hospital for the Insane raised their board rates, reduced the number of free patients, and solicited charitable donations. Limited in their ability to pursue similar options, state hospitals slowly filled up with chronic patients and experienced severe financial difficulties. As conditions in state and corporate institutions diverged more and more dramatically, the superintendents' support for Kirkbride's asylum philosophy slowly began to erode.[28]

Officially, the superintendent's association refused to condone the growing disparity between the different forms of hospital provision for the insane. In this stance, the American doctors differed from their English colleagues, who by this time had organized their profession much more explicitly along public versus private lines and accepted class-specific forms of architecture and management.[29] In contrast, although the Americans acknowledged that the men in state employ had fewer financial resources and less administrative freedom than their peers in corporate hospitals, they stubbornly refused to recognize that a different set of standards should apply to public hospitals. State asylums need not be as elegant or luxurious as private hospitals, the professional leadership argued, but in design, administration, and regimen, the public institution should be a faithful replica of its private counterpart. The AMSAII militantly resisted any suggestion that American hospital design diverge along clear-cut class lines, either by the introduction of private madhouses for the elite or separate public facilities for the indigent.

The congruence the early superintendents expected to see between corporate and public institutions reflected their assumption that both types of hospitals would have a mixed clientele. The early asylum's architecture and regimen were explicitly designed with this proposition in mind. Isaac Ray explained to a Butler Hospital trustee in 1844, "the form of construction ought to have reference to the character of the patients, the manner of conducting the service, etc." An institution for paupers did not need the arrangements that would be "indispensable," in Ray's words, in a hospital designed for "persons in affluent circumstances or a mixture of both." The mixed plan, he concluded, had much to recommend it: "This union of rich and poor... affords much greater advantages to the latter, than an institution adapted alone for them could do, and with fewer disadvantages, under a proper method and facilities of classification than would perhaps be expected." The ideal mental hospital, the early asylum doctors believed, should definitely be mixed in character. Superintendents liked Kirkbride's linear plan precisely because it could accommodate a patient population heterogeneous in both mental and social condition with a relatively confined space. Similarly, the specialty never sought to obliterate class distinctions in the asylum regimen, but rather expected many aspects of care, such as accommodations and amusements, to correspond to differential board rates.[30]

Thus, the Kirkbride plan and its variants represented the specialty's conviction that the mental hospital, whether corporate or public in funding, should serve a varied constituency. By offering the same basic treatment, if not exactly the same accommodations, to all who desired it, the asylum appropriately reflected the classless nature of American society as the superintendents viewed it: classless in the sense that it provided equality of opportunity rather than equality of condition. In espousing such a viewpoint, the early superintendents did no more than express, in institutional terms, the dominant social philosophy of the mid-nineteenth century, which widely asserted that equality of opportunity made America an open and just society.[31]

Dissidents within the association

Increasingly, some physicians began to question the wisdom of the AMSAII's stance, however. Given the vast numbers of the indigent insane still languishing in almshouses and jails, they saw a need for some form of institutional provision between an almshouse and a regular hospital. The Kirkbride plan, the dissidents argued, simply necessitated too great an outlay of funds; legislatures would not build enough hospitals of such advanced design for all the state's insane. Less expensive alternatives had to be found for the sake of the indigent and incurable. So, Kirkbride's critics argued, economy had to become the chief imperative of hospital construction.

The first superintendent to criticize the Kirkbride plan openly was John Galt, superintendent of the Eastern State Lunatic Asylum and a member of the original thirteen. In 1855, Galt published an article in the *American Journal of Insanity*, "The Farm of St. Anne," which openly criticized the AMSAII's leadership for their preoccupation with asylum design. Although Galt mentioned no one by name, his remarks were clearly directed at Kirkbride, Bell, and Ray, among others. So long, wrote Galt, as "those entrusted with the supervision of the insane, and particularly those at the head of the most richly endowed asylums, shall deem the true interests of their afflicted charges not to consist in aught on their part but tinkering gas-pipes and studying architecture, in order merely to erect costly and at the same time most unsightly edifices . . . so long may we anticipate no advancement in the treatment of insanity as far as the United States is concerned." For all the money they spent on design, Galt continued, the American superintendents had produced dysfunctional buildings, whose prisonlike features belied their therapeutic function. As an alternative model, he proposed the farm colony of Gheel, where the chronic insane lived in ordinary cottages and worked among the villagers. Instead of "tinkering," Galt concluded, his countrymen might better devote their energies to implementing the principles of employment and nonrestraint in American hospitals.[32]

"The Farm of St. Anne" aroused considerable indignation among the brethren, who condemned the journal's editor, John Gray, for even publishing Galt's "wholesale slanders," as D. T. Brown characterized the piece. At the next AMSAII meeting, Brown took the floor specifically to defend Kirkbride's reputation "as one of the most pertinacious 'tinkerers of gas pipes.' " If the Philadelphia superintendent's interest in asylum design was so misguided, Brown asked rhetorically, how had the Pennsylvania Hospital for the Insane become such a model institution? From a recent number of the *American Journal of Medical Science*, Brown quoted Pliny Earle's homage to Kirkbride: "The hospital under his superintendence already approximates so near to perfection, that there is some danger of his becoming the Alexander of his sphere, and weeping that there are no more realms to conquer." In the ensuing discussion, Galt was roundly condemned, although a few members ventured to suggest that the specialty might benefit by some healthy criticism. At the time, the clashes of opinion underlying the Galt controversies seemed to set northern against southern doctors, and the "Utica Gang" against the rest of the brethren. (Kirkbride's allies accused Gray of doctoring the transcript of the debate, so as to make it seem more critical of the tinkerers than it actually was.) In retrospect, Galt's critique seems even more noteworthy as the first open questioning of the AMSAII's allegiance to Kirkbride's asylum philosophy.[33]

In the 1860s, Galt's iconoclasm was taken up by other, younger physicians who felt dissatisfied with the specialty's propositions concerning hospital construction and design. Chief among those breaking with the asylum orthodoxy were John B. Chapin and George Cook, the proprietors of Brigham Hall, a small private asylum in upstate New York; Edward Jarvis, a Massachusetts physician who boarded a small number of insane patients in his home and played an active part in asylum affairs; and Merrick Bemis of the Worcester State Hospital.[34] Of the dissident group, the men running private homes criticized the AMSAII most vehemently, undoubtedly because they lacked the shared bond of institutional experience that inclined the superintendents toward Kirkbride's viewpoints.

Like John Galt, the younger generation of critics considered American asylums to be too expensive as well as ill-adapted for treating the different forms of insanity. The chronically ill did not need the impressive bulk or the means for constant observation built into the Kirkbride plan. As George Cook wrote in 1866, the propositions "look only to the erection of small hospitals, and the organization is mainly adapted to the treatment of recent cases." Although the linear plan had been appropriate for the era in which it was developed, Cook argued, "the intervening years have wrought many changes," particularly an increased number of chronic patients and pressures of overcrowding, which necessitated new strategies in hospital design. The dissidents also objected to the prisonlike features and overreliance on restraint they considered typical of American hospitals. The asylum's forbidding mass and barely concealed means of confinement created a fearful penal milieu hardly conducive to cure.[35]

To remedy the deficiencies of the linear plan and the oppressive regimen associated with it, the AMSAII's critics proposed to import certain features of European asylum design: the cottage or farm colony plan for poor chronic patients; extensive employment programs for public hospitals; the nonrestraint system advocated by the English physician, John Conolly; and small private "homes" or asylums for convalescent patients, especially the wealthy or refined. Taken together, these innovations would produce a more effective and economical system of asylum care. Farm colonies for incurable paupers would be inexpensive to build, and the proceeds of systematic patient labor would keep the costs of maintenance low. Living in a more domestic setting and working regularly, the chronic patients would become more manageable, thereby allowing the abandonment of mechanical restraint. Cottage residences would also benefit the more refined convalescent patients. Such small, detached units could easily be combined with existing hospital buildings to form a more eclectic style of architecture. Recognizing his colleagues' entrenched hostility to private asylums, Edward Jarvis proposed that convalescent homes be built on the grounds of the big hospitals, out of sight of the main building but under the superintendent's direct supervision. As a similar compromise, some reformers argued that farm colonies for the chronic insane could be built in conjunction with already established public institutions, reserving the regular hospital building for the curable patients.

Between 1865 and 1875, a few institutions actually implemented some of these new ideas about asylum design. In 1865, Merrick Bemis, whose Worcester State Hospital was sorely troubled by overcrowding, convinced his trustees to purchase a few cottages adjacent to the hospital for the use of convalescent, chronic, and paying patients. Over the next few years, the Worcester superintendent tried to win support for an even more ambitious plan to replace the old asylum building with an extensive cottage hospital. In 1865, Cook and Chapin convinced the New York State legislature to appropriate funds for an institution for incurables with the capacity to house 1,500 patients. As members of the planning commission, the two doctors worked to have the new Willard Asylum built as a farm colony. Even such stalwarts as Andrew McFarland and D. T. Brown considered the cottage plan for their own institutions in the late 1860s.[36]

These radical departures from the established propositions touched off a controversy within the AMSAII. After a heated debate in 1866, the membership voted on an additional set of propositions to combat the Worcester and Willard heresies. The new guidelines affirmed the majority's viewpoint that state provision for the insane had to follow the established Kirkbride plan. Overcrowding should not be solved by building separate institutions for the chronic insane, but rather by creating a district system of mixed hospitals, that is, one with facilities for curable and chronic patients, built along the usual lines. The superintendents strongly condemned any plan to separate the two classes of the insane. As a concession to the overcrowding problem, the AMSAII did agree (but only by a narrow majority) to raise the approved size of mental hospitals from 250 to 600 patients.[37]

In addition to the AMSAII's public declaration of faith in Kirk-bride's propositions, the most influential of the brethren used their political power to discourage experimentation in hospital design. In 1873, Pliny Earle, among others, convinced the Massachusetts legislature to reject Merrick Bemis's cottage plan; Bemis left the Worcester State Hospital soon afterward. Kirkbride persuaded D. T. Brown to have the new Bloomingdale Asylum constructed like the Pennsylvania Hospital for the Insane, with a linear building for each sex. In New York State, John P. Gray failed to scuttle the plan for a chronic facility, but succeeded in having the new Willard Asylum scaled down to the approved 600-patient limit and designed in the usual linear style, much to Chapin's and Cook's disgust. The Willard conflict took on a particularly personal tone, with both parties openly accusing one another of corrupt politicking.[38]

Although the orthodox superintendents appeared to be winning the battle over "congregate" versus "separate" design, as the linear and cottage plans came to be known, controversy still plagued the AMSAII. The "growing disposition to wander off from the true faith," as Kirkbride termed it, could not be so easily contained. At the AMSAII's yearly meetings, the interrelated issues of chronic care, employment, restraint, and hospital design continued to cause conflict. Throughout the continuing debate, Ray and Kirkbride, the most influential of the older superintendents, spoke with one voice to condemn any deviation from the linear plan, including the compromise scheme of combining cottages with regular hospitals. As the two doctors frequently reminded their brethren, Kirkbride had tried the cottage experiment in the 1840s and found it wanting on the grounds of insufficient supervision. The elder statesmen of the profession also argued that American patients were too violent to be placed under the nonrestraint system and too fractious to be regularly employed. In a more moderate way, most of the other superintendents, including Gray, Earle, Nichols, and Brown, leaned toward a more eclectic style of architecture and felt that both rigorous employment and the nonrestraint system had much merit. They also tended to think that the American state hospitals had been too closely influenced by practice in the corporate institutions. Earle wrote to Jarvis in 1860, "We are looking too much toward *comfort*, and too little toward labor; we are running after luxury, and away from work." Yet, at the same time, the moderate superintendents as a group backed Ray and

Kirkbride on the two most important propositions under attack: that chronic and curable patients be treated in the same institution, and that hospitals remain relatively small in size.[39]

In defending the AMSAII's consensus on these last two points, the superintendents repeatedly referred to the lessons of asylum practice. The proposed departures from the linear plan, they insisted, would only add to the already overwhelming problems of asylum practice. Six hundred patients represented the maximum that one doctor and his assistants could care for properly; given any more to attend to, the doctor would lose the ability to detect and encourage the subtle changes in behavior that often preceded recovery. Detached buildings would further complicate the chore of surveillance; the cottage plan necessarily placed more responsibility on attendants, a group in which the superintendents had little confidence. As a result, escapes, suicides, and accidents would increase under the segregate system. Likewise, separate facilities for incurables would lead to greater neglect and abuse. Inevitably, the best-intentioned physician would lower his standards in such an institution. Without the influence of a therapeutic regimen and the beneficent company of curable patients, chronic patients would descend to an inhuman condition. Moreover, the orthodox superintendents did not see how chronic care could be made any more economical than that provided by a regular hospital without sacrificing essential prerequisites of humane treatment. "Why they have got to have the same amount of air, – fresh air, I mean and warmth, – the same amount of clothing and the same amount of food. How then are you to keep them cheaper?" asked Kirkbride rhetorically. True economy, his friend Isaac Ray agreed, consisted of the hospital design that brought all the residents of the institution "within the smallest possible compass." The linear plan worked best, Ray concluded, because "the nearer our patients are to us, the better we can look after and see them, and with the greater facility we can supervise all their actions."[40]

The orthodox superintendents also invoked the family's expectations of asylum treatment in their defense of Kirkbride's propositions. Facilities for the chronic insane, they argued, would be acceptable only for paupers, who had no relatives to visit or care for them. No family, however impoverished, would consent willingly to see a loved one consigned to such a hopeless, demeaning institutional fate. Similarly, the diminution of privacy, restraint, and supervision associated with the cottage plan ran contrary to the patrons' wishes. D. T. Brown wrote of the Gheel plan that it negated the principles of "family guardianship" underlying American asylum practice. It could not be replicated in the United States, he concluded, because the "friends of patients exact *individual* responsibility in the guardians of their patients, and would hardly be satisfied to have them run about loose through a whole town or neighborhood." Similarly, Kirkbride criticized the nonrestraint system on the grounds that it would mean "mixing up all colors and all classes," a situation he was sure his asylum patrons would find repugnant.[41]

At the same time that the older superintendents objected to the segregate plan's lack of structure, they also condemned it as representing an unacceptable degree of class differentiation. Whereas the linear plan accommodated all classes in one uniform building, the segregate plan placed the very rich and the very poor in separate facilities. As such, the latter scheme threatened the ideal of the mixed, or classless, institution that had for so long guided American asylum medicine. To the older doctors, the innovations proposed by the dissidents smacked of the rigid class distinctions and intractable poverty characteristic of European society. D. T. Brown wrote of Chapin's cottage scheme for Willard, the "theory and spirit [of the Ovid plan] are opposed to the inclinations and social usages of our people." In essence, separate facilities for the chronic insane implied acceptance of a stratified society with a permanent pauper class, a development few Americans of Kirkbride's generation wished to accept.[42]

In sum, the proposed innovations in asylum design seemed too much like a retrogression to eighteenth-century institutional standards. Having worked for more than a century to differentiate the asylum from the poorhouse, medical men could hardly muster enthusiasm for any sort of mental institution designed exclusively to serve an almshouse clientele. If built only with economy in mind, to the neglect of its therapeutic features, "a hospital will lose those distinctive traits that mark the difference between a hospital and a poorhouse," wrote Ray to Dix in 1851. "The public must be taught that an insane hospital receiving patients at pauper prices can necessarily be but little better than a poor house."[43]

Had the Young Turks within the association remained the only critics of the linear plan, Kirkbride and Ray's defense of the asylum orthodoxy might have stilled their dissent, at least for a time. But in the late 1860s and 1870s, two groups arising outside the specialty and laying claim to expertise on insanity adopted a highly critical stance toward the old-line superintendents: the state boards of charity and the neurologists. These new experts combined forces with the dissident superintendents to wage a concerted and eventually successful campaign to repudiate the linear plan and the asylum philosophy associated with it.

The state boards of charities and the neurologists

The State Board of Charities, first adopted in 1863 in Massachusetts and speedily copied throughout the country, developed as a means to coordinate the state's increasingly large expenditures on welfare subsidies and institutions. As appointees of the governor, the Board of Charities undertook the supervision of public institutions, including almshouses, orphanages, asylums for the blind and feebleminded, prisons, and state mental hospitals. An agent hired by the board visited the facilities and prepared an annual report on their condition. Not surprisingly, the board's members viewed the state asylum as but one component of an extensive welfare system serving the indigent poor, a viewpoint that conflicted with the older superintendents' desire to distance the asylum from the poorhouse. Within a few years of its foundation, the State Board of Charities had emerged as a highly vocal opponent of the superintendents' administrative policies and popularized the argument that regular hospitals cost too much money to build and operate.[44]

The neurologists, who entered asylum politics at about the same time, criticized the asylum from a scientific rather than an administrative perspective. Their medical specialty, which first developed in the 1860s and grew rapidly in the 1870s, was modeled self-consciously on the new clinical medicine being practiced in Germany. Neurologists studied the pathology of the nervous system and its role in causing mental disease with new instruments, as enumerated by Edouard Séquin in 1876: "clinical study, pathological anatomy, anatomical investigation and physiological experimentation." Although on the whole pessimistic about insanity's curability, neurologists did a brisk office trade in treating mild or incipient forms of mental disease with diet, tonics, electricity, and bed rest.[45]

Like the State Boards of Charities, the neurologists developed a thorough and sometimes savage critique of the old-fashioned superintendents such as Kirkbride, accusing them of a variety of crimes. In the first place, such superintendents did no clinical research and therefore had no real scientific knowledge, as far as the neurologists could see. Their much-vaunted asylum experience consisted of no more than the "contemplation of belittling routine duties," as Edward C. Spitzka, a noted neurologist, wrote. Their cherished hospital plan was not only expensive but ill suited to the complex nature of mental disease. The AMSAII, the neurologists concluded, had become a monopoly of narrow-minded old men out of touch with scientific medicine and modern welfare practices. It was time that the superintendents allowed those with real expertise to exploit the rich clinical materials housed in the nation's mental institutions and produce some real scientific research on insanity.[46]

As their critique of the asylum superintendents evolved, both the Boards of Charities and the neurologists adopted an argument being made in yet another context, the crusade against asylum abuses. Throughout the 1870s, the indefatigable Elizabeth Packard continued her efforts to reform commitment laws. In Illinois, Rhode Island, and Massachusetts, Packard forced legislative consideration of such measures as jury trials before commitment; circulars posted in hospitals, apprising patients of their legal rights; mailboxes in the wards; and inspections by outside authorities. In Iowa and Illinois, legislatures actually enacted so-called Packard laws. Even Congress considered a national version of her bill in 1875, much to the superintendents' distress, but eventually rejected it. In addition to Packard's autobiographical exposés, which she sold as part of her reform effort, several other popular books pressed the issue of patient abuse. Charles Reade's novel *Hard Cash* detailed in highly melodramatic form the sufferings of an honest young man incarcerated in a series of lunatic asylums by his corrupt father. Less famous, but still widely read, was the anonymous autobiographical account of a former woman patient entitled *Behind the Bars*, which, like Packard's books, made a strong argument for asylum reform.[47]

The clamor over patient abuse not only spread public distrust of asylum doctors but furnished their most influential critics, the neurologists and charities, with more ammunition. Many long-standing patient complaints about restraint, the monotony of hospital life, and attendants' violence were taken up by these groups as part of their critique of American asylum medicine. To prevent patient abuse, along with economic mismanagement, the asylum critics began to campaign for the adoption of a commission system, such as had been established in England in 1845. They reasoned that only by giving a governmental agency "having as an essential characteristic, an interest antagonistic to that of the Trustees," as well as the asylum superintendent, the power to examine and license *all* mental hospitals, including private and corporate ones, could the evils of American asylum medicine be rectified.[48]

Until the late 1870s, the AMSAII's inner circle presented a united front to its increasingly vociferous critics. In particular, the extremely close friendship between Kirkbride and Ray, perhaps the two most influential men in the specialty, made the asylum monopoly appear unbreachable.[49] But changes in the AMSAII membership itself eventually brought about an end to their control of the specialty. The early association's policies had reflected the numerical balance of private and state hospital men, as well as their relative similarity in institutional interests; the original thirteen included the heads of seven municipal or state hospitals, four corporate institutions, and two small private asylums. But after the 1840s, few corporate hospitals were built, whereas the state hospital system expanded rapidly; by the 1870s, Kirkbride and Ray found themselves at the head of an organization composed largely of doctors in the state's employ. And increasingly, as conditions in public institutions diverged dramatically from those in asylums such as the Pennsylvania Hospital for the Insane, innovation became more and more compelling. It is in fact rather remarkable that the influence of the corporate hospital men lasted so long; in relation to their numbers, they played a disproportionately important role in the AMSAII's affairs throughout the 1870s.

The illusion of solidarity finally shattered in 1877 with the public defection of Pliny Earle to the heretics. Earle, a member of the original thirteen, whose professional writings and activities had gained widespread respect, especially among the iconoclasts, had in fact long been a doubter on some points of asylum orthodoxy. But not until 1877 did the Northampton superintendent take a public stand against his old friend Kirkbride. Earle's *Annual Report* for that year contained a strongly worded, statistic-laden argument against the central supposition of moral treatment: the belief in insanity's curability. Using the published tables available in every asylum's annual reports, Earle argued that the superintendents inflated the cure rate by counting periodic recoveries as cures. A patient repeatedly readmitted to the hospital would be released each time as cured, thereby deceptively increasing the institution's apparent success. Earle also claimed that pioneer doctors such as Samuel Woodward had deliberately overemphasized the positive prognosis for mental disease so as to build public support for asylum medicine. Not only had the cure rate never been as high as the first enthusiasts asserted, it had also declined precipitously over the last forty years. In light of these facts, Earle concluded, the nature of state provision for the indigent insane had to be completely reevaluated.[50]

After publication of his 1877 *Report*, Pliny Earle became a rallying point for the anti-AMSAII forces. His statements were widely publicized as proof that the cast-iron creed of the other superintendents was illusory. John Chapin congratulated Earle for his courage, averring, "it has been a wonder to me that members of the profession have not spoken as plainly before as you have done in your Report last issued." Other dissident superintendents, members of the state boards, and neurologists praised Earle's "unsparing exposure" of the "traditional and deceptive modes of reporting recoveries" that had been used to make insanity seem curable. The "river God" Woodward, wrote one of Earle's admirers, had been dethroned. In sum, the professional credibility of Kirkbride and his supporters had been severely damaged by one of their own brethren. Referring to Kirkbride's 1875 *Report*, a New Jersey doctor wrote to Earle, "I am sure you are right about the question of the curability of insanity, but your views are not the *expressed* ones of asylum specialists." In light of Earle's findings, he concluded, "it becomes an important social problem, whether the large and costly modern asylum is not a mistake if four-fifths of the insane are incurable."[51]

Ray and Kirkbride struggled to refute Earle's heresies, but with little success. Ray tried to explain the statistical trend in terms of the changing patient population and the natural aging of institutions, but he ultimately admitted that the disease itself appeared to have become more intractable. Kirkbride never publicly or privately wavered in his conviction that insanity might be cured if quickly and properly treated. No doubt his wife's case history strengthened his personal commitment to the curability doctrine. Both men were now in their seventies, and although their faith in moral treatment was undiminished, their physical and mental capacity to defend it had weakened.[52]

But it was not its adherents' old age or internal discord that finally discredited moral treatment. Rather, the obvious failure of the state mental hospital to replicate the therapeutic success of its corporate model diminished the persuasiveness of Kirkbride's asylum philosophy. The internal failures of asylum practice greatly hastened the curtailment of the superintendent's autonomy, the increase in state control over hospital management, and the establishment of a custodial standard of institutional care for the state hospital. Given the scale of economic and social change in the late nineteenth century, the growing extremes of poverty and wealth, the rationalization of welfare policies, and the pace of changing medical ideas, the rejection of moral treatment was no doubt inevitable. Yet, for all the abstract, complex forces at work against it, the demise of the old-style asylum medicine involved a very personal dimension of conflict.

THE DECLINE OF THE MIXED STATE HOSPITAL

The convergence between the internal problems and external critiques of moral treatment is amply illustrated in the asylum politics of Pennsylvania, Kirkbride's home state. In particular, the career of John Curwen, Kirkbride's most successful protégé, illustrates the way in which the demise of moral treatment was bound up with the decline of the state hospital. Curwen's superintendency at the State Lunatic Asylum at Harrisburg forms a natural comparison with Kirkbride's asylum practice due to the strong personal and professional ties between the two men and their hospitals. The contrast between their careers not only throws into relief the growing dichotomy between practices in corporate and public hospitals but also illuminates the changing dynamics of asylum politics in the 1870s and 1880s.

In 1838 and again in 1841, reformers petitioned the Pennsylvania state legislature to build a public asylum for the indigent insane.

Their efforts formed but one part of a nationwide movement aimed at creating a "widening circle of benevolence" for all dependent groups, including criminal, orphaned, aged, disabled, and impoverished citizens. The public insane asylum appealed to lay reformers in Pennsylvania, as well as other heavily populated states, on the grounds that it promised to be both humane and economical. In their appeals to the legislators, especially those written by Dorothea Dix, reformers emphasized the providential fit between the value of work in the moral treatment of insanity and the asylum's capacity to finance itself. While curing themselves by labor, the inmates would maintain the hospital and thus relieve the state of the burden of their support.[53]

Although Kirkbride played no part in the initial legislative campaign to establish a public asylum, which finally succeeded in 1845, he soon came to have an important role in shaping the new institution, first as a member of its building committee and then as a trustee for more than eleven years. Kirkbride's influence was further amplified by the appointment of John Curwen, his old assistant physician, as the first superintendent of the state hospital. (Curwen served his asylum apprenticeship at the Pennsylvania Hospital for the Insane from 1844 to 1849; see Chapter 4.) With Kirkbride's assistance, he won the highly coveted Harrisburg post over the claims of some well-qualified competitors, including H. A. Buttolph and Charles Nichols. Curwen and Kirkbride remained close personal friends and professional colleagues until the latter's death in 1883. The several hundred letters Curwen wrote to Kirkbride between 1849 and 1883 reveal the extent to which the younger man continued to rely on his elder's advice and attempted to follow the philosophy of hospital management he had first learned at the Pennsylvania Hospital for the Insane.[54]

Both Kirkbride and Curwen hoped to model the Pennsylvania State Lunatic Asylum as closely as possible on the already successful Philadelphia institution. Despite its growing affluence, the Pennsylvania Hospital for the Insane in the 1840s was a prototype of the public mental hospital. The asylum remained closely identified with the Pennsylvania Hospital's long tradition of caring for the worthy poor. The only other available model for a public hospital was the almshouse, and needless to say, physicians had no intention of allowing its undesirable features to be duplicated in the new state asylum. Rather, as the superintendents envisioned it, the Pennsylvania State Lunatic Asylum was to be a scaled-down version, in both architectural plan and clientele, of the corporate hospital. Although clearly not intended for the well-to-do, the public asylum would serve families of moderate means who could not afford the higher rates of the private institution. It would also provide chronic care for the indigent, who could "nowhere be properly taken care of at less cost," according to Kirkbride.[55]

Although John Curwen shared Kirkbride's vision of a multi-class, multipurpose state hospital, he found that concept very difficult to implement. His administration at the Harrisburg hospital was plagued by the basic problems all state superintendents faced in their practice of moral treatment: insufficient resources, accumulation of chronic patients, and constant political problems with trustees and legislators. Curwen's career is particularly significant because of his close relationship to Kirkbride and their cooperation as political lobbyists in Pennsylvania. Not only were Kirkbride's formulations concerning the state hospital profoundly influenced by his connection with the Pennsylvania State Lunatic Asylum; the failure of Curwen's mixed state asylum to replicate the administrative success of its corporate model contributed to the overall decline of Kirkbride's professional influence.

Curwen's problems in asylum practice

Curwen's asylum practice foundered on precisely the points Kirkbride emphasized in his prescriptive writings. The original building of the Harrisburg hospital was so poorly constructed that in order to make it habitable, Curwen was forced to ask for huge sums from the legislature. In 1854, only three years after its opening, the state legislature demanded a review of Curwen's accounts. He was eventually cleared, but for a time his problems were the talk of the profession. "Do you know how much the changes Curwen has been obliged to make, on account of the ignorance and interest of the architect, have cost?" inquired Charles Nichols of Dorothea Dix.[56]

In addition, Curwen had endless trouble with his trustees, for the most part political appointees who viewed the asylum as a partisan property. They rarely visited the hospital, yet were willing endlessly and rancorously to debate over details of Curwen's management, whether the amount of a food bill or the placement of an outhouse. The hospital's proximity to the capital made its affairs a staple of Harrisburg gossip. Curwen told Dix that he had to have the books she donated to the asylum bound in Philadelphia, for if it were done locally, it "may be the cause of a great deal of unnecessary talk among those who in this town know more about our business than we do ourselves." Inevitably, the asylum's proximity to the state legislature made it a convenient target for partisan attacks; the party out of power found the institution a convenient source of ammunition with which to attack the reigning administration.[57]

Unfortunately, continual financial problems made Curwen a convenient target for attack. Already vexed by the huge appropriations needed to repair the original building, the Harrisburg superintendent had great difficulty collecting the money due him from the local poor law authorities. Many townships and counties sent their indigent lunatics to the Harrisburg asylum, yet failed to pay the agreed-upon board rates. Up to a point, Curwen had sympathy with the local officials, who in many sparsely populated areas of the state had trouble collecting the poor tax used to support the insane in the asylum. But eventually, his chronic inability to pay the hospital's expenses forced the superintendent to go to court to secure the back payments. After a legal settlement in 1861, the hospital's financial condition improved, but the cost of supporting the indigent poor remained a constant drain on its resources.[58]

Only one administrative expedient kept the Pennsylvania State Lunatic Asylum from depending on state appropriations for all its expenses: Curwen's practice of admitting paying patients. In the early 1860s, inmates contributing some portion of their board comprised about half of the asylum's clientele; by the early 1870s, it was almost 60 percent. Although they generally paid board rates substantially below the actual cost of support (and much lower than those Kirkbride charged at the Pennsylvania Hospital for the Insane), the state hospital's patrons of moderate means still were Curwen's only dependable source of revenue. They provided other sources of satisfaction as well, for the paying patients tended to be more recent, promising ones than the indigent lunatics sent by the local authorities. As Curwen remarked to Kirkbride, it was unfair to expect anyone, even a physician, to show as much interest in "those who are to all human appearance incurable as in those who are keeping his mind active by changes and improvements from day to day." Thus, the superintendent could not help but be partial to his more affluent clients for professional as well as financial reasons.[59]

Still, even with the revenues generated by its paying patients, the Pennsylvania State Lunatic Asylum could hardly begin to support itself, as its original supporters had promised. Instead, every year Curwen found himself compelled to ask the legislature for some $10,000 to $20,000 in appropriations, an astronomical sum by mid-nineteenth-century standards of state spending.[60] Not surprisingly, the legislators grew increasingly indignant about these repeated requests and demanded to know why the asylum was costing the state so much money. Believing that the asylum had ample funds to support itself, they could only conclude that its superintendent was either incompetent or dishonest. Although frequent investigations of the Harrisburg hospital's management never revealed any wastefulness on Curwen's part, the same charges of extravagance surfaced year after year, especially among the representatives "fresh from the ranks of the people." The mere repetition of suspicions, however unfounded, spread the conviction that there was "something rotten out there," as one legislator said of the hospital. Although not himself familiar with the asylum, he knew that it had been "an object of suspicion" for years. "As the same charges have been repeated year after year, I have begun to entertain some suspicions myself," he stated.[61]

Significantly, in their frequent criticisms of Curwen's asylum practice, legislators rarely mentioned the quality of medical care he provided. Even his detractors consistently described him as a man of the highest medical character. Occasionally, individual legislators brought up cases of alleged patient abuse at the Harrisburg asylum, but their accusations roused little response from their colleagues. It was Curwen's appropriations requests, not his standards of patient care, that furnished the evidence that he lacked administrative ability. If anything, legislators felt that the doctor concerned himself *too* much with the welfare of his patients. Impressive buildings and commodious accommodations struck them as extravagant indulgences for a state institution. One legislator quipped that with all the money Curwen spent for furniture, he would soon have "a very grand building" with "very little room for its inmates." Legislators persistently complained about the patient amusements, which were purchased with private donations, as if they represented a wasteful expenditure of public money.

Such a "willful perversion of truth," as Curwen indignantly termed it, led one senator to vote against the asylum appropriations because "they take the money to build ten pin alleys with."[62]

Ironically, Curwen's failure to convince the legislature of his managerial ability eventually jeopardized the one sure source of income he possessed, the asylum's paying patients. If the state had to pay out huge sums to support the asylum, legislative critics concluded, the least the institution could do was to receive all the state's indigent lunatics. As it was, they claimed, Curwen had been turning these patients away on the grounds that he had no room for them, while filling the hospital with "private boarders." Tired of hearing "complaints made all over the state by parties desiring to place patients in that hospital," Curwen's critics decided to put a stop to his discretionary admissions policy. As Senator George R. Smith of Philadelphia said, "The institution was intended for the use of the poor of the Commonwealth, and the State commenced its erection with that original intention...yet in practice, its use is now perverted to the prejudice of that class of the community."[63]

The legislators' increasingly hostile scrutiny of the Harrisburg asylum received powerful reinforcement from the Pennsylvania State Board of Charities, which was founded in 1869 to bring some order to the state system of public assistance. The board's primary responsibility was to monitor welfare expenditures so as to ensure their wisest use. At least once a year, their general agent inspected all "charitable and correctional institutions" funded by the state. On the basis of the agent's report, the board recommended the amount of appropriations that each institution should receive from the state. In addition, the board attempted to "disseminate information on the best treatment of pauperism, disease, insanity and crime," so as to reduce the growing number of dependents on the state.[64] For example, if right principles concerning insanity's treatment could be universally observed, they reasoned, then the state would not be burdened with so many indigent, incurable citizens.

The asylum superintendents versus the State Board of Charities

Within a few years of its foundation, the Pennsylvania State Board of Charities and the medical superintendents came into open conflict. To begin with, the board claimed authority over a preserve that the medical men felt belonged to them exclusively, that is, asylum management. Moreover, the board viewed the state asylum as but one of many institutions designed for the indigent, a perspective that inevitably clashed with the physicians' preference for a mixed clientele. Overlapping spheres of authority and markedly different concepts of the state asylum's function soon had the lay reformers and the medical men in heated disagreement. Starting in 1873, the board began to attack Curwen's management of the Pennsylvania State Lunatic Asylum, specifically challenging the superintendents' vision of the asylum as a multiclass institution.[65]

The State Board of Charities' criticism of Curwen, its members asserted, did not involve charges of extravagance. As they stated in an 1873 pamphlet entitled *A Plea for the Insane*, "We make no personal charges of corrupt intentions but rather of mistaken proceedings. We attack a system, not men nor motives." The system the board objected to was the medical superintendents' definition of the state asylum as a multiclass institution. "The original design of the hospital," the board pointed out, was "what that of any such hospital ought, in all reason, to be, to provide for *the insane poor*." But by the "personal system" introduced at the Pennsylvania State Lunatic Asylum, the "State had...been drawn away from her clear duty, to enlist in a scheme of charity which is never recognized as the proper function or duty of the state": the subsidy of asylum care for the middle classes and the respectable poor.

Using crude but effective rhetoric, the board dramatized the inhumanity of the state asylum's preference for paying patients, picturing Curwen addressing a miserable almshouse inmate with these words: "This hospital was not established especially for such as you, those who can pay must have precedent over those who cannot, you must return to your poorhouse or prison and die there."[66]

The State Board of Charities proved equally ruthless in denouncing the professional concerns that they sensed underlay the doctors' interest in paying patients. Of course, the asylum doctors preferred the more affluent clientele, for they made "much more decent, quiet, gentlemanly and agreeable inmates, giving the Superintendent much less distasteful and repulsive work and trouble than those...from the foul dens of poorhouses or cells of prisons." But to those such as Kirkbride who argued that paying patients gave a necessary respectability to the asylum and attracted a better class of doctors into state service, the board responded, "We can scarcely listen to the suggestion with patience, or answer it with calmness." It was not the state's purpose to let the poor suffer so that the asylum's "superintendents and officers may not find themselves in charge of an institution of mere paupers."[67]

To prevent the misuse of state funds, the State Board of Charities determined to limit the superintendent's discretion in admitting patients. This was necessary, they claimed, because a superintendent "should not be exposed to the danger of abusing an enormous power of *personal patronage*, of consulting his personal convenience, or being influenced by the special solicitations of anybody's friends in dispensing the bounty of the state." In other words, by making admissions policy, which necessarily implicated the state's whole welfare system, the superintendents had strayed out of their area of expertise. From now on, the board insisted, their role should be to advise rather than rule on asylum matters. The state's interest in the poor necessitated that asylums be "SUBJECTED TO SUPERVISION OF SOME PARTY NOT CONNECTED WITH THEIR IMMEDIATE MANAGEMENT." Asserting that "THE AUTHORITY OF EXPERTS IS LIMITED," the board advanced its own claims as an agency with no "personal interest or convenience" at stake to regulate asylum affairs. Medical men had no monopoly on the insane, for "any intelligent and disinterested layman, who by personal observation, and thorough study, has made himself acquainted with the condition of the insane...is as well (perhaps better) qualified [to] judge...the broad features of any plan proposed for ameliorating their condition – to judge what is consistent with or demanded by the dictates of justice, humanity and the public good."[68]

The State Board of Charities attempted to demonstrate their new authority by proposing two fundamental alterations in Kirkbride's asylum philosophy. First, the board decided that the criminally insane should not be cared for in penitentiaries, but in state hospitals. In a letter to Kirkbride, George Harrison, the president of the board, explained that this proposition arose out of the members' conviction that it was unfair to class those not responsible for their misdeeds with the truly criminal. Second, the board expressed concern about the growing number of indigent insane accumulating in the local almshouses and jails. To the laymen on the board, it seemed obvious that not enough hospitals of the type preferred by the superintendents could be constructed to house all those poor; the only sensible solution seemed to be the construction of several inexpensive detached buildings for quiet chronic patients on the state hospital grounds, thus freeing the more liberal asylum accommodations for those patients who could still benefit from its therapeutic features.[69]

To the superintendents, the State Board of Charities' propositions appeared to be rank heresies that struck at the very heart of their conception of asylum practice. In the first place, the plan to put criminals in the state hospitals threatened to undo all the physicians' efforts to dissociate the asylum and the prison. Given the thought that Kirkbride had devoted to masking the restraints that no hospital could do without, he could hardly approve such an overt reminder of the asylum's repressive capabilities. As the Pennsylvania superintendents pointed out in a memorial to the legislature, many in the community had already protested against the asylum's use of any restraint; the prisonlike features of the convicts' wing would only increase public misgivings. Furthermore, any association with criminals would deepen the "moral odium" already attached to insanity by breaking down the "distinction between virtue and vice," as the memorial put it. Families would be even more reluctant to commit relatives, causing treatable patients to be neglected and eventually swelling the number of incurable ones. The only proper place for the criminally insane, concluded the superintendents, was a separate hospital on the grounds of a state prison, where those "unfortunates" could be kindly but securely confined without ruining the regular asylum's therapeutic character.[70]

The charities' proposition concerning the chronic insane likewise struck at an essential tenet of Kirkbride's asylum philosophy: that whether curable or not, all patients benefited from the asylum's therapeutic environment. Kirkbride and Curwen fought the charities' plan with the same arguments being used by the AMSAII as a whole. As Curwen wrote, separate asylums for the insane would inevitably degenerate into "simple receptacles for the safe-keeping of an afflicted class...rather than [function as] a curative institution." To encourage true progress rather than retrogression in the treatment of the insane, the state government simply had to commit itself to building enough hospitals for all the indigent insane.[71]

In pressing on the state legislature their opposing views of the provision to be made for the criminally and chronic insane, neither the asylum superintendents nor the State Board of Charities won a clear-cut victory. The physicians managed to block the legislation authorizing a wing for insane criminals at the new Pennsylvania State Hospital for the Insane at Danville and successfully lobbied against the concept of separate facilities for the chronic insane.[72] But the State Board of Charities succeeded in gaining more power over the admissions policies of the state mental hospitals. In 1874, they secured acts giving them the authority, first, to examine all insane criminals and transfer those whom they felt might benefit from treatment to a state hospital, and second, to move indigent patients from the almshouse to the hospital. Two years later, the Harrisburg hospital's appropriations bill was passed with a provision forbidding Curwen to take paying patients as long as he had any outstanding applications from indigent persons, whether recent or chronic.[73] So, although the doctors prevented any alteration in the asylum's form, they lost the power to mold its population. If the State Board of Charities could not expand provisions for the criminal or indigent by securing separate institutions for them, they were determined to find other means to remake the state hospital according to their own specifications.

The legislative struggles involving the asylum doctors and the State Board of Charities had a very personal tone almost from the outset, with both sides taking a dim view of their opponents' aims and methods. The board deeply resented Kirkbride's use of his authority to block their plans. Referring to a letter the superintendent sent to the chairman of the Judiciary Committee and other key legislators regarding their Danville asylum bill, the board spoke bitterly of the "higher advice" and "opposition from interested parties that led to defeat." But due to Kirkbride's national standing, the board's attacks on him remained relatively oblique. It was John Curwen, the more accessible and vulnerable opponent, who took the full brunt of the charities' displeasure. In their *Annual Reports*, the board used the Pennsylvania State Lunatic Asylum as the chief example of what a state asylum should *not* be. In administering policies affecting the Harrisburg asylum, they seemed to take pleasure in discomfiting Curwen. After their victory concerning the insane convicts, an ally reported to Curwen, the board had a "hearty chuckle" and began talking "about a patient they would send to you and see whether you would take proper care of him and not let him get out." Curwen later heard from another source that the board had sought to have appropriations from the Warren State Hospital for the Insane reduced simply because he was on its planning commission. "The plain truth," Curwen wrote to Kirkbride, "is that they have determined to make a fight on me...No matter what my name is connected with the fact is cause for them to find fault with it and oppose it." For his part, Curwen felt just as strong an animosity toward the board. " 'The poor' about whom they have made such a hue and cry may suffer if they can only make a point against me," he complained to Kirkbride. Realizing their determination to best him, Curwen concluded that he would have "to keep close at home."[74]

Curwen found himself in a weak position to resist the charities' onslaught, due to the poor state of his own institutional affairs. After almost three decades of hard use, the hospital building was once again in serious disrepair and needed large sums for its refurbishment. Meanwhile, at the height of his involvement in both state and national asylum politics, Curwen was spending more and more time away from the asylum. To make matters worse, the Western Hospital at Dixmont consistently undercut the Pennsylvania State Lunatic Asylum's appropriations bill, while at the same time taking no paying patients. Curwen claimed that in fact the Dixmont superintendent, J. A. Reed, had patrons pay the directors of the poor (the local poor relief officials) to have their relatives committed as state patients. Whether or not Reed practiced such a subterfuge, the State Board of Charities still used his record to disparage Curwen's asylum practice. In the care of the indigent, the board stated in 1873, the Western Hospital "comes much nearer to our idea of the duty and the intention of the state...than that at Harrisburg."[75]

The State Board of Charities' hostility toward Curwen's methods in asylum practice, coupled with his weak institutional position, eventually cost Kirkbride's protégé the Harrisburg post. The chief agent in his downfall was Hiram Corson, a country doctor with a special interest in asylum matters. As Corson explained to Pliny Earle in 1877, he had become a member of the State Board of Charities in 1869, hoping "to have some supervision over these secret institutions, which to most people represented somewhat strongly the Bastille." First as a board member of the State Board

of Charities and later as a trustee of the Pennsylvania State Lunatic
Asylum, Corson stated his opposition to the AMSAII's principles,
especially their insistence on what he felt to be "large expensive
hospitals." Like most asylum critics, he believed in "greater freedom from seclusion and restraint, and the importance of employment as a remedial measure and means of discipline." Corson's
strong views led him into conflict with both Kirkbride and Curwen, whom he criticized for having "exerted themselves to oppose
change." Corson found Curwen's asylum practice particularly rep-
rehensible. After his appointment as a trustee, Corson urged the
other board members to criticize Curwen publicly and force the
superintendent to change his methods. More specifically, Corson
charged that sexual misconduct had occurred among the Harrisburg patients. To rectify this deplorable situation, Corson proposed that a female medical superintendent be appointed to take
charge of the women patients, on the assumption that she would
be more attentive to the moral conditions prevailing in the wards.
Curwen, not surprisingly, strongly resisted such a notion, not
only because he had little sympathy with the cause of women
physicians but, more importantly, because he believed that his
authority would be irretrievably undermined by such an
appointment.[76]

Although his opposition to a female superintendent was the chief
reason the board gave for firing Curwen in late 1880, the incident
reflected an ongoing struggle over his institutional autonomy.
Curwen told Dorothea Dix that the trustees gave as their real
reason for firing him that "Dr. Curwen wanted to have things
too much his own way." Curwen himself believed that the incident
reflected "a squabble on their part for the patronage of the hospital." Kirkbride echoed his protégé's complaints in a letter to
Dix, claiming the firing to be an "outrage of no ordinary kind
and disgraceful to all concerned with it." Curwen's problems at
Harrisburg, he concluded, had been the "fault of others, much
more than his own. For years, he had been thwarted in all his
plans, and the men, who have now removed him, have been doing
all they could to annoy him, till his position of late has been most
uncomfortable." Curwen soon obtained another post at the new
Warren, Pennsylvania, state hospital, where he remained until his
retirement in 1911. But his well-publicized difficulties, combined
with Kirkbride's increasing infirmities, greatly diminished the su-

perintendents' power to resist their critics' schemes for change. Thus, the failures of the Pennsylvania State Lunatic Asylum helped to usher in a new era of hospital politics in which the asylum doctors had much less influence and autonomy.[77]

The Pennsylvania State Lunacy Commission

The starting date for this new era was 1883, when the forces opposed to Curwen and Kirkbride won their most important victory: the foundation of a State Lunacy Commission, which gave the State Board of Charities the supervisory powers it had so long desired. Governor Henry Hoyt had appointed a committee in May 1882 to investigate the charges of patient abuse and asylum mismanagement so frequently leveled against the state's mental hospitals. The composition of the committee reflected the convergence of interests opposed to the dominant asylum philosophy; it included S. Weir Mitchell, a prominent Philadelphia neurologist and an outspoken critic of the asylum superintendents; L. Clarke Davis, the reputed author of the "Modern Lettre de Cachet," as well as numerous editorials attacking the Harrisburg hospital; and George L. Harrison of the State Board of Charities. The governor placed neither Curwen nor Kirkbride on the commission, an omission that reflected the decline in their political influence. J. A. Reed of the Dixmont hospital, a superintendent sympathetic to the cause of asylum reform, represented the superintendents' interests. After several months of deliberation, the group returned a report highly critical of the fiscal and therapeutic practices prevailing in Pennsylvania's mental hospitals. Taking their inspiration from the English Lunacy Commission, the committee recommended a bill giving the state the power to inspect and license all mental institutions, private as well as public, and guaranteeing patients the right to legal counsel and mailing privileges. Furthermore, the law made any superintendent violating the Lunacy Commission's regulations liable to civil prosecution.[78]

Despite his age and infirmity, Thomas Story Kirkbride attempted to ward off this last, most crushing blow to his asylum philosophy. The bedridden seventy-two-year-old doctor wrote a passionate letter to the joint legislative committee considering the bill, urging them to reject it. Such a bill, he argued, would repay the humanitarian efforts of the men in charge of institutions such as the Pennsylvania Hospital for the Insane by unjustly accusing them of a pecuniary interest in their admissions policies. The committee had to believe that superintendents and their trustees were men "utterly devoid of principle...ready to connive with wicked relations to keep the unfortunate confined, to secure possession of their estates." The committee, Kirkbride complained, seemed to regard the features of moral treatment as mere "novelties" in caring for the insane, when in fact they formed the foundation of the asylum's therapeutic regimen. Furthermore, unfettered mailing privileges would cause endless harm to both patients and their families by allowing the often embarrassing delusions of the insane to be broadcast without check. The end result would be increased "suspicions and anxieties" about asylum care that were "already too prevalent in the community," thereby delaying commitment until the patient could no longer benefit by treatment. Ultimately, the Lunacy Commission plan would cause the whole specialty to decline, Kirkbride concluded, because it destroyed the autonomy that made the superintendent's work most effective and rewarding. "The result of such proceedings," he wrote, "will ultimately be to prevent the highest order of medical men from accepting such positions in any of our hospitals, and the results must be that their places will be filled by persons who are tempted simply by the salaries given for their services."[79]

Neither Kirkbride's personal prestige nor "the great social influence of the Pennsylvania Hospital for the Insane," as one of the bill's advocates termed it, proved strong enough to defeat the Lunacy Commission's plan. After a heated debate, the bill became law in 1883. The governor did make one concession to Kirkbride; he appointed to the first Lunacy Commission Thomas G. Morton, Kirkbride's son-in-law, whose only qualification for the job, according to a sarcastic editorial note in the *Journal of Nervous and Mental Diseases*, was his personal tie to a "doctrinaire" member of the Superintendents' Association.[80]

Even with a sympathetic presence among its members, the Lunacy Commission brought about a radical change in the superintendent's position within the asylum. Many important aspects of asylum practice formerly left to the chief physician's discretion became subject to the commission's regulation: the filing of commitment papers, the format of case records, the admission and discharge of individual patients, and the use of restraint and seclusion. In all these vital matters, the asylum superintendent stood in a new relationship to a powerful, often hostile external authority. Thus, by the time of his death, the cornerstone of Kirkbride's asylum philosophy, that is, the superintendent's control over the great whole, had been effectively destroyed.

In some respects, the conflict between the asylum superintendents and the State Board of Charities in Pennsylvania was not typical of the nation as a whole. The close personal and professional relationship between the Pennsylvania State Lunatic Asylum and the Pennsylvania Hospital for the Insane had no counterpart elsewhere; for example, the McLean Asylum had no such decisive influence on the Worcester State Hospital in Massachusetts, or the Bloomingdale Asylum on the state hospital at Utica, New York. A unique conjunction of circumstances created the Pennsylvania debate over the proper character of the state mental hospital. In the first place, the long-established image of the Quaker-dominated Pennsylvania Hospital as an institution for the worthy poor tempered the elite tendencies of the asylum. More importantly, due to Kirkbride's personal reputation and professional renown, his distinctive vision of the corporate hospital as a model for the state institution remained dominant in Pennsylvania asylum politics for several decades. Thus, in no other state did the concept of a multiclass state mental hospital gain such influence or suffer so explicit a defeat.

Yet, the fundamental issues involved in the Pennsylvania debate did not pertain to that state alone. As late as the 1880s, many state asylums still had paying clients along with indigent patients. The legitimacy of these mixed state institutions (mixed in the social and mental condition of the patients) fueled controversies in states other than Pennsylvania. Certainly, the long-standing antagonism between the Utica and Willard state hospitals in New York involved the issue of mixed versus indigent patients, as did the debate over the proper character of the new Danvers State Hospital in Massachusetts. In an even broader sense, the recurrent controversy over the care of the chronic insane involved the question so explicitly debated in Pennsylvania: Should the state mental hospital serve first the indigent, who made up the bulk of incurable patients, or strive to remain a multiclass facility with both a therapeutic and a custodial function?[81]

Those late-nineteenth-century reformers who asserted that the state mental hospital's overriding duty was to the poor certainly had the force of numbers behind their contentions. The inhuman conditions suffered by the insane in almshouses and jails made for a compelling argument against Kirkbride's philosophy of asylum construction and design. His critics were undoubtedly right in asserting that the nineteenth-century taxpayer would never pay for the system of regular hospitals that Kirkbride demanded. Furthermore, in changing the direction of American asylum medicine, the asylum's critics focused on very real defects in moral treatment. The principle of restraint had indeed shaped the asylum's design, as Kirkbride's own writings demonstrate. For the noncompliant patient involuntarily confined there, the mental hospital had an undeniably punitive character. And as the neurologists so volubly argued, the American superintendents were isolated from the newest developments in medical science.

On the other hand, the doctrinaire superintendents who so bitterly resisted change also perceived a vital truth: that a hospital containing none but the poorest, least influential, and most incoherent members of society would inevitably degenerate into a structure no better than its almshouse predecessor. In the eighteenth century, reformers had set the asylum on a course distinct from the almshouse by catering to a more affluent clientele and securing the physician a greater degree of institutional power. When the state mental hospital's right to serve a more attractive set of patients and patrons was denied in the late nineteenth century, the institution inevitably returned to almshouse standards of care.

In light of the failure of subsequent generations of physicians to cure insanity, the scientific knowledge that the old superintendents lacked also seems less critical. The neurologists' gospel of medical progress, which urged the treatment of diseases rather than individuals and viewed the asylum as a source of clinical material rather than a therapeutic facility, undoubtedly accelerated the objectification of the mental patient. After a century of such "progress," one can better appreciate the wisdom of Kirkbride's remarks on the benefits of science. "I do not belong to that school that believes the chief object of institutions for the insane is to furnish an abundant supply of subjects for post-mortem examinations and for the use of the microscope," he once said. Although expressing his "high appreciation" for scientific research, Kirkbride concluded, "We must not expect too much aid in treatment from the microscope or other modern modes of investigation, interesting as they are."[82]

Given the scale of late-nineteenth-century social problems, it is difficult to imagine a satisfactory resolution to the dilemmas involved in the state care of the insane. In many respects, the transformation of the classless asylum of the mid-nineteenth century into a rigid two-tier system of mental hospitals (private, therapeutically oriented ones for the wealthy and public, custodial care for the poor) paralleled the larger changes in American society. Thomas Story Kirkbride's asylum philosophy reflected mid-century confidence about American society, confidence that its communities would be able to expand and mature without creating the intractable social problems and ingrained class distinctions apparent in European society. Kirkbride's linear plan, which allowed all levels of society to be brought together within a small, rigidly structured compass, served as an architectural metaphor for his vision of mid-nineteenth-century Philadelphia: still a walking city, despite its increase in population, with the different classes sorting themselves into distinct neighborhoods but still possessed of common social knowledge. In such an organic community, the personal character of good and benevolent men represented the only defense needed against social chaos.

But by the 1880s, Kirkbride's metaphor for American society no longer seemed applicable. Just as increasing residential segregation and the growing impersonality of social relations hastened a new concept of urban order, the accumulation of a vast population of the incurably insane poor necessitated a more differentiated and stratified system of mental hospitals. Asylum order came to depend not upon the "personal character of its chief," as Ray termed it, but on the more abstract quality of state guardianship.[83] In many respects, the transformation of the asylum presaged the hard realities of turn-of-the-century American society, with its increasing isolation of the classes and its massive social problems. And like other Progressive era reforms, the new asylum order reflected the mixed blessings of state intervention and scientific advance.

CONCLUSION: A GENEROUS
SYMPATHY

In the last years of his life, Thomas Story Kirkbride enjoyed little of the public acclaim that a man of his experience and reputation might reasonably have expected. His asylum philosophy, the work of a lifetime, was under attack in every quarter: the courtroom, the press, the state legislature, even the superintendents' association. Yet, Kirkbride's devotion to his principles of asylum practice never wavered. Stricken in October 1879 with an "obscure and serious illness" that brought him close to death, he recovered, and used his convalescence to complete a long-intended task: the revision of his 1854 treatise on asylum design. The new edition of *On the Construction, Organization and General Arrangements of Hospitals for the Insane* appeared in late 1880, with extensive new architectural plans and additional technical suggestions, but with the substance of its argument unchanged. In defiance of his critics, Kirkbride stubbornly maintained that insanity was usually curable if quickly and properly treated; that state hospitals should be built and administered like their corporate counterparts; that mental institutions should ideally have 250 patients and, even under the most pressing circumstances, never more than 600; and that restraint had to be an integral part of asylum treatment. As the book made evident, the debates of the last decade had left hardly a dent in Kirkbride's cast-iron creed.[1]

This restatement of Kirkbride's views did not still the growing dissent against his style of asylum practice, however. Despite the respect many superintendents and reformers had for him, Kirkbride was widely perceived as an obstacle to progress, that is, the development of psychiatry as a clinical specialty, and the remodeling of the state mental hospital. The young physicians entering the field, committed to new, essentially European visions of medical research, resented the personal influence that a physician so ignorant of modern developments attempted to (and often did) wield. It was not simply that Kirkbride's ideas were hopelessly outdated, but that he continued to insist upon their scientific and moral correctness. Despite his old-fashioned approach to asylum medicine, his opinions still influenced the thinking of younger, active superintendents such as Charles Nichols and John Curwen, not to mention many politicians and reformers. Perhaps inevitably, a "more or less personal feeling" against Kirkbride grew up among the newest generation of asylum doctors. They could not understand the "deep and fervent veneration" Kirkbride felt for the propositions that to them seemed "outgrown and no longer necessary." For his part, Kirkbride was angered by the criticism coming from superintendents he regarded as inexperienced and irresponsible about asylum matters. "It is lamentable," the English alienist D. H. Tuke commiserated with Kirkbride in 1880, "to hear of those who have borne the burden and heat of the day being vilified by upstarts who had scarcely seen the light when they began their work."[2]

Ill health and discouragement eventually weakened Kirkbride's resolve to press the fight for the "old-time wisdom," as his critics patronizingly referred to the propositions. In late March 1881, he lost the encouragement and companionship of his beloved friend Isaac Ray, who died at the age of seventy-four.[3] Over the next two years, the debates in the state legislature and the activities of the Hoyt Commission weighed heavily upon him. As solace, Kirkbride threw himself into his work at the hospital, spending long hours on the wards; there was "a certain anxiety in his desire to be there," Eliza Butler Kirkbride thought, almost as if he sought reassurance in the familiar routines of asylum life. In mid-March 1883, the seventy-four-year-old doctor came down with a bad cold, which rapidly developed into pneumonia. Near death in April, he rallied once again to regain some measure of strength during the summer months, only to worsen as winter approached. In mid-December, Kirkbride slipped into a coma and died peacefully at 11:45 P.M., Sunday, December 16. After a service at the Twelfth Street Meeting House, he was buried in the South Laurel Hill Cemetery by the side of his first wife, Ann, on December 20.[4]

Thomas Story Kirkbride's death occasioned many public tributes to his character and achievements, but none so eloquent as the memorial written by Eliza Butler Kirkbride, published in the hospital's *Report* for 1883. In this lengthy account of Kirkbride's career, Eliza attempted to refute the charge that her husband had not been progressive in his views. She detailed the countless improvements in amusements and occupations that had constituted his life's work. Yet, the best testimony to Kirkbride's accomplishments, Eliza insisted, was not to be found in the institutional structure he had built, but in the lives of the cured patients he left behind. Kirkbride's real genius as a physician had been manifest in his "power over the afflicted"; the "personal ministry" he pursued with his patients had been "more potent, perhaps, in itself than the many remedial agencies gathered within this Institution." Eliza felt that Kirkbride had gained that power over the insane not by clinical expertise or architectural innovation, pursuits he respected but knew to be limited; rather, the secret of his success had been the "generous sympathy for all who suffer" manifested in his every thought and action. What made Kirkbride a great doctor, according to his wife and former patient, was his character.[5]

Evaluating Kirkbride's contribution to the field, the brethren also stressed his "unswerving and untiring professional and administrative labor" on behalf of the insane. At the AMSAII meeting in June 1884, John Gray praised him as a "natural leader" who had done much to advance the cause of asylum medicine. "Men followed him, listened to him, recognized him as a man of thought and reflection with a power of formulating his ideas distinctly and clearly, and of presenting them . . . plainly." Gray observed, "Even before the Association existed, Kirkbride had commenced the work of development of the structure of psychological medicine in this country – building from within and building from without – not alone a physical structure, but laying down principles for the guidance of those who might come after him." The details of Kirkbride's plans might become obsolete, but the principles underlying them would never lose their relevance, he claimed.[6]

Yet, even as they paid tribute to their departed colleague, Kirkbride's associates acknowledged that his ideas had outlived their usefulness. "We must not estimate him," urged Gray, in a remark obviously directed at Kirkbride's youthful critics in the audience, "not as though we judged him today, as though he had arisen now or within the last quarter of a century. It must be borne in mind he came upon the stage at a time when there was little that could be said in regard to the treatment of the insane." Despite such pleas for charity, not a single young superintendent rose to pay homage to Kirkbride. The President of the AMSAII, Orpheus Everts, who had been an outspoken critic of the propositions, felt compelled to defend their silence "as a more satisfactory expression of their feelings than anything else." Whatever respectful sentiments some may have entertained, the young doctors surely felt a sense of relief that the uncompromising, self-righteous figure of Kirkbride would no longer be there to obstruct their pursuit of progress.[7]

Kirkbride's propositions on asylum construction and design survived him by only a few years. At the AMSAII's 1888 meeting, William W. Godding of the Government Hospital moved that they be abandoned, since no one any longer mistook for "living cannon" what had long since become mere historic truth and "innocuous desuetude." He offered two resolutions: first, that the AMSAII vote "Not to affirm" rather than reject the old propositions outright, and second, that the group not adopt any new guidelines in their place. By this strategy, asylum doctors could show their respect for the historic resolutions while making it clear that the specialty need no longer be bound by a uniform set of institutional standards. Although Godding's compromise struck some doctors as forced, the AMSAII voted 21 to 13 to accept the first resolution and unanimously passed the second.[8]

The end of an era did not pass without reference to Kirkbride. Immediately after the vote, John Curwen rose to challenge the younger generation, who had so summarily rejected his old mentor's beliefs, to improve upon his accomplishments. "No man living today nor no man ever did live who insisted more on everything which could be made available for the purpose of improving in every way, the condition of the insane...This is the point we must all aim at and to strive to surpass," Curwen stated. But the sentiments of those present probably came closer to Pliny Earle's estimation of the propositions:

I most fully believe that they have constituted the principal factor among those agencies which, in some sections of the country, have greatly impaired the prestige which the Association once enjoyed, by engendering a belief that it is practically averse to progress in improvement; that it is running in the "cast-irons ruts" of precedent, that it is indissolubly bound to the faith of the father, despite the enlightenment of

more recent observation and thought. It is to be feared that the direct
benefit of the Propositions to the cause, which they were intended to
promote, has been more than counterbalanced by the indirect detriment
thus produced.[9]

Over the next three decades, the new trends in asylum medicine
already evident by Kirkbride's last years became even more pronounced. The late-nineteenth-century specialty concerned itself
increasingly with the somatic as opposed to the psychological
factors producing mental disease. Hereditarian explanations for
insanity (which Kirkbride had always opposed) became much more
popular. Influenced by a new conception of disease as the product
of cellular pathology, asylum doctors or psychiatrists, as they
began to call themselves, tried to identify the physiological processes or disturbances associated with disordered mental states. The
trend toward equating insanity with cellular pathology reinforced
the widespread pessimism concerning its curability. Brain tissues
and nerve cells, it was assumed, did not easily regenerate; thus,
physicians had relatively little impetus to develop new therapeutic
modalities. Instead, prevention of insanity became their highest
priority, and psychiatrists gave renewed emphasis to mental hygiene measures.

For those so unfortunate as to become insane, medical men felt
they could do little but administer custodial institutions in the least
expensive, most humane fashion possible. To accommodate the
rising population of the chronic insane, state hospitals expanded
in size to hold more than 1,000 patients. Huge new institutions
built according to the cottage plan became commonplace in the
more densely populated states. Concurrently, many small private
asylums or sanitaria were established to serve affluent families
eager to avoid the bleak prospect of state care. In sum, the developments Kirkbride had most feared – the abandonment of moral
treatment, a purely clinical approach to patients, huge custodial
hospitals, and a sharply class-differentiated system of mental health
care – all came to pass in the late nineteenth century. What might
be styled a "cult of pessimism" thoroughly supplanted the old cult
of curability.[10]

The asylum practice of Kirkbride's successor at the Pennsylvania
Hospital for the Insane, John B. Chapin, exemplified the changing
perspective of the late-nineteenth-century specialty. In the mid-
1860s, while associated with Brigham Hall, a small private asylum

in Canandaigua, New York, Chapin had been among the first members of the AMSAII to challenge the cult of curability and argue for less expensive, more varied state facilities for the indigent insane. After leading the campaign to found the Willard State Hospital in Ovid, New York, he became its first superintendent. As head of the 1,800-patient institution for the insane, then by far the largest state hospital in the country, Chapin earned a "solid reputation as an economist," and became a leader of the Young Turks within the superintendents' association. His administration at Willard, an admiring newspaper account stated in 1884, had disproved "some of the most cherished theories of the American superintendents of the insane on the subject of hospital architecture, the maximum hospital population, and the cost of hospital support."[11]

The Pennsylvania Hospital managers hired Chapin because of his reputation as an economist rather than an iconoclast. After a visit to Willard, the board was convinced that he had the kind of executive ability needed to keep their institution in the front ranks. To secure Chapin's services, they gave up their resolution to hire two physicians for the Male and Female departments, the plan Kirkbride had preferred but Chapin refused to accept. For a salary of $6,000 and sole authority over both branches of the asylum, John Chapin left Willard in the summer of 1884, and took charge of the Pennsylvania Hospital for the Insane on September 1, 1884.[12]

Under Chapin's administration, the hospital took on a new, more up-to-date look. To relieve the monotony of the linear plan, he added more varied forms of accommodation, including a stylish villa for the wealthy and a cottage near the hospital farm for those in need of systematic labor. He also arranged for a house in the seaside resort of Cape May, New Jersey, to be used for convalescent patients. Showing the neurologists' influence, Chapin's medical practice emphasized strengthening measures such as a rich diet, enforced bed rest, and soothing tonics. As an aid to clinical observation, he had his assistants keep detailed case records, noting the results of neurological examinations, blood pressure readings, and the like. In keeping with the specialty's heightened interest in prophylaxis, Chapin convinced the managers to establish a new outpatient department for nervous and mental diseases at the Eighth Street hospital, which dispensed free advice and treatment for incipient disorders in order to prevent their degeneration into more intractable forms of insanity.[13]

In many other respects, Chapin modernized the mental hospital by making it more efficient and regimented. He had the attendants uniformed, improved the food service, and overhauled the re-cordkeeping system. Following the dictates of the 1883 Lunacy Law, the superintendent admitted no patient without the proper certificates, and kept a daily record of the number of patients confined or in seclusion. The institution also stopped admitting opium eaters and chronic alcoholics, except as voluntary patients, in an attempt to rid itself of that litigious clientele. Although maintaining complete control of the asylum's operation, Chapin allowed his assistant a freer hand on the wards, acting more as an administrator than a physician and apparently taking little direct responsibility for patient care. Altogether, Chapin's asylum took on the character of many Progressive era institutions, with their greater degree of bureaucracy and impersonality.[14]

Yet, in many respects, Chapin did not depart from his prede-cessor's practice at the Pennsylvania Hospital for the Insane. In his medical practice, he never abandoned physical restraint and used narcotics, particularly sulfanol, as extensively as Kirkbride had. Because patrons still appreciated the building's appearance, he de-voted considerable money and attention to the ward furnishings and hospital grounds. To advertise the asylum's homelike com-forts, Chapin's *Reports* carried photographs of the patients' parlors and rooms (a ploy Kirkbride would surely have approved). The elaborate round of occupations and amusements that had been the mainstay of the old moral treatment still formed the centerpiece of the hospital day. Like his predecessor, Chapin prided himself on introducing new activities, among them a gymnastic pavilion, art classes, and a hospital orchestra. For all his efforts to streamline the hospital's administration, Chapin also encountered the perils of asylum practice: family disputes over commitment, disobedient attendants, patient suicides, and writs of habeas corpus. Perhaps because he came to recognize the continuity between their careers, Chapin proved surprisingly eager to invoke the Kirkbride tradi-tion, a tradition he had once derided, to legitimate his own su-perintendency. Praising Kirkbride in the *Report* for 1891 as a man of "experience and wise judgment" whose writings formed a "compendium of knowledge upon every phase of hospital admin-istration," Chapin announced his resolve to "follow and preserve the wholesome traditions of administration" that his predecessor had established. The older he got, the more Chapin moved away from his youthful iconoclasm to embrace the spirit if not the substance of Kirkbride's asylum practice.[15]

Chapin's mellowing was indicative of a process of professional self-evaluation and myth making taking place within the larger specialty. As the memories of past conflicts faded and they themselves became the target of youthful criticism, even the most intransigent of Kirkbride's foes grew more kindly in their estimation of him. The historical retrospects prepared for the AMSAII's semicentennial in 1894 revealed their need to create a heroic past for their profession, a past in which all the members of the original thirteen, no matter how wrong-minded, were enshrined. Presiding as president over the 1894 meeting, John Curwen delivered an exceedingly long address that gave his old mentor the lion's share of praise. His younger colleague, G. Alder Blumer of the Utica hospital, not surprisingly, gave higher marks to Pliny Earle and John Gray, whom he presented as farsighted advocates of "scientific psychiatry," but Kirkbride received a short but respectful mention in his historical paper. The same tone characterized the first major history of the specialty, the four-volume *Institutional Care of the Insane in the United States and Canada*, edited by Henry Hurd and published in 1916-17. Hurd portrayed Ray and Kirkbride's attempt to prevent change as the kind of mistake "often made by elderly men who seek in vain to arrange the world and to set it in order for all future time." But unlike the harsh judgment Pliny Earle had expressed in 1888, Hurd concluded that Kirkbride's propositions had given the specialty a firm foundation in its earliest, most precarious years.[16]

Ironically, more recent histories of American psychiatry have tended to reverse Hurd's order of estimation and rate the original thirteen much higher than their late-nineteenth-century successors. Norman Dain and Gerald Grob have suggested that Kirkbride's generation of superintendents were far more talented, committed, and charismatic figures than the small-minded office seekers who followed them. The cult of curability, J. Sanbourne Bockoven and Eric Carlson have pointed out, produced a higher standard of patient care than did the somaticism of the later period. From a psychological standpoint, they have argued, the principles of moral treatment seem hardly as old-fashioned as the Young Turks of the 1870s and 1880s made out. Furthermore, scholars concerned about the deterioration of the state mental hospital system cannot so easily agree with Hurd's conclusion that the "weight of argument" favored the younger men in their advocacy of large chronic-care institutions. From a post-1950s perspective, Kirkbride's warnings about custodialism, patient abuse, and the decline of professional standards seem remarkably prescient.[17]

Even with the renewal of interest in the original thirteen, Thomas Story Kirkbride's reputation has not worn particularly well, however. Although during his own lifetime considered one of the foremost if not the best American asylum superintendent, he has generally been less admired by twentieth-century scholars than Samuel Woodward, Amariah Brigham, Isaac Ray, or even John Gray. In comparison to them, Kirkbride did little medical research, trial work, or professional writing, that is, the types of activities medical historians find easiest to evaluate. What little he did publish concerned asylum construction and design, matters of no immediate interest to contemporary observers. Historians have been tempted to see in the gas-tinkerers' obsessive concern with building details a foreshadowing of the narrow administrative focus that would characterize the late-nineteenth-century specialty. As for Kirkbride's other claim to excellence, his ability as an asylum practitioner, that too has not worn well. Many of his patients spoke highly of him, and his fellow doctors admired his work with the insane: This much the historical record shows. But the force of character, the bedside manner that made Kirkbride's asylum practice so exemplary in his own time cannot be easily recaptured.[18]

In many respects, the transient quality of Kirkbride's reputation reflects a tendency among both contemporary and historical observers to see medical research as more important than medical practice. Medicine progresses, it is assumed, not by the provision of excellent patient care but by scientific investigation. Physicians and historians alike tend to revere the scientific pathfinders more than the practical men of medicine. Still, there has always been a tradition, albeit a sentimental one, that acknowledges the importance of inspired bedside medicine to the profession's advance. Theoretically, improved patient care is the final object of all medical progress; in more concrete terms, physicians draw enormous social authority from their ability to relieve pain, and cannot stray too far from that aspect of their professional enterprise without losing public support. Thus, in every generation of physicians, a few inspired practitioners have been singled out for notice, so as to prove medicine's unswerving devotion to the patient. For seventeenth-century English physicians, one such figure was Thomas Sydenham; for the late-nineteenth-century American profession, it was William Osler.[19]

This was the role Thomas Story Kirkbride played in mid–nineteenth-century American asylum medicine. At a time when the newly established specialty desperately needed social legitimacy, he infused it with a special sense of mission. Of all the brethren, he best exemplified "all that is lovely in the character of the good physician," to quote one admirer. To fulfill the specialty's need for moral leadership, Kirkbride did not need intellectual prowess, but only a deep and unquestionable concern for his patients. The excellence of the Pennsylvania Hospital for the Insane, along with the superintendent's obvious sympathy for its inmates, served as the best kind of proof that medical men were the proper caretakers of the mentally disturbed. In this respect, Kirkbride played much the same role for the American specialty as John Conolly did in the English profession; their names became synonymous with the humanitarian aims of asylum work.[20]

To conclude that Kirkbride furnished early asylum medicine with a moral justification it desperately needed does not necessarily mean that it deserved vindication. The exacting nature of Kirkbride's conscience may have served only to cover the multitude of sins committed by his less scrupulous brethren. John C. Bucknill implied as much concerning Kirkbride's public statements on restraint. "I am very certain," he wrote to the Philadelphia superintendent, "that with your gentle and tender heart you would never abuse restraint or any other means of treatment – but it is just the advocacy of such a man as you are, the honesty of which cannot be suspected, that throws a shield over the misdoings of others at the Philadelphia Almshouse, for instance."[21] At a more fundamental level, some would question the moral legitimacy of any mental hospital, past or present, no matter how well administered. Certainly, Kirkbride's asylum practice involved some of the same moral dilemmas concerning involuntary confinement and treatment that still trouble our society. The paternalism, the coercion, and the almost fearful emphasis on restraint were as integral a part of Kirkbride's attitude toward his patients as his much vaunted sympathy.

Notwithstanding the limitations apparent to a modern observer, Kirkbride's approach to patient care was certainly far superior to our own in one crucial respect: the care of the chronic insane. The mid-nineteenth-century asylum doctor, with his curious blend of religious and scientific values, was on balance well suited to such work. His devotion to science made him exacting and observant, yet he had not as yet developed the impersonal view of patients as clinical material that would ultimately facilitate the objectification and neglect of hopeless cases. Victorian society rewarded the physician for selfless devotion to an intellectually and therapeutically unrewarding class of patients, a reward by and large denied to later generations. The end result was a high standard of care for the chronic insane. Thus, in this respect, the mid-nineteenth-century asylum, at least the leading corporate institutions, might be viewed as a peak in medical achievement rather than as one point on an upward line toward scientific enlightenment. In our own times, when the qualities Thomas Story Kirkbride brought to asylum practice are in short supply, his ability to sustain "a generous sympathy with all who suffer" still commands respect.

APPENDIXES

1. THE PATIENT POPULATION, PENNSYLVANIA HOSPITAL FOR THE INSANE

When compared with the pre-1840 patient population at the old Eighth Street hospital, the data in Tables A. 1 to A. 5 suggest several interesting trends. First, the ratio of male to female admissions evened out in the new asylum: Whereas at the old eighteenth-century hospital (c. 1780–1830) men had outnumbered women by 70 to 30 percent, at the new asylum the sexes were divided more evenly, 55 to 45 percent. Second, the striking differences in the patients' marital status observed in the old hospital disappeared. In Malin's 1828 survey,[1] single men had outnumbered the married by 58 to 35 percent. Between 1841 and 1883, single male patients declined in number from 56 to 47 percent of the total male admissions; married men climbed from 39 to 46 percent of the total. The number of widowed men remained the same, 6 percent. The female patients showed an opposite trend. The number of single and married female patients in the old hospital had been 31 and 50 percent, respectively. Between 1841 and 1883, single women formed 40 to 43 percent of the patients; the married women remained at around 46 percent of the total. The number of widows fell from 19 percent in 1830 to approximately 12.5 percent in the new asylum. The two new trends most apparent between 1841 and 1883 – the rise in admissions of women, especially single ones, and married men – both indicate that the asylum gained in social respectability after its relocation. The increased number of women patients, especially young unmarried ones, suggests that the social custom Rush observed in the 1790s had changed; families no longer viewed the hospital as an improper place for ladies. The greater willingness to commit married men, economically the most val-

Table A.1. *Sex differences in marital status* (N = 8,852)

Marital status	Men (%)	Women (%)
Married	46	47
Single	49	41
Widowed	5	12

Source: AR 1883, p. 15.

Table A.2. *Age at time of admission*
(N = 8,852)

Under 20	6%
20–29	28%
30–39	27%
40–49	20%
50–59	11%
60 and over	8%

Note: There were only slight differences (1–2%) in the ages of men and women at the time of admission.
Source: AR 1883, p. 12.

Table A.3. *Nativity of foreign-born patients*
(N = 2,154)

Irish	51%
German	22%
English	16%
Other	11%

Source: AR 1883, p. 16.

Table A.4. *Residence of out-of-state patients*
(N = 1,667)

South	49%
North	35%
Midwest and West	12%
Outside United States	4%

Source: AR 1883, p. 17.

Table A.5. *Diagnoses upon admission, by sex (in percentages; N = 8,832)*[a]

Diagnosis	Men (N = 4,748)	Women (N = 4,084)
Mania	42.5	48
Melancholia	23	33
Monomania	15.5	11
Dementia	19	8

[a]This figure does not include patients admitted for delirium.
Source: AR 1883, p. 18.

uable family members, perhaps also reflects an increased faith in asylum therapy.

Some aspects of the patient population changed less dramatically. The age of patients at admission rose only slightly between 1830 and 1880. The number of patients over fifty at admission increased from 13 to 20 percent. This increase probably reflects the changing age structure of the population as a whole rather than a change in admissions policy, since there is little evidence that Kirkbride encouraged the commitment of aged patients.[2] The nativity of the patient population showed no change; the proportion of foreign-born patients remained 25 percent of the total admissions, with the Irish, English, and Germans predominating.

2. CURE RATES AT THE PENNSYLVANIA HOSPITAL FOR THE INSANE

It must be remembered that the percentage of patients discharged as cured compared to the number under treatment at any given time was much lower than the figures indicated in Table A.6. In 1850, for example, 215 patients were discharged or died and 213 remained in the hospital; of the 428 patients under treatment during the year, 106, or 25 percent, were cured. Kirkbride, not surprisingly, preferred to emphasize the ratio of cures to discharges rather than the number under treatment. Table A.7 shows the treatment rate expressed in the latter form for selected years.

Pliny Earle accused the early asylum superintendents of falsifying their statistics so as to make mental disease appear more

Table A.6. *Treatment outcomes, by decade, Pennsylvania Hospital for the Insane, 1841–80 (in percentages)*

Outcome	1841–50 (N = 1,593)	1850–60 (N = 1,704)	1860–70 (N = 2,155)	1870–80 (N = 2,472)
Cured	53	53	46	41
Much improved	8	10	7	8
Improved	15	16	18	19
Stationary	13	8	15	16
Died	11	13	14	16

Source: Data calculated from statistics presented in *AR* 1850, pp. 5, 26; *AR* 1860, pp. 10–11, 20; *AR* 1870, pp. 5–6, 14; and *AR* 1880, pp. 5–6, 14.

Table A.7. *Treatment outcomes, by total percentage of patients treated, Pennsylvania Hospital for the Insane, for selected years*

Outcome	1850 (N = 428)	1860 (N = 465)	1870 (N = 574)	1880 (N = 590)
Cured	25	21	16	15
Improved	14	9	11	9
Stationary	5	5.5	7	11
Died	6	5.5	6	5
Remain in hospital	50	59	60	60

Source: Data calculated from statistics presented in *AR* 1850, pp. 5, 26; *AR* 1860, pp. 10–11, 20; *AR* 1870, pp. 5–6, 14; and *AR* 1880, pp. 5–6, 14.

curable.[3] In particular, he claimed that counting periodic cases as cured inflated recovery rates. As can be seen in Chapter 6, Earle's arguments were widely taken as proof that moral treatment had failed. Upon reviewing the statistics controversy, several scholars have concluded that Earle's judgments were too harsh. Bockoven not only questioned Earle's calculations but presented data from a follow-up study on former patients from the Worcester State Hospital that threw doubt on Earle's pessimistic estimate that only 4 percent of all insane patients were curable. This study, done between 1882 and 1893, showed that of the individuals discharged as cured between 1833 and 1846, 48 percent had remained well all their lives; 6 percent had one recurrence and then stayed well; 30

Table A.8. *Treatment outcomes, by sex, Pennsylvania Hospital for the Insane, 1860–80 (in percentages)*

	1860–70		1870–80	
Outcome	Men (N = 1,165)	Women (N = 990)	Men (N = 1,377)	Women (N = 1,095)
Cured	43	51	37	46
Improved	22	27	25	28
Stationary	21	9	20	11
Died	14	13	18	15

Source: Data calculated from statistics presented in *AR* 1850, pp. 5, 26; *AR* 1860, pp. 10–11, 20; *AR* 1870, pp. 5–6, 14; and *AR* 1880, pp. 5–6, 14.

percent had relapsed; and 6 percent could not be located.[4] Norman Dain estimates that one-third of all patients admitted to the Eastern State Hospital in a year recovered.[5] Treatment outcomes by sex, for selected decades, at the Pennsylvania Hospital for the Insane, are presented in Table A.8.

3. PAYING PATIENTS IN STATE HOSPITALS

As a whole, state hospital annual reports are highly uneven in their inclusion of statistics for paying versus poor patients, as well as board payments as a source of revenue. These data are not reported consistently for the same hospital over time, nor are comparable data given for all institutions. But the figures are given in enough cases to conclude that many of the older state hospitals in the South and North took in sizable numbers of paying patients, or *boarders*, as they were sometimes called, and that the revenue they supplied made a substantial contribution to the asylum's treasury. Table A.9 shows the breakdown for paying versus poor patients in twelve state institutions.

Often, even if *Reports* did not give figures for the paying/poor categories, they did list in the treasurer's or steward's report the amount received in board payments for private patients, along with the amounts paid by public authorities (city, county, and state) for indigent cases and state appropriations for the asylum. The number of paying patients in the state hospital might be quite small, yet their share of the asylum's revenues quite substantial.

Table A.9. *Paying versus poor patients in selected state hospitals (in percentages)*

Institution	Date	Paying	Poor
Worcester State Hospital	1864*a*	33	67
Taunton State Hospital	1853–60*b*	24	76
Northampton State Hospital	1870*c*	27	73
New Hampshire State Lunatic Asylum	1872*d*	71	29
New York State Lunatic Asylum	1843–65*e*	38	62
Western Pennsylvania Hospital for the Insane	1856–70*f*	52	48
Danville State Hospital for the Insane	1873*g*	34	66
Pennsylvania State Lunatic Asylum	1862*h*	50	50
Maryland Hospital for the Insane	1867*i*	46	54
Tennessee Hospital for the Insane	1857–9 *j*	53	47
Mississippi Lunatic Asylum	1872*k*	31	69
South Carolina Lunatic Asylum	1859*l*	45	55

*a*32nd *AR* 1864, p. 49. *e*AR 1865, p. 20. *i*AR 1867, p. 14.
*b*7th *AR* 1860, p. 43. *f*AR 1870, p. 19. *j*4th *Biennial Report*, 1857–9, p. 4.
*c*15th *AR* 1870, p. 29 *g*AR 1873–4, p. 24. *k*AR 1872, p. 42.
*d*AR 1872, p. 16. *h*AR 1862, p. 5. *l*AR 1859, p. 8.

Table A.10 compares the percentage of revenue from private boarders to that of all other sources of income for eleven state institutions.

The Maine Hospital for the Insane in 1870 listed $77,000 in revenue from patient board and $6,000 in state appropriations.[6] It is not clear whether the board monies included public support of the indigent. The Vermont Asylum for the Insane in 1859 reported almost $60,000 from "board of patients, etc." and made no mention of any state appropriation.[7] I suspect that both of these hospitals had a high percentage of paying patients, as did the New Hampshire State Lunatic Asylum.

Even as late as 1883, when the practice of taking paying patients in state mental hospitals had attracted public criticism, many of the older institutions still had 5 to 15 percent of their patient population paying board. The Commission on Lunacy included a chart giving the paying versus poor categories for all American mental hospitals.[8] Table A.11 lists the state hospitals having more than 5 percent of paying patients.

Table A.10. *Sources of asylum revenue, private versus public sources (in percentages)*

Institution	Date	Private	Public
Worcester State Hospital	1875[a]	41	59
Taunton State Hospital	1860[b]	16	84
Northhampton State Hospital	1870[c]	40	60
New York State Lunatic Asylum	1860[d]	21	79
Western Pennsylvania Hospital for the Insane	1859[e]	28	72
New Jersey State Lunatic Asylum	1860[f]	29	71
New Hampshire State Lunatic Asylum	1862[g]	54	46
Maryland Hospital for the Insane	1867[h]	62	38
Tennessee Hospital for the Insane	1857–9[i]	38	62
North Carolina Asylum for the Insane	1860[j]	29	71
South Carolina Lunatic Asylum	1872[k]	17	83

[a]42nd *AR* 1875, p. 11. [e]*AR* 1859, p. 13 [i]4th *Biennial Report*, 1857–9, p. 19.
[b]7th *AR* 1860, p. 8. [f]*AR* 1860, p. 21 [j]*AR* 1859–60, pp. 42–3.
[c]15th *AR* 1870, p. 7. [g]*AR* 1862, p. 39. [k]*AR* 1872, p. 17.
[d]18th *AR* 1860, p. 48. [h]*AR* 1867, p. 5.

Table A. 11. *Paying patients in state hospitals, 1883*
(in percentages)

Institution	Paying patients
Alabama Hospital for the Insane	8
Maryland Hospital for the Insane	12
Worcester, State Hospital (Mass.)	15
Taunton State Hospital (Mass.)	9
Northampton State Hospital (Mass.)	12
Danvers State Hospital (Mass.)	15
Michigan Insane Asylum	12
Eastern Michigan I.A.	12
Missouri Lunatic Asylum No. 1	17
Missouri Lunatic Asylum No. 2	13
New Hampshire State Lunatic Asylum	71
New Jersey State Lunatic Asylum (Trenton)	19
New Jersey State Lunatic Asylum (Morristown)	21
New York State Lunatic Asylum (Utica)	20
Hudson River State Hospital (N.Y.)	26
Buffalo State Hospital (N.Y.)	9
Pennsylvania State Lunatic Asylum	48
State Hospital (Pa.)[a]	16
State Hospital (Pa.)[a]	6
State Hospital (Pa.)[a]	11
South Carolina Lunatic Asylum	6
Tennessee Hospital for the Insane	8
Vermont Asylum for the Insane	31
Eastern Lunatic Asylum (Va.)	7
Western Lunatic Asylum (Va.)	13

[a]No further identification was supplied in the chart. These must be the Danville, Norristown, and Warren State Hospitals.
Source: Commission on Lunacy, PSBC, 1ST *AR* (Harrisburg, Pa., 1884), PP. 85–90.

NOTES

The following abbreviations are used in the notes:

AJI   *American Journal of Insanity*
AJMS   *American Journal of Medical Science*
AR   Thomas Story Kirkbride, *Report of the Pennsylvania Hospital for the Insane* (published annually), Philadelphia, Pa.
AS   Pliny Earle, Samuel Woodward, and George Chandler Papers, American Antiquarian Society, Worcester, Mass.
BC   Bucks County Historical Society
BH   Isaac Ray Papers, Butler Hospital, Providence, R.I.
BHM   *Bulletin of the History of Medicine*
CB-FD   Casebook, Female Department, Pennsylvania Hospital for the Insane, Philadelphia, Pa.
CB-MD   Casebook, Male Department, Pennsylvania Hospital for the Insane, Philadelphia, Pa.
CB-OS   Casebook, Old Series, Pennsylvania Hospital for the Insane, Philadelphia, Pa.
CL   Edward Jarvis Papers, Countway Library of the Harvard Medical School, Boston, Mass.
EB Diary   Diary of Eliza Butler
FD   Female Department, Pennsylvania Hospital for the Insane, Philadelphia, Pa.
GC   General Correspondence, Pennsylvania Hospital for the Insane, Philadelphia, Pa.
HC   Friends Hospital Collection, Haverford College, Haverford, Pa.
HL   Dorothea Dix Papers, Houghton Library, Harvard University, Cambridge, Mass.
IPH   Institute for the Pennsylvania Hospital Archives (at the Forty-Ninth Street hospital), Philadelphia, Pa.
JB   Butler Hospital Papers, John Carter Brown Library, Brown University, Providence, R.I.
JHM   *Journal of the History of Medicine and Allied Sciences*
JNMD   *Journal of Nervous and Mental Diseases*
JSH   *Journal of Social History*
LP   Letterpress
LR   *Legislative Record*, Pennsylvania legislature
MD   Male Department, Pennsylvania Hospital for the Insane, Philadelphia, Pa.
MH   *Medical History*
MM   Board of Managers' Minutes, Pennsylvania Hospital for the Insane, Philadelphia, Pa.
MR   Thomas Story Kirkbride's Monthly Report to the Board of Managers, Pennsylvania Hospital for the Insane, Philadelphia, Pa.
NA   St. Elizabeth's Papers, Department of Interior Record Group 418, National Archives, Washington, D.C.
NY   New York Historical Society

PC   Patient Correspondence, Pennsylvania Hospital for the Insane, Philadel-
                phia, Pa.
PCA   Philadelphia City Archives, Philadelphia, Pa.
PH   Pennsylvania Hospital Archives (at the Eighth Street hospital), Philadel-
                phia, Pa.
PL   Butler Family Papers, Firestone Library, Princeton University, Princeton,
                N.J.
PMHB   *Pennsylvania Magazine of History and Biography*
"Proceedings"   "Proceedings of the Association of Medical Superintendents of American
                Asylums for the Insane"
PSBC *AR*   Pennsylvania State Board of Charities, *Annual Report*
PSLA *AR*   Pennsylvania State Lunatic Asylum, *Annual Report*
Rous Diary   Diary of Lucy Rous, companion, Pennsylvania Hospital for the Insane,
                Philadelphia, Pa.
TU   Eliza B. Kirkbride Papers, Temple Urban Archives, Philadelphia, Pa.

Unless otherwise noted (see the preceding list of abbreviations), all manuscript materials
cited in the notes are in the Institute of the Pennsylvania Hospital Archives. See the listing
of manuscript sources at the end for full references to materials in the Institute and Pennsylvania Hospital Archives.

To preserve confidentiality of patient records, citations of patient-related materials give
only the initials of the individual involved. These initials, if used in conjunction with other
identifying information, make it possible to locate the manuscript items cited.

Preface

1 Gerald Grob uses the phrase "treatment–incarceration dichotomy" in "Reflections on the History of Social Policy in America," *Reviews in American History*
  7 (1979):293–306.
2 Gerald Grob, *The State and the Mentally Ill: A History of the Worcester State Hospital
  in Massachusetts, 1830–1920* (Chapel Hill, N.C., 1966).
3 I use the term "corporate" rather than "public" to distinguish the nonprivate,
  charitable institutions, such as the Pennsylvania Hospital for the Insane, Hartford
  Retreat, and McLean Hospital, from private establishments run for profit, such as
  Brigham Hall, Sanford Hall, and the Woodbrook Retreat. This was a crucial distinction to the asylum doctors, and therefore one I have preserved in my own
  discussion.
4 John K. Wing, *Reasoning about Madness* (New York, 1978). Thomas Scheff,
  Mental Illness and Social Processes (New York, 1967), p. 9, defines an agnostic
  scholar as one who "seeks to describe the behavior of members of a society
  without necessarily sharing [or, I might add, rejecting] the assumptions that are
  made in that society about illness."
5 Thomas Story Kirkbride, *On the Construction, Organization and General Arrangements of Hospitals for the Insane* (Philadelphia, 1854), p. 74.

Introduction: The historian and the asylum

1 John Bucknill, *Notes on Asylums for the Insane in America* (New York, 1973; reprint
  of 1876 ed.), p. 4, described the hospital buildings as "architecturally unpretentious."
  The two branches of the Pennsylvania Hospital for the Insane were renamed the
  Department for Nervous and Mental Diseases in 1918. The Institute of the Pennsylvania Hospital opened in 1930 on the grounds of the Forty-ninth Street hospital
  as a separate outpatient clinic and short-term hospital facility. At the same time,
  the male patients in the old Forty-ninth Street hospital were moved back to the
  original building at 4401 Haverford Street. The Forty-fourth Street hospital was
  closed in 1959 and its remaining inhabitants returned to the Forty-ninth Street
  hospital, which had been enlarged by the completion of the six-story North Build-

ing. The City of Philadelphia bought the Forty-fourth Street property and tore down the original asylum building to make way for a housing project. See "Pennsylvania Hospital Opens Modern Psychiatric Unit," *Modern Hospitals* 92 (1959):36–42; and *The Pennsylvania Hospital Bulletin* 14:1 (1957):1.

2 David Mechanic, *Mental Health and Social Policy* (Englewood, Cliffs, N.J., 1980), pp. 87–8. For overviews of the de-institutionalization question, see Leona Bachrach, *De-Institutionalization: An Analytic Review and Sociological Perspective* (DHEW Pub. No. ADM 76-351; Washington, D.C., 1976); and Paul Lehrman, *Deinstitutionalization and the Welfare State* (New Brunswick, N.J., 1982).

3 Carl Taube and Richard Redick, "Provisional Data on Patient Care Episodes in Mental Health Facilities," *Mental Health Statistical Note 139* (1977):1–6; Lehrman, *Deinstitutionalization*, pp. 1–6.

4 The hospital founders' petition is reprinted in Thomas G. Morton, *A History of the Pennsylvania Hospital* (Philadelphia, 1895), p. 6.

5 Albert Deutsch, *The Mentally Ill in America*, 2nd ed. (New York, 1949), pp. 55–71; Samuel Coates, "Cases of Several Lunatics in the Pennsylvania Hospital," mss. notebook, PH, p. 129; Manasseh Cutler, quoted in Morton, *History*, p. 163.

6 Benjamin Rush, *Medical Inquiries and Observations upon the Diseases of the Mind* (Philadelphia, 1812), p. 175.

7 Deutsch, *The Mentally Ill in America* (New York, 1937 and 1949); quotations are from the second edition, pp. 206 and 189.

8 J. Sanbourne Bockoven, *Moral Treatment in American Psychiatry* (New York, 1963); Eric Carlson and Norman Dain, "The Psychotherapy That Was Moral Treatment," *American Journal of Psychiatry* 117 (1960):519–24; Dain and Carlson, "Milieu Therapy in the Nineteenth Century," *JNMD* 131 (1960):277–90; idem, "Social Class and Psychological Medicine in the United States, 1789–1824," *BHM* 33 (1959):454–65; Dain, *Concepts of Insanity in the United States, 1789–1865* (New Brunswick, N.J., 1964).

9 Christopher Lasch, "The Origins of the Asylum," in *The World of Nations* (New York, 1973), pp. xii, 5. For review articles on the social control interpretation in American history, see William Muraskin, "The Social Control Theory in American History: A Critique," *JSH* 9 (1976):559–69; Peter Sterns, "Toward a Wider Vision: Trends in Social History," in *The Past Before Us*, edited by Michael Kammen (Ithaca, N.Y., 1980), pp. 205–30.

10 Michel Foucault, *Madness and Civilization* (New York, 1965). Quotations are from pp. 278 and 8.

11 David Rothman, *The Discovery of the Asylum* (Boston, 1971). Quotations are from pp. 151 and 266.

12 Lasch, "Origins," pp. 3–17; Michael Katz, "Origins of the Institutional State," *Marxist Perspectives* I (1978):6–22. Lasch, "Origins," p. 16, uses the phrase "single standard of citizenship."

13 Richard Fox, *So Far Disordered in Mind: Insanity in California, 1870–1930* (Berkeley, 1978). Quotations are from pp. 14, 186, and 13.

14 Gerald Grob, *The State and the Mentally Ill: A History of the Worcester State Hospital in Massachusetts, 1830–1920* (Chapel Hill, N.C., 1966); *Mental Institutions in America: Social Policy to 1875* (New York, 1973).

15 For representative examples of the interactionist perspective, see Thomas Scheff, "The Labeling Theory of Mental Illness," *American Sociological Review* 39 (1974):44–52; idem, *Being Mentally Ill: A Sociological Theory* (Chicago, 1966); and Walter Gove, ed., *The Labelling of Deviance*, 2nd ed. (New York, 1975). Other scholars associated with the labeling school are Howard Becker, Edwin Lemert, and Edwin Shur. Although Thomas Szasz is a psychiatrist, his work is often associated with this sociological school. His best-known works are *The Myth of Mental Illness* (New York, 1961) and *The Manufacture of Madness* (New York, 1970). Erving Goffman, *Asylums: Essays on the Social Situation of Mental Patients and Other Inmates* (New York, 1961), presents the "total institution" concept.

16 Gerald Grob, "Reflections on the History of Social Policy in America." *Reviews in American History* 7 (1979):293–306. See also his historiographic essay "Redis-

covering Asylums: The Unhistorical History of the Mental Hospital," *Hastings Center Report* (August 1977), 33–41.

17 New work is being done along these lines. See, for example, Barbara Rosenkrantz and Maris Vinovskis, "The Invisible Lunatics: Old Age and Insanity in Mid-Nineteenth Century Massachusetts," in *Aging and the Elderly*, edited by Stuart F. Spicker et al. (Atlantic Highlands, N.J., 1978), pp. 95–125; Barbara Rosenkrantz and Maris A. Vinovskis, "Caring for the Insane in Ante-bellum Massachusetts: Family, Community and State Participation," in *Kin and Communities: Families in America* edited by Allan J. Lichtman and Joan R. Challinor (Washington, 1979) pp. 187–218; and Ellen Dwyer, "Varieties of Female Deviance," unpublished paper delivered at the Social Science History Association Meeting, Boston, November 1979.

18 Delores Hayden, *Seven American Utopias: The Architecture of Communitarian Socialism, 1790–1975* (Cambridge, 1976), p. 33. Rothman, *Discovery*, p. 84, uses the term "moral architecture." Kirkbride uses the phrase "generous confidence" in Thomas Story Kirkbride, *On the Construction, Organization and General Arrangements of Hospitals for the Insane* (Philadelphia, 1854), p. 11.

19 Charles Nichols to Dorothea Dix, 4 July 1869, HL.

20 Charles Rosenberg has described this transformation of the hospital in several articles: "Florence Nightingale on Moral Contagion: The Hospital as Moral Universe," in *Healing and History*, edited by Charles Rosenberg (New York, 1979), pp. 116–35; "And Heal the Sick: The Hospital and The Patient in Nineteenth Century America," *JSH* 10 (1977):428–47; and "Inward Vision and Outward Glance: The Shaping of the American Hospital, 1880–1914," *BHM* 53 (1979):346–91.

CHAPTER 1. *From hospital to asylum*

1 This account of the asylum's first months of operation is drawn from Thomas Story Kirkbride, "Journal, 1841," and *AR* 1841, esp. pp. 34–6.

2 Quotations are taken from *AR* 1841, p. 36; Kirkbride, "Journal, 1841," entry for 31 January; and *AR* 1841, p. 34.

3 Surprisingly, there is no short, comprehensive survey of European moral treatment. Richard Hunter and Ida Macalpine, eds., "Introduction," *Description of the Retreat* (London, 1964), pp. 1–25, provide a solid description of the York Retreat. For more recent interpretations of Tuke's work, see Anne Digby, "Moral Treatment at the Retreat, 1796–1846," and Roy Porter, "Was There a Moral Therapy in the Eighteenth Century?" both unpublished papers presented at the Wellcome Institute, 1980.

4 See Thomas G. Morton, *A History of the Pennsylvania Hospital* (Philadelphia, 1895), esp. pp. 3–13, for an account of the hospital's founding. The 1756 hospital is now called the Pine Building.

5 For accounts of the English voluntary hospital movement, see Wilbur K. Jordan, *The Charities of London, 1480–1660* (New York, 1960), pp. 186–90; Brian Abel-Smith, *The Hospitals, 1800–1948* (London, 1964), pp. 5–6; W. H. McMenemey, "The Hospital Movement of the Eighteenth Century and Its Development," and Alexander Walk, "Mental Hospitals," in *The Evolution of Hospitals in Britain*, edited by Frederick H. Poynter (London, 1964), pp. 43–71, 123–46.

The various social and political needs served by the Pennsylvania Hospital are suggested by William H. Williams, *America's First Hospital: The Pennsylvania Hospital, 1751-1841* (Wayne, Pa., 1976), pp. 8–14, and Sydney James, *A People Among Peoples: Quaker Benevolence in Eighteenth Century America* (Cambridge, Mass., 1963), pp. 205-14.

According to Williams, more than two-thirds of the men who signed the original petition for the Pennsylvania Hospital were Friends. The first Board of Managers included seven practicing Friends, one lapsed Friend, and four members of other denominations. Before the Revolution, 57% of the managers were

Quakers. Of the managers who served for five years or more – the real leadership, in other words – 80% were Friends. With the exception of Benjamin Franklin, the president, secretary, and treasurer of the board were always Friends.

6 On Philadelphia's medical preeminence, see Leonard K. Eaton, *New England Hospitals, 1790-1833* (Ann Arbor, Mich., 1957), p. 14; Carl Bridenbaugh, *Rebels and Gentlemen* (New York, 1942), pp. 263-72; and Richard Shyrock, *Medicine and Society in America, 1660-1860* (Ithaca, N.Y., 1960), pp. 22-31.

7 Morton, *History*, p. 6, reprints the petition.

8 Ibid.

9 For surveys of medical thinking on insanity before the mid-1700s, see Erwin Ackerknecht, *A Short History of Psychiatry*, 2nd rev. ed. (New York, 1968); Franz Alexander and Sheldon Selesnick, *The History of Psychiatry* (New York, 1966); Thomas Graham, *Medieval Minds* (London, 1967); Bennett Simon, *Mind and Madness in Ancient Greece* (Ithaca, N.Y., 1978); Richard Hunter and Ida Macalpine, *Three Hundred Years of Psychiatry* (New York, 1963); and Gregory Zilboorg, *A History of Medical Psychology* (New York, 1941).

   Michael MacDonald, *Mystical Bedlam: Madness, Anxiety and Healing in Seventeenth-Century England* (Cambridge, 1981), provides an excellent exposition of popular concepts of madness. MacDonald's analysis of the practice of Richard Napier, an astrological physician, shows that his services were sought by all classes of English society. In the early 1600s, explanations of insanity still combined magical, religious, and scientific concepts. But by the eighteenth century, the governing elite had rejected the religious or supernatural elements of traditional thinking, and medical rationalism gained considerable ground among the upper classes. See esp. pp. 1–12, 229–31.

10 Edward O'Donoghue, *The Story of Bethlehem Hospital From Its Foundation in 1247* (New York, 1915), pp. 224-5; Walk, "Mental Hospitals," pp. 124-5. Patricia Allderidge, "Management and Mismanagement at Bedlam, 1547-1633," in *Health, Medicine and Mortality in the Sixteenth Century*, edited by Charles Webster (New York, 1979), pp. 141-64, states that O'Donoghue's history must be used with caution (see p. 141, note 1). Unfortunately, her own careful reconstruction of Bethlehem's early history does not go up to Tyson's administration. No doubt his claims were much exaggerated, but the fact remains that the Pennsylvania Hospital managers believed them, and included lunatics in the new institution in hopes of replicating Tyson's supposed success. See also Allderidge, "Hospitals, Madhouses and Asylums: Cycles in the Care of the Insane," *British Journal of Psychiatry* 134 (1979):321–34. As she points out here, lunatics were being brought to Bethlehem to be cured, rather than simply confined, as least as early as the mid-fifteenth century (323).

11 Benjamin Franklin, *Some Account of the Pennsylvania Hospital* (Baltimore, 1954; reprint of 1754 ed), p. 3. See Robert J. Hunter, "The Origin of the Philadelphia General Hospital," *PMHB* 57 (1933):32-57; and Charles Lawrence, *History of the Philadelphia Almshouses and Hospitals* (New York, 1976; reprint of 1905 ed.), for the early history of the almshouse.

12 The distinction comes across clearly in contemporary comparisons of the two institutions. See, for example, the remarks of the Overseers of the Poor, quoted in Hunter, "Origin," 41.

13 My observations on the early treatment of the insane are based primarily on Morton, *History*, and MM, PH.

14 Examples are taken from Samuel Coates, "Cases of Several Lunatics in the Pennsylvania Hospital," mss. notebook, PH, p. 66; Mayor of Philadelphia to managers, n.d. (re. SB), Patient Correspondence, PH; "List of Patients from House of Employment," 6 March 1789, Managers Papers, PH.

15 Samuel Rhoads to "Any Constable," 22 December 1763, Patient Correspondence, PH; "Warrant to apprehend J.E. and convey him to the Pennsylvania Hospital," 29 July 1788, Patient Correspondence, PH. Generally, my observations on commitments to the early hospital are based on Boxes 1961-9, Patient Correspondence, PH.

16 Quotations are from Coates, "Cases," p. 129; Edward Cutbush, *An Inaugural Dissertation on Insanity* (Philadelphia, 1794), p. 15.

17 See Myra C. Glenn, "Changing Attitudes Toward Corporal Punishment," Ph.D. dissertation, State University of New York at Buffalo, 1979.

18 These conclusions are based on my analysis of the Admission and Discharge Books, 1804–33, PH. See also Robert Downie, "Pennsylvania Hospital Admissions, 1751–1850," *Transactions and Studies of the College of Physicians of Philadelphia* 32 (1964–5):21–35.

19 Expense Report, 1790, Managers Papers, PH.

20 Benjamin Rush, *Medical Inquiries and Observations upon the Diseases of the Mind* (Philadelphia, 1812), p. 60, attributed the lower number of female insane patients to the "want of accommodations suited to female delicacy." Comparative rates for male and female patients are as follows:

	Cured	Relieved	No improvement	"Eloped"	Died
Men	36.2	20.4	20.4	8.4	14.6
Women	32.0	26.4	22.4	4.4	14.8

21 Cutbush, *Inaugural Dissertation*, p. 8; Rush, *Medical Inquiries*, pp. 56–57; William Malin, *Some Account of the Pennsylvania Hospital* (Philadelphia, 1828), pp. 39–40.

22 Malin, *Some Account*, p. 40. The high percentage of single persons in the hospital reflects two social facts: the comparatively large number of unmarried individuals in preindustrial societies, and the greater likelihood that a single person would have no relatives nearby to provide home care.

23 Williams, *America's First Hospital*, p. 59, gives figures on paying and poor patients. Morton, *History*, p. 138, discusses the Girard case. Statistics on patient occupations are from Downie, "Pennsylvania Hospital Admissions," 29.

24 WW to Israel Pemberton, 8 December 1763, Patient Correspondence, PH. MM 3:213 records that the western wards were being finished in "a stile of superior consequence for the accommodation of Lunatic Patients."

25 MM 6:390–6; 7:34.

26 Rush noted in his commonplace book on 1 March 1792 that the Assembly had allotted the money to build a "mad house," suggesting that the West Wing was seen as an asylum rather than an extension of the general hospital. See George Corner, ed., *The Autobiography of Benjamin Rush* (Princeton, N.J., 1948), p. 216.

27 Rush is usually given the entire credit (or blame, depending on the scholar's politics) for introducing reform at the Pennsylvania Hospital. Yet, his authority over the lunatic patients was limited. As was the universal custom in the general hospitals of the day, no one physician had complete responsibility for the patients. Like all attending physicians, Rush served there for only four months out of the year. While on duty, he visited the institution only twice a week, and had to examine all the sick and injured patients as well as the insane on those days. Rush did ask for and receive certain privileges in treating the lunatics. During 1787, he had permission to treat all the "maniacal" patients, that is, those admitted in a violent state. See Benjamin Rush to John C. Lettsom, 28 September 1787, in Herbert Butterfield, ed., *Letters of Benjamin Rush*, 2 vols. (Princeton, N.J., 1951), vol. 1, p. 443. Ten years later, Rush and Philip Syng Physick assumed responsibility for all the lunatic patients not under another doctor's care (see MM 7:155). But throughout this period, other attending physicians prescribed treatment for their private patients among the insane. The daily medical attendance devolved upon the resident medical physicians. So, in practice, a number of doctors cared for the insane during the years when new medical measures were introduced at the Pennsylvania Hospital. Rush's work is best seen as part of a broader consensus about the proper treatment of the insane that emerged in this period.

28 Rush, *Medical Inquiries*, pp. 181–2, 222–5, describes these various experiments.

For a later example of heroic treatment, see Hospital Cases 1:256–8 (1827), PH. I have found only one reference to the use of Rush's tranquilizer chair in the early hospital records, in Coates, "Cases," p. 43. At the 1870 meeting of the asylum superintendents, Kirkbride mentioned receiving six "restraining chairs" when he opened the West Philadelphia asylum, "of which I had the pleasure of making a bonfire," he added, but did not explicitly state that they came from the old hospital. See "Proceedings," *AJI* 27 (1870):206.

29 Rush, *Medical Inquiries*, p. 106. For other examples, see ibid., pp. 182–3; Coates, "Cases," pp. 129–31.

30 William Malin to managers, quoted in Morton, *History*, p. 159. See pp. 157–60 for Malin's review of employments and amusements in the West Wing.

31 Corner, *Autobiography*, p. 262; MM 8:202–3, 485. See also MM 4:205, 224, 345, 483, 509.

32 See note 14 for the full reference to Coates's notebook. I describe Coates's account more fully in my article, "The Domesticated Madman: Changing Attitudes Toward Insanity at the Pennsylvania Hospital, 1780–1830," *PMHB* 56 (1982):271–86.

33 These figures are based on my calculations from the Admission and Discharge Records.

34 Quoted in Morton, *History*, pp. 155–6; see also Malin, *Some Account*, pp. 19, 22.

35 Quotations are taken from Morton, *History*, p. 156; Ann Warder, "Extracts from the Diary of Mrs. Ann Warder," *PMHB* 18 (1894):53; Morton, *History*, p. 156. The managers were constantly trying to cut down on the traffic through the lunatics' quarters. See, for example, "Committee on the Condition of the House," 29 June 1812, and "Committee Report on Visiting," 24 June 1822, both in Managers' Papers, PH. Thomas Cope, a prominent Quaker merchant, also took friends on excursions to see the lunatics. See *Philadelphia Merchant: The Diary of Thomas P. Cope, 1800–1851* (South Bend, Ind., 1978), p. 183. I am convinced that the patrons' desire for more privacy was a central issue in the decision to build a new asylum.

36 MM 8:479.

37 Morton, *History*, pp. 154–7, reprints Malin's tract, entitled "Remarks on the Present State of the Pennsylvania Hospital and a Plea for the Necessity of Providing a Separate Asylum for the Insane."

38 MM 9:34–5, 37–42. The contributors' role in pushing for the more remote location for the new asylum is intriguing; perhaps as representatives of the class of potential patrons, they had a strong desire for a more isolated site. Thomas Story Kirkbride in *AR* 1881, pp. 13–14, credits the hospital physicians with convincing the managers to remove the asylum to the country and to appoint a single medical man to be its head.

39 I base my conjectures concerning the independent development of reform at the Pennsylvania Hospital on the following reasoning. By the mid-1790s, the hospital managers had already shown a definite interest in innovation by allowing Rush to pursue his experiments and by raising funds to build a separate insane department. The new West Wing was completed in 1796, the same year William Tuke founded the York Retreat. Throughout the years from 1780 to 1815, the hospital archives contain no reference (at least that I have found) to either Pinel or Tuke. Judging from their accession numbers, the library copies of Philippe Pinel, *Treatise on Insanity* (Sheffield, England, 1806) and *Traité Medico-Philosophique Sur L'Alienation*, 2nd ed. (Paris, 1809), both arrived around 1810. Samuel Tuke, *Description of the Retreat* (Philadelphia, 1813), arrived in 1813; the English edition (York, England, 1813) apparently arrived in 1815. Rush mentions Pinel's work in *Medical Inquiries*. Since by 1811 Philadelphia Friends had begun to plan for the construction of the Friends Asylum, which opened in 1813, the Pennsylvania Hospital officers must surely have heard of Tuke's work by the early 1810s. Norman Dain, *Concepts of Insanity in the United States, 1789-1865* (New Brunswick, N.J., 1964), p. 219 (note 5), states that a Philadelphia Friend, Thomas

Scattergood, visited the York Retreat in 1797. Scattergood undoubtedly spoke of the Retreat upon his return, but there is no evidence that the hospital officers heard of his visit.

Other scholars have pointed out that the reforms associated with Pinel and Tuke actually developed simultaneously in many places. See Albert Deutsch, *The Mentally Ill in America*, 2nd ed. (New York, 1949), pp. 94-5; William Parry-Jones, *The Trade in Lunacy* (London, 1972), pp. 171-4; and Porter, "Was There a Moral Therapy?"

40 Dora Weiner, "Health and Mental Health in the Thought of Philippe Pinel," in *Healing and History*, edited by Charles Rosenberg, (New York, 1979), pp. 75-6, notes that Jean-Baptiste Pussin, the "keeper" of the insane at the Bicêtre, had a decisive influence on Pinel's conception of moral treatment. Here again, one might argue that common institutional concerns informed the medical rationale for asylum reform.

The only other eighteenth-century general hospital in America, the New York Hospital (founded 1776, opened 1791), followed a pattern of development similar to that of the Pennsylvania Hospital. A separate hospital for the insane was built on the grounds of the general hospital in 1808, and a rural asylum opened in 1821. The Massachusetts General Hospital skipped over the intermediary state and established a separate rural asylum (McLean) in 1818; the general hospital opened in 1821. See William Russell, *The New York Hospital: A History of the Psychiatric Service 1771-1936* (New York, 1945), esp. pp. 49, 65-75, 119-30; and Deutsch, *The Mentally Ill*, 2nd ed., pp. 102-5.

41 For recent overviews of American social history c. 1790-1840, see Paul Boyer, *Urban Masses and the Moral Order in America 1820-1920* (Cambridge, Mass., 1978), esp. pp. 1-120; Richard Brown, *Modernization: The Transformation of American Life 1600-1865* (New York, 1976): James Henretta, *The Evolution of American Society, 1700-1815* (Lexington, Mass., 1973); and Ronald Walters, *American Reformers* (New York, 1978).

42 Stephen Thernstrom, *The Other Bostonians* (Cambridge, Mass., 1973), p. 256. See also idem, *Poverty and Progress* (Cambridge, Mass., 1964), esp. pp. 33-79.

43 Compare the Pennsylvania Hospital's development with the account of W. David Lewis, *From Newgate to Dannemora: The Rise of the Penitentiary in New York, 1796-1848* (Ithaca, N.Y., 1965), esp. pp. 59-67. A crisis in prison management caused by recurrent problems of overcrowding, administrative laxity, and poorly designed buildings led to increasing emphasis on classification, separation, and more intense institutional discipline.

On the whole, historians have accorded little weight to internal or administrative pressures for change in early nineteenth century institutions. David Rothman, *The Discovery of the Asylum* (Boston, 1971), points to similarities in institutional design and routine, but presents them as a generalized cultural response to change, rather than measures adopted to relieve specific internal tensions within unspecialized eighteenth century institutions. Similarly, Christopher Lasch, "The Origins of the Asylum," in *The World of Nations* (New York, 1973) and Michael Katz, "Origins of the Institutional State," *Marxist Perspectives* 1 (1978):6-22, relate the same phenomenon to the uncertainties of early nineteenth-century capitalism.

44 Walters, *American Reformers*, has included chapters on temperance and health reform that suggest the self-regulatory aspects of the impulse for order, although he himself does not emphasize that aspect. See also Boyer, *Urban Masses*, pp. 30, 61-2. His discussion of the Sunday School movement, pp. 34-53, touches on the self-regulation theme. Mary Ryan, *Cradle of the Middle Class: The Family in Oneida County, New York 1790-1865* (New York, 1981), esp. pp. 104-44, highlights the reformers' emphasis on family protection. Brown, *Modernization*, suggests a framework for relating the self-culture and self-control themes in nineteenth-century reform.

45 Deutsch, in *The Mentally Ill*, 2nd ed., p. 132, makes use of the phrase "cult of curability."

CHAPTER 2. *Christian and physician*

1 Samuel Woodward to Pliny Earle, 11 October 1840, Earle Papers, AS, mentions the Pennsylvania Hospital for the Insane offer. See also Alfred Stille to Samuel Woodward, 19 October 1840, Woodward Papers, AS, for the reference to Woodward's refusal of the post.

2 Thomas Story Kirkbride to James Greeves, 22 February 1845, LP 2:40. Albert Deutsch, *The Mentally Ill in America*, 2nd ed. (New York, 1949), p. 206, writes, "A prominent British psychiatrist, Dr. T. S. Clouston, recalling a visit he once made in Philadelphia, remarked that a street car conductor whom he approached could not tell him where the Pennsylvania Hospital for the Insane was, but readily directed him to 'Kirkbride's'."

3 Howard S. Becker, *Outsiders: Studies in the Sociology of Deviance* (New York, 1963), pp. 147-63, defines the "moral entrepreneur" as a "role creator." Andrew Scull, "From Madness to Mental Illness: Medical Men as Moral Entrepreneurs," *Archives Européenes de Sociologie* 16 (1975):218-59, applies the term to nineteenth-century asylum doctors.

4 Thomas Story Kirkbride, "Autobiographical Sketch Dictated...in 1882" (Philadelphia, 1882), pp. 1-2. Earl D. Bond, *Dr. Kirkbride and His Mental Hospital* (Philadelphia, 1947), is a short, very laudatory biography of Kirkbride. Bond, a prominent American psychiatrist, was physician-in-chief of the Department of Mental and Nervous Diseases. His account seems accurate, but whenever possible, I have cited the original sources rather than his book, which has no footnotes. In a few instances, he gives facts that I have not been able to verify; in these cases, I cite him.

"Farm Map of Lower Makefield Township, Bucks County, Pa., Surveyed, Drawn and Published by Thomas Hughes 1858," BC, shows the size and location of John Kirkbride's farm. The Bucks County Tax Records for Lower Makefield, 1819 and 1828, BC, list the plaster mill and ferry, respectively. "Marriages and Deaths in Bucks County, 1804-34," BC, p. 22, records the marriage of John Kirkbride and Elizabeth Story on 12 October 1808.

William Wade Hinshaw, *Encyclopedia of American Quaker Genealogy*, 6 vols. (Ann Arbor, Mich., 1938), vol. 2, p. 962, lists the following information for Kirkbride's family:

John Kirkbride, b. 5 October 1777; d. 14 January 1864.
Elizabeth Curtis, b. 18 November 1787; d. 12 March 1860. (Elizabeth Curtis was John Kirkbride's mother's maiden name; Hinshaw or the meeting made an error here; John's wife was Elizabeth Story.)
Children of John and Elizabeth Kirkbride:
Thomas Story, b. 31 July 1809; [d. 16 December 1883].
Mahlon S., b. 3 March 1811; d. 24 January 1887.
Mary, b. 14 February 1813; d.?
William, b. 1 April 1815; d. 18 September 1827.
Elizabeth, b. 24 May 1817; d.?
Rachel, b. 1 March 1820; d?
Rebecca, b. 3 July 1826; d. 24 January 1890.
Anna, b. 27 October 1829; d. 27 July 1830.
Kirkbride's sister Elizabeth married a Mr. Carlisle. Her daughter Elizabeth, better known as "Lizzie" Carlisle, made her home with Kirkbride and his family.

5 The "farm product" quotation comes from an article in the *Times and Dispatch*, 15 November 1871, clipping in AM file, GC.

6 "Domestic Portraiture of Our Ancestors Kirkbride 1650 to 1824" [pamphlet in genealogical file], BC, pp. 1-6, 20-7. Quotations are from pp. 23, 22.

7 Kirkbride, "Autobiographical Sketch," p. 3; Bond, *Dr. Kirkbride*, p. 9. A "guarded" education is one consistent with the society's religious principles.

8 My discussion of the Hicksite schism is based on Philip S. Benjamin, *The Philadelphia Quakers in the Industrial Age 1865-1920* (Philadelphia, 1976), esp. chap. 1; and Robert W. Doherty, *The Hicksite Separation* (New Brunswick, N.J., 1967). Hinshaw, *Encyclopedia*, vol. 2, p. 1075, lists John, Mahlon, Elizabeth, and Mary Kirkbride as being disowned by the Hicksites for joining the Orthodox meeting. Many years later, Mahlon Kirkbride did join the Hicksites (vol. 2, p. 1054).

9 *AR* 1883, p. 148. See also p. 72 for a reference to Kirkbride's religious principles. Chapter 5, note 88, discusses his efforts to remain a member of the society after marrying a non-Quaker in 1866.

10 Sidney Mead, *The Lively Experiment* (New York, 1963), esp. chaps. 2 and 7, discusses Protestant denominationalism. Joan Brumberg, "The Feminization of Teaching," *History of Education Quarterly* (forthcoming): refers to the debate over denominational politics in public education. Leonard Eaton, "Eli Todd and the Hartford Retreat," *New England Quarterly* 26 (1953):444, notes that Amariah Brigham's nomination for the Retreat position drew criticism because his theological soundness was in doubt.

11 Mrs. C, MH, 10 July 1860, PC. Two other early asylum doctors, Pliny Earle and Charles Nichols, were also Friends.

12 Bond, *Dr. Kirkbride*, p. 14.

13 Ibid., pp. 9-11. William Allinson, "Memorials of the Life and Character of John Gummere" [available in pamphlet file, Historical Society of Pennsylvania], comments on Gummere's style of authority, a style much like that attributed to the adult Kirkbride. He was "theoretically sound in Christian faith" and inspired a "filial confidence" in his students. Allinson recalled that "his school was remarkably well-drilled – and kept in order without any severity...His power over his pupils was absolute, because he ruled alike the judgment and the affections. So strong was the sentiment of affection that he was repeatedly known to quell disaffection by the moral power of a grieved look." Perhaps Kirkbride learned some of his persuasive techniques from Gummere.

14 William Rothstein, *American Physicians in the Nineteenth Century: From Sects to Science* (Baltimore, 1972), pp. 115-20, discusses the prevailing standards of education for physicians. The exact number of college graduates in the 1820s is difficult to determine, but it was certainly a tiny fraction of male youths. According to Burton J. Bledstein, *The Culture of Professionalism: The Middle Class and the Development of Higher Education* (New York, 1976), p. 241, the thirty-seven best-known colleges produced a combined total of 413 graduates per year in that decade.

15 Statistics on rural–urban residence can be found in the U.S. Bureau of the Census, *Historical Statistics of the United States*, 2 vols. (Washington, D.C., 1975), vol. 1, p. 12. On the rising standard of living in the early nineteenth century, see James Henretta, *The Evolution of American Society, 1700-1815* (Lexington, Mass., 1973), pp. 188-206. Rolla Tryon, *Household Manufactures in the United States, 1640-1860* (New York, 1966; reprint of 1917 ed.), documents the spread of consumer goods. Maris Vinovskis, "Angels' Heads and Weeping Willows: Death in Early America," in *The American Family in Social-Historical Perspective*, edited by Michael Gordon, 2nd ed. (New York, 1978), pp. 546-63, discusses the relatively low levels of mortality in America.

16 Charles Rosenberg, *The Cholera Years: The United States in 1832, 1849 and 1866* (Chicago, 1962), provides an overview of health conditions in the antebellum city. The health problems and cultural concerns I discuss in the following section were only beginning to emerge in the 1820s, but were well articulated by the time Kirkbride entered asylum practice in the 1840s, and continued to dominate the popular health literature throughout the nineteenth century. See Rosenberg, "The Place of George M. Beard in Nineteenth Century Psychiatry," *BHM* 36 (1962):245-59, for a discussion of contemporary views of "civilization and its

discents," or the link between modern life and ill health, both mental and physical. John Haller and Robin Haller, *The Physician and Sexuality in Victorian America* (New York, 1974), pp. 252-70, discuss venereal disease.

17 On domestic medicine and popular health manuals, see Guenther B. Risse, "Introduction," and John B. Blake, "From Buchan to Fishbein: The Literature of Domestic Medicine," in *Medicine Without Doctors*, edited by Guenther Risse, Ronald Numbers, and Judith Leavitt (New York, 1977), pp. 1-9, 11-30.

18 On the connection between personal morality and health, see Stephen Nissenbaum, *Sex, Diet and Debility in Jacksonian America: Sylvester Graham and Health Reform* (Westport, Conn., 1980); Charles Rosenberg, "Sexuality, Class and Role," in *No Other Gods: Science and American Social Thought*, edited by Rosenberg (Baltimore, 1976), pp. 71-88; Regina Morantz, "Nineteenth Century Health Reform and Women," in *Medicine Without Doctors*, pp. 73-93.

19 On the popular health movement in antebellum America, see the essays in Risse et al. eds., *Medicine Without Doctors*; Martha Verbrugge, "The Social Meaning of Personal Health: The Ladies Physiological Institute of Boston and Vicinity in the 1850s," in *Health Care in America*, edited by Susan Reverby and David Rosner (Philadelphia, 1979), pp. 45-66. On the growth of resorts, see Harry B. Weiss and Howard Kemble, *The Great American Water-Cure Craze: A History of Hydropathy in the United States* (Trenton, N.J., 1967), and Marshall Legan, "Hydropathy in America," *BHM* 45 (1971):267-80. Lee Soltow and Edward Stevens, *The Rise of Literacy and the Common School in the United States* (Chicago, 1981), pp. 153, 155, estimate that the illiteracy rate among men fell from around 25% (North) and 40%-50% (South) in 1800 to 3% (Northeast), 9% (Northwest), 19% (Southeast), and 17% (Southwest) in 1840. The rates for women appear to have been significantly lower than those for men, but the disparity was greatly reduced by 1860.

20 On medical sectarianism, see Ronald Numbers, "Do-It-Yourself the Sectarian Way," in Risse et al., *Medicine Without Doctors*, pp. 49-72; Rothstein, *American Physicians*, pp. 125-74; and Martin Kaufman, *Homeopathy in America* (Baltimore, 1971). On patent medicine, see James H. Young, "Patent Medicines and the Self-Help Syndrome," in Risse et al., *Medicine Without Doctors*, pp. 95-116; Young, *The Toadstool Millionaires* (Princeton, N.J., 1961). On diet reform, see Nissenbaum, *Sex, Diet and Debility*. On hydropathy, see Numbers, "Do-It-Yourself the Sectarian Way," and works on hydropathy cited in note 19.

21 Charles Rosenberg has influenced my thinking on this point.

22 Rothstein, *American Physicians*, pp. 85-7; and Henry Shafer, *The American Medical Profession* (New York, 1936), pp. 33-4, discuss the function of the preceptorial relation in medical education.

23 Kirkbride, "Autobiographical Sketch," pp. 3-4. My information on Kirkbride's preceptor comes from Fred B. Rogers, "Dr. Nicholas Belleville (1753-1831), Aristocratic Physician," *Journal of the Medical Society of New Jersey* 55 (1958):71-7. Kirkbride had cause to be grateful that his preceptor devoted so much time to him. Medical apprentices frequently complained of neglect. See Samuel Rezneck, "The Study of Medicine at the Vermont Academy of Medicine...," in *Theory and Practice in American Medicine*, edited by Gert H. Brieger (New York, 1976) p. 16.

24 For discussions of nineteenth-century concepts of disease, see Richard Shryock, *Medicine and Society in America, 1660-1860* (Ithaca, N.Y., 1960), pp. 68-9; Charles Rosenberg, "The Therapeutic Revolution," *Perspectives in Biology and Medicine* (Summer 1977):487-9; and Joseph Kett, *The Formation of the American Medical Profession* (New Haven, Conn., 1968), pp. 156-61.

25 Rogers, "Dr. Nicholas Belleville," 74-5. Erwin H. Ackerknecht, *Medicine at the Paris Hospital, 1794-1848* (Baltimore, 1967), p. xi, discusses the traits of the Paris School referred to here and later in this chapter. Charles Rosenberg, "The Practice of Medicine in New York a Century Ago," *BHM* 41 (1967):241-2, provides a good discussion of physical examination and prognostic skills before the introduction of auscultation, the laryngoscope, or blood and urine tests. Few of these

latter methods were in wide use in the late 1860s. Kirkbride was evidently using a stethoscope in the late 1830s. See H. Lippincott to Kirkbride, 5 March [1836?], GC.

26 Rogers, "Dr. Nicholas Belleville," 75-6. Descriptions of Belleville's practice are taken from Kirkbride, "Notes on the Practice of Dr. N. Belleville, 1830," pp, 5, 12, 22, IPH.

27 Rogers, "Dr. Nicholas Belleville," p. 75. See Kirkbride, "Notes on the Practice...," pp. 11, 13-14, 18-19, 20, 27, for drug recipes.

28 For a discussion of medical school and medical careers, see Barnes Riznick, "The Professional Lives of Early Nineteenth Century New England Doctors," *JHM* 19 (1964):11-12.

29 Irwin Richman, *The Brightest Ornament: A Biography of Nathaniel Chapman* (Bellefonte, Pa., 1967), p. 5. Although a convincing case for Chapman's mediocrity, this is a weak biography. Chapman may have had some interest in Parisian pathological methods, but the evidence on this point is contradictory. Richard Shryock, "The Advent of Modern Medicine in Philadelphia, 1800-1850," *Yale Journal of Biology and Medicine* 13 (1941):727-8, 732, presents Chapman as a source of Parisian viewpoints in the city; Richman, *The Brightest Ornament*, esp. p. 100, portrays Chapman as cognizant of but hostile to the work of Francois J.-V. Broussais and Francois Magendie. Whatever the case, it seems certain that Kirkbride got no real introduction to the Paris School from Chapman.

For comparisons of American and European medical education, see Shryock, *Medicine and Society*, pp. 141-2; Russell M. Jones, "American Doctors and the Parisian Medical World," *BHM* 47 (1973):49-50; and Shafer, *The American Medical Profession*, pp. 36-7, 88-9.

30 Lester King, *The Medical World of the Eighteenth Century* (Chicago, 1958), provides an overview of medical thinking in this period.

31 The shortest and clearest exposition of these medical systems can be found in Shryock, *Medicine and Society*, pp. 67-70. See also Guenther G. Risse, "The History of John Brown's Medical System in Germany During the Years 1790-1806," Ph.D. dissertation, University of Chicago, 1971; idem, "The Bruonian System," *Clio Medica* 5 (1970):45-51; and Whitfield Bell, "Some American Students of 'That Shining Oracle of Physic,' Dr. William Cullen of Edinburgh, 1755-1766," *Proceedings of the American Philosophical Society* 94 (1950):275-81.

32 Rosenberg, "The Therapeutic Revolution," 496-500, offers a broad perspective on this shift in therapeutics. See also Kett, *Formation*, pp. 157-60. For Kirkbride's list of drugs, see Kirkbride, "Notebook, 1831," p. 114.

33 See Courtney R. Hall, "The Rise of Professional Surgery in the United States, 1800-1865," *BHM* 26 (1952):231-62, for a discussion of antebellum surgery. On midwifery, see Jane Donegan, *Women Midwives and Medical Men* (Westport, Conn., 1978).

34 Kirkbride, "Notes on the Practice...," pp. 39-43, has a series of quotations from Rush; see ibid., pp. 109-24, for notes on George Burrows, *Commentaries on the Causes, Forms, Symptoms, and Treatment, Moral and Medical, of Insanity* (London, 1828). The review of Burrows's book is quoted in Richard Hunter and Ida Macalpine, *Three Hundred Years of Psychiatry* (New York, 1963), p. 778.

35 Kirkbride, "An Essay on Neuralgia for the Degree of Doctor of Medicine in the University of Pennsylvania...16 January 1832." Copy of mss. in IPH. On Chapman's interest in neuralgia, see "Remarks on Tic Dôuloureaux; with cases," *AJMS* 14, no. 28 (1834):289-320.

36 See Ida Macalpine and Richard Hunter, *George III and the Mad Business* (London, 1969), pp. 287-90, for a discussion of this trend in the eighteenth century; Rosenberg, "The Place of George M. Beard," for the same in the second half of the nineteenth century.

37 Kirkbride, "Autobiographical Sketch," p. 4. Williams, *America's First Hospital*, p. 136, discusses service at the Pennsylvania Hospital as a means of enhancing one's professional status.

38 Kirkbride, "Autobiographical Sketch," p. 4. Kirkbride does not give his uncle's

name here, but the letter, which is preserved in the IPH archives, was from Jenks. See J. R. Jenks to Kirkbride, 10 April 1832, Documents Relating to Kirkbride's Career, No. 11. See note 60 in this chapter for more about Kirkbride's marriage to Jenks's daughter, Ann. The Friends Hospital is now within the city limits of Philadelphia, on City Line Avenue.

39 See Chapter 1, note 3, for general references on moral treatment.

40 Samuel Tuke, *The Description of the Retreat Near York* (Philadelphia, 1813). An abridged version of the account appeared in the *Account of the Rise and Progress of the Asylum Proposed to Be Established Near Philadelphia . . .* (Philadelphia, 1814). For a general discussion of Tuke's influence in America, see Deutsch, *The Mentally Ill*, 2nd ed., pp. 95-9.

41 See Dain and Carlson, "Milieu Therapy in the Nineteenth Century," *JNMD* 131 (1960):277-90.

42 Friends Asylum, Managers' Minutes, 2:352-3, HC. These comments were also reprinted in the *Sixteenth Annual Report on the State of the Asylum for the Relief of Persons Deprived of the Use of their Reason*, 1833, pp. 3, 5. Anne Digby, "Moral Treatment at the Retreat, 1796-1846," unpublished paper presented at the Wellcome Institute, 1980, pp. 19-21, states that in the late 1830s, a similar shift toward more reliance on medical men and medical therapeutics took place at the York Retreat. The Friends Asylum had approximately fifteen to thirty patients between 1817 and 1830 and forty to fifty in the 1830s. After 1834, admission was not limited to the Society of Friends. After the 1827-8 schism, it was controlled by the Orthodox Meeting. See Benjamin, *The Philadelphia Quakers*, p. 11. Kirkbride resided at the asylum for one year "without other compensation than his board and washing." See Friends Asylum, Managers' Minutes 2:232-3.

43 MM 9:41. See Deutsch, *The Mentally Ill*, 2nd ed., pp. 104, 112, for references to McLean and the Hartford Retreat; William Russell, *The New York Hospital: A History of the Psychiatric Service 1771-1936* (New York: 1945), p. 190, on Bloomingdale. See MM 9;41, 44-7, for a discussion of medical attendance at the Pennsylvania Hospital's asylum. The quotation comes from the minority report of Manager Charles Robert. The board did not at first accept his argument, and it is unclear at what point between 1835 and 1840 they reversed their position. (At the Bloomingdale Asylum and the Hartford Retreat, the lay superintendent continued to have considerable administrative power and a certain independence of the medical superintendent's authority, a situation the asylum doctors deplored. See pp. 113-14 for further discussion of this point.)
   The early public mental hospitals moved to the single superintendent plan more slowly than their corporate counterparts. Norman Dain, *Disordered Minds* (Williamsburg, Va., 1971), p. 66, states that the Eastern State Hospital did not get a superintendent until 1841. According to John Curwen, *History of the Association of Medical Superintendents of American Institutions for the Insane from 1844 to 1874* (Harrisburg, 1875), the Eastern State Lunatic Asylum in Kentucky, founded in 1824, did not get a genuine medical superintendent until 1844; the South Carolina Lunatic Asylum, founded in 1828, got one in 1836.

44 Friends Asylum, Managers Minutes 2:352-3, HC. See also Charles Evans, *Account of the Asylum for the Relief of Persons Deprived of the Use of their Reason, Near Frankford, Pennsylvania* (Philadelphia, 1839), p. 9.

45 Cases in the next few paragraphs are taken from the Friends Asylum, Managers Minutes 2:356-9, HC. The attending managers said that the cases had been "condensed . . . from the medical journal of the House, kept by the Resident Physician," i.e., Kirkbride.

46 Examples are taken from the Friends Asylum, Visiting Committee Minutes, 8 December and 9 June 1832; 12 January 1833, HC.

47 Friends Asylum, *Sixteenth Annual Report*, p. 5; Kirkbride, "Autobiographical Sketch," pp. 4-5.

48 For a description of the resident's duties at the Pennsylvania Hospital, see Williams, *America's First Hospital*, pp. 137-8. Kirkbride entered cases of puerperal fever, tetanus, strangulated femoral hernia, and dislocated humerus upon the dorsum scapula in Hospital Cases 1, PH. He later published a series of case

histories in *AJMS* 15, no. 29 (Nov. 1834):64-80; 15, no. 30 (Feb. 1835): 342-61; no. 31 (May 1835):13-34; 16, no. 32 (Aug. 1835):309-32; and 17, no. 33 (Nov. 1835):39-56.

49 Hospital Cases 1, also labeled "Journal of Cases Observed by Dr. Kirkbride in 1833-34 at the Pennsylvania Hospital," and "Hospital Cases Continued, 1834." Eaton, "Eli Todd," p. 440, states that Todd wrote very little. Perhaps Kirkbride got the recipes from the *Annual Reports* of the Hartford Retreat.

50 Kirkbride, "Autobiographical Sketch," pp. 5-6. For more on Gerhard and Louis, see Jones, "American Doctors," esp. 187. Gerhard later served at the Philadelphia General Hospital, and became famous for distinguishing typhoid from typhus fever on the basis of pathological evidence.

51 Kirkbride, "Autobiographical Sketch," p. 6.

52 Jones, "American Doctors," provides a good discussion of this career pattern in Kirkbride's generation. For a surgical specialty, an American would probably have gone to London or Edinburgh; see Hall, "The Rise of Professional Surgery," pp. 238-9.

53 Kirkbride, "Autobiographical Sketch," pp. 7-9. See Riznick, "Professional Lives," 4, for a discussion of the difficulties young doctors often encountered in setting up a practice.

54 All information on Kirkbride's private practice comes from his Casebook for Private Patients, 1836-7, and Account Books, vol. 1 (1835-9) and vol. 2 (1839-40). His apparent success in clearing up a man's syphilitic skin eruption with the nonmercurial plan prompted Kirkbride to write in the Casebook, p. 24, "This fact shows how easy it is to be deceived with respect to the good effects of mercury administered under such circumstances."

55 Rosenberg, "The Practice of Medicine," 229.

56 On medical care in the nineteenth-century general hospital, see Charles Rosenberg, "And Heal the Sick: The Hospital and The Patient in Nineteenth Century America," *JSH* 10 (1977):428-47; Rosenberg, "Inward Vision and Outward Glance: The Shaping of the American Hospital, 1880-1914," *BHM* 53 (1979):346-91; and Morris Vogel, *The Transformation of the Modern Hospital* (Chicago, 1980).

57 These estimates of Kirkbride's income are derived from his Account Books, vols. 1 and 2. On the state of medical practice at this time, see Edward Atwater, "The Medical Profession in a New Society, Rochester, New York, 1811-1860," *BHM* 47 (1973):22-3, 228; Shryock, *Medicine and Society*, pp. 143-9. Riznick, "Professional Lives," 6, gives $500.00 as an average income for a New England physician in the late 1830s. For New York in the 1860s, Rosenberg, "The Practice of Medicine," 229, gives $400.00 as an average beginning income and $1,500.00-2,000.00 as a successful physician's income. These figures suggest that Kirkbride was doing well in private practice. His career does not seem to conform to the general pattern Constance McGovern reports in " 'Mad Doctors': American psychiatrists, 1800-1860," Ph.D. dissertation, University of Massachusetts, 1976.

58 Kirkbride, "Autobiographical Sketch," pp. 9-10.

59 Ibid., pp. 9-11. The board did not record why they preferred Kirkbride to the other candidates eager for the job. Certainly, they knew him and respected his work; perhaps they also judged him to be a safe candidate, since they were worried about losing control over the new rural asylum (see MM 9:37-8). Also, Kirkbride had not been involved in the controversy over where to locate the new mental hospital. Benjamin Horner Coates, probably his chief rival for the job (see "Autobiographical Sketch," p. 10; his father, Samuel Coates, had been an influential manager), had written some rather critical letters to the managers concerning the care of the lunatic patients. See B. Coates to Alex Johnston and Charles Watson, 26 July 1828, Managers Papers, PH.

60 Ibid., p. 11. Kirkbride married Ann West Jenks on 4 June 1839. She was the daughter of Joseph Richardson Jenks, a flour merchant ranked in 1845 as one of Philadelphia's wealthiest citizens. Jenks served as a manager at the Pennsylvania Hospital from 1827 to 1828. See Thomas G. Morton, *A History of the Pennsylvania Hospital* (Philadelphia, 1895), p. 427, for a short biographical sketch of him.

Kirkbride's account of his reaction to the unexpected job offer in the "Autobiographical Sketch" is consistent with a much earlier version of his decision-making process, given in a letter to one of the managers (Kirkbride was complaining about a salary reduction). See Kirkbride to James Greeves, 22 February 1845, LP 2:4. When asked once if he regretted abandoning his interest in surgery, Kirkbride replied, "I remembered Lot's wife. I never looked back." *AR* 1883, p. 152.

61 Kirkbride, "Autobiographical Sketch," p. 11.

62 Rosenberg, "And Heal the Sick," 434, 437, discusses the factors diffusing medical authority in the general hospital.

63 Besides corresponding with other superintendents, Kirkbride familiarized himself with the state of American asylum practice on two asylum tours; on the first, in November and December 1841, he examined the "most noted" institutions in New York and New England; on the second, in June 1845, he visited the Blackwell's Island Asylum, Bloomingdale, Sanford Hall, New York State Hospital at Utica, Worcester State Hospital, Boston City Lunatic Hospital, McLean Asylum for the Insane, New Hampshire Hospital, and the Hartford Retreat. See Kirkbride, "Journal, 1841," entry for 1 January; and "Journal of a Visit to Nine Institutions for the Insane, 1845."

64 For overviews of American psychiatric thought, see Grob, *Mental Institutions in America: Social Policy to 1875* (New York), 1973, pp. 151-71; Grob, *The State and the Mentally Ill: A History of the Worcester State Hospital in Massachusetts, 1830-1920* (Chapel Hill, N.C., 1966), pp. 51-4; Norman Dain, *Concepts of Insanity in the United States, 1789-1865* (New Brunswick, N.J., 1964), esp. chaps. 1, 3, and 4; and David Rothman, *The Discovery of the Asylum* (Boston, 1971), pp. 110-29.

65 I base these observations on biographical information given in the superintendents' obituaries in the *AJI*: 18 (1862):421-34 (Bell); 6 (1849):185-92 (Brigham); 47 (1890):92-5 (Butler); 50 (1893):127-9 (Earle); 6 (1849):71-92 (Macdonald); 37 (1881):480-3 (Ray); 31 (1874):134-7 (Rockwell); 31 (1874):274-5 (Stribling); 1 (1845):384 (White); and 8 (1851):117-32 (Woodward).

66 Grob, *Mental Institutions in America*, pp. 132-74, gives a summary of the profession's early development. For more recent studies of the specialty, see Constance McGovern, " 'Mad-Doctors,' " and John Pitts, "The Association of Medical Superintendents of American Institutions for the Insane," Ph.D. dissertation, University of Pennsylvania, 1979.

67 See Chapter 5, note 102, for more on private asylums.

68 Quotations are from "Manuscript Notes of the Medical Lectures of Nathaniel Chapman," taken by Dr. Wilmer Worthington, in two volumes, vol. 1, pp. 125, 79-81. On humoralism, see Ackerknecht, *A Short History*, 2nd rev. ed., pp. 36-7; Shryock, *Medicine and Society*, pp. 68-9; and Macalpine and Hunter, *George III*, p. 288.

69 See the references cited in note 30.

70 William Cullen, *First Lines on the Practice of Physic*, went through ten editions between 1781 and 1816. The section on insanity, which first appeared in the fourth Edinburgh edition, was included in all but the first of the American editions. See Robert M. Austin, *Early American Medical Imprints* (Washington, D.C., 1961), pp. 62-3.

71 This tendency to emphasize somatic factors can be seen in the relative length of the discussions concerning the physical and mental causes of insanity. Robert Whytt, *Observations on the Nature, Causes, and Cure of Those Disorders Which Have Been Commonly Called Nervous, Hypochondriac or Hysteric* (Edinburgh, 1765), for example, gives five categories of physical causes and only one for psychological causes.

72 See Whytt, *Observations*, and George Cheyne, *The English Malady, Or a Treatise on Nervous Diseases of All Kinds* (London, 1733).

73 The first edition of Pinel's major work was *Treatise on Insanity*, tr. D. D. Davis (Sheffield, England, 1806). My discussion of Pinel relies heavily on Kathleen

Grange, "Pinel and Eighteenth Century Psychiatry," *BHM* 35 (1961):442-53; Evelyn A. Woods and Eric Carlson, "The Psychiatry of Philippe Pinel," *BHM* 35 (1961):14-25; and Walther Riese, *The Legacy of Philippe Pinel* (New York, 1969). Grange, pp. 442-3, discusses Pinel's use of the term "moral" to denote psychological faculties. See also Lester King, "A Note on So-Called 'Moral Treatment', *JHM* 19 (1964):297-8; and Eric Carlson and Norman Dain, "The Meaning of Moral Insanity," *BHM* 38 (1962):134. For background on the Scottish philosophy, see S. A. Grave, *The Scottish Philosophy of Common Sense* (Oxford, 1960); Anand C. Chitnis, *The Scottish Enlightenment* (Totowa, N.J., 1976); and Gladys Bryson, *Man and Society* (Princeton, N.J., 1945).

74 See Scull, "From Madness to Mental Illness," 225-6 and William Bynum, "Rationales for Therapy in British Psychiatry," *Medical History* 18 (1974):322-5, for discussions of the medical modification of Pinel and Tuke's antimedicine implications. See Dain and Carlson, "Milieu Therapy," 285, for a discussion of the immaterial–incurable problem.

75 Pliny Earle, "Bloodletting in Mental Disorders," *AJI* 10 (1854):390-1, 386-7. The historical argument Earle used also allowed the superintendents gracefully to repudiate Rush. Earle wrote that it was far easier to believe that the disease had changed character than to suppose that "such an acute and sagacious observer, a learned and profound medical philosopher" as Rush had reached a wrong conclusion (397). This same line of argument was used in general medicine as well. See Rosenberg, "The Therapeutic Revolution," 497–504, and Rothstein, *American Physicians*, pp. 177–97.

76 John Curwen, quoted in "Proceedings," *AJI* 11 (1854):52.

77 Pliny Earle, "On the Causes of Insanity," *AJI* 4 (1848):185-211.

78 Dain, *Concepts*, pp. 59–63.

79 See John Davies, *Phrenology: Fad and Science* (New Haven, Conn., 1955), for a general account of phrenology.

80 On phrenology and its impact on psychiatry, see R. A. Cooter, "Phrenology and British Alienists, c. 1825–1845," *Medical History* 20 (1976), esp. 140–6; Dain, *Concepts*, esp. pp. 61–3; Bynum, "Rationales," 331; Davies, *Phrenology*, pp. 89–97; Robert M. Young, *Mind, Brain and Adaptation in the Nineteenth Century* (Oxford, 1970), pp. 9–53; and Eric Carlson, "The Influence of Phrenology on Early American Psychiatric Thought," *American Journal of Psychiatry* 115 (1958):535–8.

81 John Fonerden, "The Brain Is Modified by Habits," *AJI* 7 (1850):59–61; Amariah Brigham, *Remarks on the Influence of Mental Cultivation upon Health* (Hartford, Conn., 1832), p. 14.

82 Earle, "Bloodletting," p. 397. See also James Bates, "Report on the Medical Treatment of Insanity. . .," *AJI* 7 (1850):100, for a similar argument.

83 Samuel Woodward, "Observations on the Medical Treatment of Insanity," *AJI* 7 (1850):62. See also Bates, "Medical Treatment," 106–9 (Bates warns his colleagues about the danger of habit formation, 108–9); John Allen, "On the Treatment of Insanity," *AJI* 6 (1850):277–83. Nathaniel Chapman, *Elements of Therapeutics and Materia Medica*, 5th ed., enl. and rev., 2 vols. (Philadelphia, 1827), vol. 2, p. 171, warned against using opium to treat mania.

David Musto, *The American Disease: Origins of Narcotic Control* (New Haven, Conn., 1973), pp. 1–3, gives the early history of morphine in the United States. According to him, one of the largest morphine-producing firms in the country, Rosengarten and Co. of Philadelphia, began manufacturing morphine salts, the usual form in which the drug was used, in 1832 (p. 2). Other forms of morphine were probably used before the 1830s. European chemists first derived morphine from opium in the 1810s. John Redmon Coxe, *The American Dispensatory*, 5th ed. (Philadelphia, 1822), pp. 461–3, discusses its therapeutic properties. Musto argues that physicians had little understanding of the drug's habit-forming propensity until the 1870s (pp. 72–5). Also, remember that asylum doctors administered morphine by mouth, which dilutes its potency; hypodermic injections did not become common practice until after Kirkbride's time.

84 Brigham, *Remarks*, p. 26; T. Romeyn Beck, *Inaugural Dissertation on Insanity* (New York, 1811), quoted in Deutsch, *The Mentally Ill*, p. 92.

85 Pliny Earle to Kirkbride, 18 August 1858, GC.

86 Remarks by Edward Jarvis, quoted in "Proceedings," *AJI* 14 (1857):81.

87 Earle, "On the Causes of Insanity," 207; Amariah Brigham, *Observations on the Influence of Religion upon the Health and Physical Welfare of Mankind* (Boston, 1835), p. 269.

88 Brigham, *Remarks*, p. 70; Edward Jarvis, "On the Supposed Increase of Insanity," *AJI* 8 (1852):363–4.

89 Fonerden, "The Brain Is Modified by Habits," 59.

90 Dr. Devay, "On the Importance of Certain Premonitory Symptoms of Severe Cerebral Disease," *AJI* 8 (1851):34; [Amariah Brigham], "Editorial," *AJI* 1 (1844):97.

The controversy over moral insanity perfectly illustrates this vulnerability. Pinel first posited the existence of a form of mental disease that affected only the "moral sentiments and affections." Although most superintendents believed that such a disorder existed, they found it difficult to distinguish it from simple wickedness. Reluctant to equate sin with insanity, they usually tried to avoid the diagnosis; as Earle complained, "this question of moral insanity borders so nearly upon religion" that it was useless to discuss it. But the legal use of the insanity plea in criminal proceedings forced them to give testimony on precisely this distinction. Many defense lawyers wanted to argue that the ability to commit a heinous crime in itself constituted proof of moral insanity. When called in to testify as expert witnesses, the asylum doctors often had great difficulty supporting their diagnoses under cross-examination, and suffered some loss of reputation as a result. For discussion of the moral insanity controversy, see Dain, *Concepts*, pp. 77–82; and Charles Rosenberg, *The Trial of the Assassin Guiteau* (Chicago, 1968); and S. P. Fullinwider, "Insanity as the Loss of Self: The Moral Insanity Controversy Revisited," *BHM* 49 (1975):87–101.

91 My reference to a commonsense psychological medicine should not be confused with Adolph Meyer's "commonsense psychiatry" of the early twentieth century.

92 Remarks of Isaac Ray, "Proceedings," *AJI* 33 (1876):278. Rosenberg, "The Place of George Beard," points out the flattering and reassuring elements of his theory.

93 See, for example, Charles Rosenberg and Carroll Smith-Rosenberg, "Piety and Social Action: Some Origins of the American Public Health Movement," in *No Other Gods*, edited by Charles Rosenberg, pp. 109–22; Charles Rosenberg, "Florence Nightingale on Contagion: The Hospital as Moral Universe," in *Healing and History*, edited by Charles Rosenberg, pp. 116–35; Barbara Rosenkrantz, *Public Health and the State* (Cambridge, 1972). William McLoughlin, *The Meaning of Henry Ward Beecher* (New York, 1970), esp. pp. 34–83, discusses a prominent Protestant minister's efforts to reconcile science and religion.

CHAPTER 3: *The burden of being their keepers*

1 Morris Vogel, *The Invention of the Modern Hospital* (Chicago, 1980), pp. 9–12, discusses popular attitudes toward the hospital.

2 Ibid., esp. pp. 97–119. I suspect that the asylum served as a model for financing and publicizing the new private pavilions. Vogel notes on p. 112 concerning the Massachusetts General Hospital, "McLean's provided a model for the trustees to draw upon in extending general hospital care beyond the poorer classes."

3 Thomas Story Kirkbride's patient-related correspondence includes several thousand letters received between 1840 and 1883. They have been sorted by the initial of the patient's last name. My citations give the initials of the patient first, the initials of the letter writer second, and then the date of the correspondence. All letters are addressed to Kirkbride unless otherwise noted. Some patient-related materials have been misfiled in his General Correspondence; they will be marked "GC." To my knowledge, the only other work using family letters to an asylum

superintendent is Dale Robison, *Wisconsin and the Mentally Ill: A History of the "Wisconsin Plan" of State and County Care, 1860-1915* (New York, 1980).

4 Using the resources of the Philadelphia Social History Project, I matched the Philadelphia-resident securities for admissions to the Pennsylvania Hospital for the Insane during 1870 with the census taken that year. Not until the mid-1880s did the hospital registers begin to list the name of the party committing the patient, so the security was my best link to the household the patient came from. I chose that census year because complete addresses for the women's securities were not available until the late 1860s. Of 137 cases, I located 63 in the census schedules.

   After completing this exercise in record linkage, I have reservations about using the security as a proxy for the family committing the patient. Of the 63 securities I located, I could find only 17 actually living with the patient for whom they had financial responsibility. With my limited information, I could not tell whether the other two-thirds of the securities were nonresident kin or employers, or whether the patient might have been in another institution at the time of the census. Despite its imperfections, my method did provide an indication of the securities' wealth, which I think can be taken as an index of community support for the asylum, if not the actual worth of the patrons themselves. (The millionaire security was in fact the patient's parent.)

5 These figures were calculated from Kirkbride's MR, 24 March 1855, Managers Papers, PH.

6 Class differences in both the prevalence and form of mental illness have been repeatedly shown in contemporary studies. August B. Hollingshead and Fredrick C. Redlich, *Social Class and Mental Illness* (New York, 1958), and Leo Srole et al., *Mental Health in the Metropolis* (New York, 1962), are only two of the best-known examinations of the association between class and mental disorders. There is little reason to doubt that the same association, although perhaps manifested in different ways, existed in the past. Unfortunately, the limited nature of the hospital records makes it impossible to measure this association in any rigorous way.

7 Michael MacDonald, *Mystical Bedlam: Madness, Anxiety and Healing in Seventeenth-Century England* (Cambridge, 1981), shows that a popular or folk concept of insanity as a disease was widespread long before the 1800s, and coexisted with supernatural or spiritual explanations for the disorder.

   I did not do a systematic analysis of terminology used in the lay letters, but can make the following observations: the first lay account I found to employ the word "nerves" was DP to Samuel Coates, 11 March 1816; "excitement" appears first in WH to the managers, 28 June 1828. Both are in PC, PH. These terms were common by the late 1840s.

8 See, for example, AB, WB 3 July 1857, PC; HB to JP, 30 November 1857, PC.

9 IG, Mrs. G, 13 July 1861, PC; Mrs. C, MMC, 26 July 1860, PC, and Charles Goestch, *Essays on Simeon Baldwin* (Storrs, Conn., 1981), pp. 252–3, 256–7, mention "derangement of the womb."

   Seeing an insane relative in the sick role had many advantages for the patrons. Besides giving them a plan of action, it helped mitigate, if not entirely abate, the anger they felt toward the disruptive individual. Simeon Baldwin made this revealing comment in his diary concerning his wife's insanity: "I say to myself: It is disease, but it hard to bear and forbear, where one apparently in as good health as anyone, – for her strength seems unabated though her good looks are gone, – abuses and hectors you and all around you, without reason, and mismanages your children most woefully" (p. 228).

10 Mrs. JC, JC, 7 October 1862, PC; JC, Dr. DC, 11 March 1849, PC; Mrs. B, EAB, 4 January 1861, PC; LB, JB, 26 June 1859, PC.

11 GT, MT, 9 July 1858, PC; RB, OB, 15 September 1845, PC.

12 SB, DD, 15 June 1848, PC.

13 Mr. A, VA, 24 March 1851, PC; AD to Kirkbride, 9 December 1865, GC; Mr. R, WP, 5 May 1871, PC.

14 Kirkbride asked how symptoms were first manifested; if the patient had any "peculiarities of temper, habits, disposition or pursuits" before its onset; used any addictive substances; had been subject to "any bodily disease," including epilepsy, suppressed eruptions, discharges, sores, or injuries to the head; what the supposed cause of the insanity was; and what treatment had been administered. See Mr. P, MP, 11 April 1855, PC; in this letter, a patron specifically mentions the list of questions in the *Annual Report* when reporting on a relative's case.
    The first diagnosis of mental illness is still usually made by family or friends. Once an individual is brought for treatment, their diagnosis is rarely challenged by medical personnel. See David Mechanic, "Some Factors in Identifying and Defining Mental Illness," *Mental Hygiene* 46 (1962):69–70. To get a sense of the striking parallels between the commitment process in nineteenth- and twentieth-century society, compare my discussion in this chapter with the contemporary view presented in Allan Horwitz, *The Social Control of Mental Illness* (New York, 1982).

15 CB-OS 1:127–8.

16 These are categories I devised while reading through the letters.

17 Mr. W, JFW, 14 February 1845, PC; Mrs. G, RRG, 6 September 1861, PC.

18 Mrs. JM, JM, 21 March 1848, PC; BB, DT, 30 November 1860, PC; Mrs. K, Dr. AM, 17 November 1846, PC; SB, HB, 7 February 1848, PC; "C's" [patient unnamed, ?misfiled], Dr. H, 1 June 1860, PC; Mrs. WHF, WHF, 31 March 1865, PC; SB, DD, 15 June 1848, PC; Mrs. JM, JM, 21 March 1848, PC.

19 Mrs. WBC, Dr. WW, 20 October 1858, PC; SB, DD, 25 May 1848, PC.

20 "W's" [patient unnamed], AW, 26 April 1853, PC; MB, Mrs. CB, 12 December 1865, PC; SB, DD, 25 May 1848, PC.

21 SB, DD, 17 November 1848, PC; LB, JB, 26 June 1859, PC; Mrs. K, Dr. AM, 17 November 1846, PC; Miss H, WC, 29 July 1858, PC; SB, DD, 25 May 1848, PC.

22 JH, JC, 24 August 1849, PC; "J's" [patient unnamed], PJ, 2 July 1857, PC.

23 AB, WB, 28 August 1857, PC; EB, LAB, 4 March 1862, PC; LB, JB, 26 June 1859, PC; AB, WB, 28 August 1857, PC; Mrs. CH, CH, 2 July 1855, PC.

24 Miss M, JM, 9 September 1848, PC; "J's" [patient unnamed], JSJ, 16 March 1851, PC; HB, JP, 30 November 1857, PC.

25 Mrs. JH, JH, 5 June 1857, PC; HC, AC, 20 March 1857, PC; JC, Dr. DC, 11 March 1849, PC; Mrs. HM, HM, 14 May 1855, PC; Miss B., HB, 8 November 1851, PC; Mrs. K., Dr. WT, 19 July 1855, PC; FT 11 June 1857, GC.

26 GC, 28 June 1864 [misfiled], GC.

27 My catalog of symptoms is consistent with Richard Fox's findings in *So Far Disordered in Mind: Insanity in California, 1870–1930* (Berkeley, 1978), esp. chap. 6, pp. 135–62. Using court commitment proceedings, he tabulated the behaviors cited as insane in a similar fashion. But the sketchiness of his data, which allow only an aggregate tabulation of symptoms, does not fully capture the *dynamics* of the labeling process, as he admits. My own reading of family accounts convinces me that we cannot reduce the social definition of insanity to a static set of characteristics; in other words, insanity is more than the sum of its symptoms – which is why I think that the distinctions I make in the next section are so important.

28 Mr. W, JFW, 14 February 1845, PC; DB, EB, 30 September 1860, PC; Miss E, JME, 21 June 1857, PC; LB, AHT, 15 June 1856, PC; JH, CH, 2 April 1855, PC.

29 Col. H, TS, 4 October 1859, PC; Mr. T, Dr. AW, 20 August 1861, PC; "W's" (patient unnamed), HW, 11 October 1865, PC; SS, WAS, 19 August 1856, PC. WW, 17 February 1848, GC. Ibid, "Trial of Wiley Williams," *The Sun*, vol. 2, No. 140, 18 December 1849.

30 See the discussion of visiting in Chapter 1, pp. 33–5.

31 Mrs. JM, JM, 21 March 1848, PC.

32 For an interesting discussion of the last resort as a sociological phenomenon, see

Robert M. Emerson, "On Last Resorts," *American Journal of Sociology* 87:1 (1981):1–22.

33 Mrs. WHF, WHF, 31 May 1865, PC; AB, ALB, 20 February 1861, PC; SB, HFB, 7 February 1848, PC. One patron actually referred to his efforts to distract his wife along this line as moral treatment; see Mrs. H, EH, 9 October 1847, PC. FT, 11 June 1857, GC, mentions a private nurse.

34 See, for example, Mrs. JM, JM, 21 March 1848, PC; Mrs. K, Dr. AM, 17 November 1846, PC; Mr. B, Dr. H, 8 March 1845, PC; AS, Dr. FH, 21 June 1850, PC.

35 Mrs. LH, Dr. JWR, 21 September 1857, PC; ED, Dr. IC, 24 August 1857, PC.

36 "T's" (patient unnamed), Dr. WHT, 28 May 1847, PC; Mrs. WBC, Dr. WW, 20 October 1858, PC.

37 Mrs. K, Dr. WT, 19 July 1855, PC; CM, Dr. IJ, 29 April 1848, PC.

38 "T's" (patient unnamed), Dr. WT, 28 May 1847, PC; WGH, Dr. TR, 18 June 1848, PC; JCH, 7 April 1846, GC.

39 Mrs. J, Dr. IT, 8 February 1848, PC; "X's" (patient unnamed), Dr. XX, 18 September 1857, PC. *AR* 1846, p. 33. Kirkbride's General Correspondence (IPH) contains numerous referrals from prominent local physicians, including D. Hayes Agnew, Robley Dunglinson, and Samuel Jackson. His ploy of inviting medical groups for visits obviously worked, for after one such tour of the Pennsylvania Hospital for the Insane with the State Medical Society, Dr. Daniel Holmes of Canton, Pa., wrote, "After visiting your admirable establishment for the treatment of insane patients I determined to send my patients there if possible." "C's" (patient unnamed), Dr. Daniel Holmes, 1 June 1860, PC.

40 S. Weir Mitchell, *Wear and Tear* (Philadelphia, 1871); idem, *Fat and Blood* (Philadelphia, 1877). Charlotte Perkins Gilman gives a sardonic view of the "rest cure" she received at S. Weir Mitchell's hands in *The Living of Charlotte Perkins Gilman* (New York, 1972; reprint of 1935 ed.). Carroll Smith-Rosenberg analyzes Mitchell's methods with women in "The Hysterical Woman: Sex Roles and Role Conflict in 19th Century America," *Social Research* 39 (Winter 1972):652–78. In the 1850s, women with mental disorders were sometimes taken to see Hugh Lenox Hodge, Sr. (1796–1873), a professor at the University of Pennsylvania Medical School who specialized in women's diseases. For references to Dr. Hodges, see Mrs. R, CMR, 12 February 1859, PC; Mrs. W, JAW, 4 March 1853, PC; Mrs. W, JW, 24 December 1855, PC. Kirkbride occasionally did some consulting work himself, advising individuals troubled by mild nervous disorders who were in no need of hospitalization. He charged $5.00 for a consultation. See LM, 21 September 1855, 25 September 1855, PC; OJ, 25 August 1857, 21 December 1857, PC. For recent histories of neurology, see Andrew Abbott, "The Evolution of American Psychiatry, 1880–1930," Ph.D. dissertation, University of Chicago, 1982; Bonnie Blustein, "New York Neurologists and the Specialization of American Medicine," *BHM* 53:2 (Summer 1979):170–83; idem, "A New York Medical Man: William Alexander Hammond (1828–1900), Neurologist," Ph.D. dissertation, University of Pennsylvania, 1979; and Charles Rosenberg, *The Trial of the Assassin Guiteau* (Chicago, 1968).

41 S. W. Mitchell, 15 March (no year), GC. The Philadelphia Neurological Society invited Kirkbride to become a founding member of their group; he evidently did not accept their offer. Philadelphia Neurological Society, 12 December 1883, GC.

42 Mr. F, GF, 31 January 1849, PC. For background on American spas, see Harry B. Weiss and Howard R. Kemble, *The Great American Water-Cure Craze: A History of Hydropathy in the United States* (Trenton, N.J., 1967), and Marshall S. Legan, "Hydropathy in America: A Nineteenth Century Panacea," *BHM* 45 (May–June 1971), 267–80.

43 Mrs. MW, SW, 4 May 1854, PC; Mr. W., HD, 15 September 1853, PC. According to Kirkbride, there were at least seven private asylums in the United States. See Kirkbride to S. Preston Jones, undated note headed "Total Applications for Writ of Habeas Corpus" [undated, probably 1868]. On the back,

there is a list in Kirkbride's hand, headed "Private Institutions in the United States; Landpen[?] Hall, Litchfield, Brigham Hall, Cutter's, Given's, Beaver [?], Paterson's." Kirkbride was probably helping Isaac Ray with his article, "A Modern 'Lettre de Cachet' Reviewed," *Atlantic Monthly* 22 (August 1868):227–43, for in that piece Ray gives the number of private asylums as seven. James Macdonald founded Sanford Hall; Robert Given, Kirkbride's former assistant, ran the Woodbrook Retreat in Kellyville, Pa. Undoubtedly, there were many other "homes" run by doctors and lay people. After the 1870s, private clinics and sanitaria became much more numerous, as the neurologists tried to break the asylum doctors' monopoly on wealthy patients.

44 The phrase "pathway to the mental hospital" comes from a well-known article by John A. Clausen and Marian R. Yarrow, "The Impact of Mental Illness on the Family," *Journal of Social Issues* 11 (1955):3–64. For a detailed account of one family's experience with insanity, see Goetsch, *Essays on Simeon Baldwin*, pp. 217–41. Using diaries and personal correspondence, Goetsch traces Baldwin's gradual recognition of his wife's insanity and search for treatment. Baldwin's writings give an intimate view of insanity's impact on the household.

45 Mrs. R, IS, 9 February 1871, PC.

46 Mr. M, JM, 25 October 1855, PC; GHK, Mrs. GHK, 22 December 1862, PC; "C's" [patient unnamed], WC, 19 March 1848, PC. In the *AR* 1842, p. 23, Kirkbride states that four patients who were brought to the asylum during that year had been chained in their own homes, and "were capable of feeling, and did not fail to express their sense of degradation."

47 Mrs. J, IT, 8 February 1848, PC; Mrs. A, JMA, 14 January 1852, PC; Mrs. C, Dr. W, 20 October 1858, PC; GT, MT, 9 July 1858, PC.

48 This revulsion against restraint appears to have been part of a larger rejection of corporal punishment. Myra C. Glenn, "Changing Attitudes Towards Corporal Punishment," Ph.D. dissertation, State University of New York at Buffalo, 1979, examines this movement in antebellum education, prison reform, and the military.

49 EB, LB, 20 August 1862, PC; Miss D. HGD, 19 August 1882, PC; SS, WAS, 19 August 1856, PC.

50 "R's" [patient unnamed], JR, 27 Feburary 1861, PC; Mrs. B, AP, 15 October 1855, PC; HC, AC, 6 July 1859, PC; SS, WAS, 19 August 1856, PC; CS, JS, 29 May 1855, PC; Mrs. W, LW, 27 May 1868, PC.

51 FF, WF, 14 January 1846, PC; MV, GL, 11 July 1861, PC.

52 Miss C, PC, 18 September 1862, PC; Mrs. G, RRG, 5 October 1861, PC.

53 *AR* 1882, p. 37; CB, GB, 25 January 1847, PC. The statistics Kirkbride kept on the duration of the disease before admission show that of 8,852 patients admitted between 1841 and 1883 (see table, *AR* 1883, p. 18), 48% had been insane for less than three months; 21% for three months to one year; 24% for one to five years; 6% for five to twenty years; and 1% for more than twenty years. These figures probably underestimate the length of time a patient was disturbed before the family sought hospital care, since as the patrons' accounts show, family members often resisted recognizing a relative's mental alienation.

54 Mr. W, HD, 15 September 1853, PC; WTT, LMP, 15 May 1860, PC; Mrs. MR, RLL, 18 December 1868, PC; "L's" [patient unnamed], JL, 26 November 1859, PC; MG, CG, 28 June 1859, PC; Mrs. M, RYM, 21 July 1857, PC.

55 GT, MT, 9 July 1858 , PC; Mr. M, CP [undated, ans. July 1855], PC; MB, SB, 15 May 1879, PC.

56 BB, Dr. DHT, 30 November 1860, PC; LB, JDB, 26 June 1859, PC; JMC, MC, 20 October 1848, PC; "M's" [patient unnamed], HM, 8 January 1861, PC.

57 "L's" [patient unnamed], JL, 26 November 1859, PC; AW, GW, 22 June 1859, PC.

58 Mrs. JC, JC, 6 December 1861, PC; HTB, STP, 20 October 1845, PC; JR, CM, 3 May 1860, PC; R. and Miss C, EYC, 28 December 1849, PC; SG, JG, 5 May 1865, PC; JC, Dr. DC, 31 July 1848 and 11 March 1849, PC.

59 EP, SC, 24 June 1857, PC; Mr. E, AR, 9 August 1861, PC: Mr. I, JFI, 28 November 1859, PC; Mrs. C, MMC, 16 July 1860, PC.

60 SB, DD, 14 February 1848, PC; Mrs. L, JL, 21 November 1848, PC; JC, Dr. JC, [April?] 1846, PC; HTB, STB, 20 October 1845, PC.

61 EM, SM, 26 August 1842, PC; WL, Mrs. L, 5 February 1866, PC; Mrs. MJB, TB, 21 September 1860, PC; AF Sr., AF Jr., 31 May 1848, PC.

62 EL, EF, 18 October 1865, PC; Judge G, GW, 13 June 1851, PC; IS, TS, 21 March 1862, PC.

63 Kirkbride to Wistar Morris and S. Morris Waln, 25 January 1867, Managers' Correspondence with Superintendent of PHI, PH. See "Proceedings," *AJI* 26 (1869):139, for Kirkbride's comment on the 1869 law. He described it as "unobjectionable," adding that it would relieve the hospital officers of legal responsibility for a patient's detention, so long as they followed the proper commitment procedure. The Pennsylvania law closely resembled the AMSAII's model bill, which was written by Isaac Ray. See Ray, "Project of a Law for Determining the Legal Relations of the Insane," *AJI* 7 (1851):215–33.

There is no way of knowing how faithfully the hospital authorities adhered to their own regulations. I have come across only one incident in which a patient was admitted without a doctor's certificate. See Mrs. JPS, JPS, 28 October 1861, PC. In that letter, the patron states that he has not yet sent the family doctor's certificate, but will do so if Kirkbride requests it. In another letter, EL to EAF, 8 October 1865, [misfiled] GC, a patient claimed that no doctor saw her before admission.

64 Mrs. W, LW, 27 May 1868, PC; FT, 11 June 1857, GC.

65 Miss D, Dr. WWH, 12 August 1882, PC.

66 Dr. AV Williams, 3 August 1852, GC; Dr. JC Hall, 7 April 1846, GC; Dr. WJM, Dr. JE, 20 May 1853, PC.

67 ATH, JH, 5 June 1857, 12 May 1858, 2 August 1858, 10 August 1858, PC; ATH, JT, 16 August 1858, PC.

68 [Amariah Brigham], "Editorial," *AJI* 1 (1844):97. See also Charles Rosenberg, "The Therapeutic Revolution," *Perspectives in Biology and Medicine* (Summer 1977), 494–6.

69 My figures on the number of mental hospitals are taken from Samuel W. Hamilton, "The History of the American Mental Hospital," in *One Hundred Years of American Psychiatry*, edited by J. K. Hall et al. (New York, 1944), pp. 153–66; and Frederick Wines, *Report on the Defective, Dependent, and Delinquent Classes of the Population of the United States, as Returned at the 10th Census (June 1, 1880)* (Washington, D.C., 1888), pp. 90–2. I arrived at the ratio of beds to adults by using statistics given in Hamilton, "The History of the Mental Hospital," 86, on the number of patients in hospitals; and statistics on the adult population given in U.S. Bureau of the Census, *Historical Statistics of the United States*, 2 vols. (Washington, D.C., 1975), vol. 1, pp. 15–18.

70 The modernization and madness argument has been made by scholars as diverse as George Rosen, *Madness in Society* (Chicago, 1968); Michel Foucault, *Madness and Civilization* (New York, 1965); and David Rothman, *The Discovery of the Asylum* (Boston, 1971).

71 James Henretta, *The Evolution of American Society, 1700–1815* (Lexington, Mass., 1973), pp. 200–5, briefly discusses this feedback model of economic development.

72 My conjectures concerning intolerance of insanity parallel Fox's work on California. Where our interpretations differ, I believe, is in the weight accorded to pull factors in asylum utilization. Simply put, I find patrons expressing hope for a cure; Fox does not. This probably reflects the different nature of the institutions involved, i.e., private vs. public facilities.

73 Much of the recent work in family history has focused on the rise of the companionate family. See Philippe Aries, *Centuries of Childhood* (New York, 1962); Lawrence Stone, *The Family, Sex and Marriage* (New York, 1977); Edward Shorter, *The Making of the Modern Family* (New York, 1975); and Randolph Trumbach, *The Rise of the Egalitarian Family* (New York, 1978). The changes

occurring in the United States between 1750 and 1850 are suggested by Nancy Cott, *The Bonds of Womanhood* (New Haven, Conn., 1977); Mary Ryan, *Cradle of the Middle Class: The Family in Oneida County New York 1790-1865* (New York, 1981); Barbara Welter, "The Cult of True Womanhood," *American Quarterly* 18 (1966):151–74; Rolla Tryon, *Household Manufactures in the United States, 1640–1860* (New York, 1966; reprint of 1917 ed.).

74 Recent historical literature on child rearing in this period would seem to support my conjecture. See, for example, Philip Greven, *The Protestant Temperament* (New York, 1977); William McLoughlin, "Evangelical Child-Rearing in the Age of Jackson," *Journal of Social History* 9 (1975):21–34.

Richard Fox, *So Far Disordered in Mind*, comes to basically the same conclusion I do concerning the connection between the family and the asylum. He finds that 57% of all San Francisco commitment proceedings were initiated by relatives rather than police or welfare agencies. He concludes that insanity was "not a threat to social order in the abstract, but in many cases to the 'public order' of their neighborhoods and the tranquility and financial survival of their families" (p. 163). The "helping professions and their ancillary institutions," he continues, "did not simply muscle the family and community aside," but rather worked with them to ensure social control. This perspective differs from that of Christopher Lasch, *Haven in a Heartless World* (New York, 1977). Lasch asserts that the rise of the "therapeutic state" has led to the deterioration of the family. He may be right that the abdication of familial responsibility for deviant and dependent members was the first step on a long road toward dissolution; but at the time, the nineteenth-century mental hospital arose as an institution designed to preserve the family order rather than destroy it.

Much more work remains to be done in linking specific changes in the family with utilization of institutions. The scholars cited in the Preface, note 18, are working on this problem.

CHAPTER 4: *The persuasive institution*

1 Thomas Story Kirkbride, "Remarks on the Construction and Arrangements of Hospitals for the Insane," *American Journal of the Medical Sciences* n.s. 13 (1847):40–56; idem, *On the Construction, Organization and General Arrangements of Hospitals for the Insane* (Philadelphia, 1854). Kirkbride also published "Notice of Some Experiments in Heating and Ventilating Hospitals and Other Buildings, By Steam and Hot Water," *AJMS* n.s. 19 (1850):298–318.

2 Kirkbride, *On the Construction*, p. 11 All citations will be to the first edition of this book unless otherwise noted.

3 See Delores Hayden, *Seven American Utopias: The Architecture of Communitarian Socialism, 1790–1975* (Cambridge, 1976), and David Rothman, *The Discovery of the Asylum* (Boston, 1971).

4 Florence Nightingale, *Notes on Hospitals* (London, 1859). Like Kirkbride's design, Nightingale's hospital plans embodied a conception of the moral universe. Compare my discussion of Kirkbride with that of Charles Rosenberg, "Florence Nightingale on Moral Contagion," in *Healing and History* edited by Charles Rosenberg, (New York, 1979), pp. 116–35." The *Index Catalogue of the Library of the Surgeon General's Office* (Washington, D.C., 1885) listed many monographs and articles under the heading "hospital construction."

Around the same time that Kirkbride was formulating his ideas, several European physicians published influential treatises on asylum construction, most notably Maximilian Jacobi, *On the Construction and Management of Hospitals for the Insane. . .*, tr. John Kitching (London, 1841), and John Conolly, *The Construction and Government of Lunatic Asylums and Hospitals for the Insane* (London, 1847). In most respects, their recommendations closely paralleled Kirkbride's work. All agreed, for example, on the therapeutic value of good building design, the importance of seemingly trivial details of construction and management to the asylum's success, and the necessity for the physician to have complete control over all asylum affairs. Their consensus on these points apparently grew out of the fundamental similarity between American and European mental hospitals, rather than any direct exchange of ideas, for there is no evidence that Kirkbride read either Jacobi or Conolly before writing his own treatise on hospital construction.

On one important issue, the type of hospital plan they recommended, the European and American asylum doctors did not agree. Jacobi favored a variant of the quadrangle plan, whereas Conolly preferred the H form. Both rejected the linear plan, which Kirkbride championed, on the grounds that although it offered the maximum degree of separation for the patients, it spread them out over too great a distance to be convenient. Without being overly speculative, it seems plausible to assume that Kirkbride's choice of the linear plan reflected certain design dilemmas peculiar to American asylum practice. Unlike Conolly, who openly expressed his disapproval of mixed hospitals (see esp. pp. 1–6, 19), Kirkbride expected his institution to serve all classes, and thus required the greater degree of separation offered by the linear plan.

5 Albert Deutsch, *The Mentally Ill in America*, 2nd ed. (New York, 1949), esp. p. 190.

6 Hayden, *Seven American Utopias*, p. 33.

7 Letters from patients' families frequently asked for copies of the *Annual Reports*. See, for example, JC, MC, 9 March 1848, PC; BB Jr., BB Sr., 16 March 1861, PC; MB, WB, 15 February 1858, PC. Kirkbride also gave copies to general practitioners in order to facilitate referrals. (See Chapter 3, pp. 104–7, for more information on referrals.) See, for example, Mr. L, WS, 25 July 1845; PC; Kirkbride to Dr. Henderson, 23 February, LP 2:326. The managers usually had several thousand copies of Kirkbride's *Annual Reports* printed. In 1844, they ordered 2,500 copies; in 1862, 3,000 copies; and in 1873, 4,500 copies. MM 9:224; 10:97, 465.

Historians have recognized asylum annual reports to be a form of propaganda used by the superintendents, but have not considered their audience very closely. Norman Dain, *Concepts of Insanity in the United States, 1789–1865* (New Brunswick, N.J., 1964), p. 121, suggests that the private hospitals may have inflated the recovery rates cited in their reports to attract patients. He does not consider in any detail, however, how other parts of the annual reports might have been written to appeal to prospective patrons. Deutsch, *The Mentally Ill*, 2nd ed., pp. 206–7, sees the reports as "mediums of beneficial propaganda, addressed to the public in hopes of creating mass backing behind the cause of the insane." Yet, his use of the word "public" does not adequately delineate the specific audience (i.e., potential patrons) that the asylum doctors wished to reach. Deutsch characterized Kirkbride's *Annual Reports* as particularly skillful in their appeal to a lay audience.

8 The asylum did accept cases of insanity attributed to excessive alcohol use. How the physicians distinguished between those suffering from mania-a-potu, or delirium tremens, and alcohol-induced insanity is unclear.

9 *AR 1853*, p. 30; *AR 1873*, p. 39; *AR 1858*, pp. 41, 37; for Kirkbride's views on heredity, see, for example, *AR 1843*, p. 29. He took the same position when discussing heredity and insanity with his professional colleagues. See, for example, his statements in "Proceedings," *AJI* 14 (1857):84; *AJI* 28 (1871):264. In my discussion of Kirkbride's *Annual Reports*, only references to the exact quotations used in the text will be given. The basic concepts outlined here reappear over and over again in Kirkbride's writings.

10 *AR 1849*, p. 26; *AR 1858*, p. 37; *AR 1852*, p. 27.

11 See, for example, *AR 1850*, pp. 18–22.

12 *AR 1858*, p. 38; *AR 1867*, p. 27; *AR 1864*, p. 29; *AR 1856*, p. 7.

13 See, for example, *AR 1867*, pp. 26–27; *AR 1865*, p. 8; *AR 1862*, p. 12.

14 *AR 1860*, p. 9; *AR 1849*, p. 26. On chronic patients, see *AR 1846*, pp. 9–13. See also *AR 1845*, pp. 9–10, for a good example of Kirkbride's attempt to portray chronic patients sympathetically. Here the superintendent refers to an incurable male patient who possesses "all the courtesy of character, polished manner, and

social disposition which eminently characterized him in youth, and which still make him one of the most welcome guests at all our parties and entertainments" (p. 10).

15 *AR* 1882, p. 37; ibid., p. 38; *AR* 1860, pp. 9–10.

16 *AR* 1860, p. 9; *AR* 1869, pp. 8, 9.

17 *AR* 1865, p. 24; *AR* 1871, p. 40.

18 *AR* 1844, pp. 25, 24.

19 *AR* 1858, pp. 33–32. See the list of lectures given in *AR* 1858, pp. 22–31. The slides used in the patient lectures, which were made by William and Frederick Langenheim of Philadelphia, are part of the institute's archives. Dr. George Layne of the institute has catalogued them and written a paper about their uses, entitled "Kirkbride–Langenheim Collaboration: Early Use of Photography in Psychiatric Treatment in Philadelphia," *PMHB* 105:2 (April 1981):182–202.

20 *AR* 1869, p. 26, *AR* 1845, p. 38; *AR* 1846, pp. 24–25.

21 *AR* 1843, p. 26. See also *AR* 1844, pp. 32–33, for Kirkbride's claims concerning the use of restraint at the Pennsylvania Hospital for the Insane.

22 Kirkbride, *On the Construction*, p. 7.

23 Ibid., pp. 13, 35–36. Kirkbride prepared the hospital plans included in *On the Construction* with the assistance of architect Samuel Sloan. Sloan was the architect for the Male Department, completed in 1859. See Thomas Story Kirkbride *On the Construction, Organization, and General Arrangements of Hospitals for the Insane*, 2nd ed. (Philadelphia, 1880), p. 102. See also "The Kirkbride Plan: Architecture for a Treatment System That Changed," *Hospital and Community Psychiatry* 27 (1976):475, for more on Sloan.

24 Kirkbride. *On the Construction*, pp. 11, 12.

25 Ibid., p. 11; Thomas Story Kirkbride to John Evans, 18 May 1845, LP 1:79.

26 Kirkbride to Dorothea Dix, 23 March 1856, IPH.

27 Thomas Story Kirkbride, "Description of the Pleasure Grounds and Farm of the Pennsylvania Hospital for the Insane, with Remarks," *AJI* 4 (1848):353.

28 Kirkbride, *On the Construction*, pp. 16–17.

29 Ibid., pp. 18, 57, 20.

30 *AR* 1878, p. 51; Kirkbride, *On the Construction*, pp. 15, 16.

31 Ibid., pp. 24, 28.

32 Ibid., pp. 20-2.

33 Ibid., pp. 41–2. Kirkbride opposed the introduction into the hospital of any personnel who would not be strictly subordinate to his authority. He considered consulting physicians an unnecessary addition to the hospital staff because they only duplicated duties that properly belonged to the chief physician. He also did not recommend having a chaplain, on the grounds that religious services should be "as much under the control of the physician as anything else connected with the care of the patients." See *On the Construction*, p. 46; "Proceedings," *AJI* 26 (1869):158.

34 *On the Construction*, pp. 42–3.

35 Ibid.

36 Ibid., pp. 44, 45, 9.

37 Ibid., pp. 38–40.

38 Ibid., p. 11. Kirkbride complained about his lack of participation in the early planning of the asylum in several letters to fellow superintendents. See Kirkbride to William Awl, 27 June 1843 and 24 July 1844; Kirkbride to Amariah Brigham, 23 November 1844, in LP 1:98, 326, 405.

39 Kirkbride, "Description of the Pleasure Grounds," pp. 347–54. Kirkbride approved of the hospital's site (if not the building), as he makes clear in *AR* 1853, pp. 34–5, 40.

40 For a description of the original building, see the "Final Report of the Building Committee," MM 9 (1842):185–86 (PH); *AR* 1841, pp. 8–19; Thomas Story Kirkbride, "A Sketch of the History, Buildings and Organization of the Pennsylvania Hospital for the Insane," *AJI* 2 (1845):99–109. Thomas G. Morton, *History of the Pennsylvania Hospital* (Philadelphia, 1895), p. 165, note 1, provides

information on the asylum's architect, Isaac Holden. Shortly after designing the Pennsylvania Hospital for the Insane, Holden returned to England; he later drew up the plans for the Prestwick County Lunatic Asylum near Manchester.

41 MM 9:149; Morton, *History*, pp. 170–1.

42 *AR* 1846, pp. 25–9; *AR* 1849, pp. 7–12.

43 *AR* 1847, p. 24; Thomas Story Kirkbride, "Remarks on Cottages for Certain Classes of Patients. . .," *AJI* 7 (1851):378. For Kirkbride's later reservations about cottages, see "Proceedings," *AJI* 28 (1871):328–9.

44 *AR* 1846, p. 30; *AR* 1848, p. 20; *AR* 1852, pp. 26, 32.

45 *AR* 1848, pp. 32–3; MM 9 (1854):503–4. Until the early 1850s, when Kirkbride had the hospital converted to gas lighting, the use of kerosene lamps must have further polluted the hospital atmosphere. See MM 9 (1855):529.

46 MR, 24 June 1854, PH; Miss V, ES, 20 December 1857; PC; MR, 23 February 1850, PH.

47 Kirkbride to Amariah Brigham, 23 November 1844, LP 1:405.

48 *AR* 1855, p. 6; *AR* 1854, p. 30.

49 *AR* 1853, p. 34.

50 Isaac Ray to John Sawyer, 11 August 1873, BH. Ray did not like the way the doors opened into the hall, however, as he stated in the same letter. He also felt that the absence of common dormitories was a "serious defect" in Kirkbride's arrangements. *AR* 1859, p. 34, gives the cost of the new building, and pp. 9–30 describe it in great detail. The two hospitals were connected by a footpath and bridge, and, after 1874, a telegraph. See MM 10 (1874):521–2. John D. Thompson and Grace Goldin, *The Hospital: A Social and Architectural History* (New Haven, Conn., 1975), p. 76, state that the linear plan was curtailed because the lot was too small, but I have not been able to verify this.

51 *AR* 1861, pp. 21–2; *AR* 1868, pp. 21–7; *AR* 1873, pp. 29–37; *AR* 1880, pp. 18–20.

52 Their transactions were recorded in the Attending Managers Minutes, vols. 1 and 2 (1841–94), and, Minutes, MD, vol. 1 (1859–93), IPH.

53 Morton, *History*, pp. 428–37, has short biographical sketches of the managers. Included were prominent Philadelphia merchants, bank presidents, directors of railroads, and mine and factory owners, who also had a long record of benevolent service in other charitable institutions. Kirkbride dedicated the second edition of *On the Construction* to the Pennsylvania Hospital's Board of Managers.

54 Samuel Welsh to Kirkbride, 27 July 1857, GC; William Biddle to Kirkbride, 12 August 1873, GC. The General Correspondence file contains some fifty to sixty letters written by Welsh to Kirkbride, which reveal his wide-ranging interest in asylum matters. Kirkbride makes his boast in *On the Construction*, 2nd ed., p. 224. After the Male Department opened in 1859, the attending managers included both hospitals on their Saturday visits, dining alternately at each. MM 10 (1859):18–20.

55 Caleb Cope to Kirkbride, 14 February 1866, GC. MM 10 (1863):124 records that a committee was convened to look into charges that a patient made against her attendant. Judging from the Attending Managers Minutes, surely the most boring set of records in the hospital archives, the managers rarely involved themselves in the asylum's day-to-day management. In Clement Biddle to Kirkbride, 26 April 1853, GC; William Biddle to Kirkbride [no day or month given], 1853, GC, Managers ask his permission to bring guests to the asylum. We can get some idea of the methods Kirkbride used with the managers from advice he once gave to his fellow superintendent, John Gray: "let the idea expressed rest until it matures and then the second person will conceive it to be his own" (JG, 11 May 1852, GC).

56 William Biddle, 16 April 1880, GC. The state of Kirkbride's finances can be deduced from the *Reports*. Compare this with John Curwen's financial problems at the Pennsylvania State Lunatic Asylum, which are discussed in Chapter 6.

57 Caleb Cope, 14 February 1866, GC; William Biddle, 16 April 1880, GC. MM 10:71, 175, refer to the financial problems caused by the Civil War.

58 Samuel Welsh, 21 November, GC. Kirkbride attended the managers' meetings to present his Monthly Reports. Some of these reports were inventoried and microfilmed at the Eighth Street hospital archives (PH) and others at the Forty-ninth Street hospital (IPH).

59 Kirkbride to attending managers, 23 September 1843, LP 1:157; MR, 27 June 1863, PH.

60 MR, 22 April 1854, PH; MR, 26 February 1859, PH. Figures on board rates have been calculated from the Monthly Reports. The number of out-of-state patients is given in the *Reports*.

61 MR, 26 February 1859, PH; MR, 26 March 1864, PH. Kirkbride to managers, 26 September 1844, LP 1:367.

62 Kirkbride to Dorothea Dix, 12 July 1847, HL; John Curwen to Dix, 26 July 1852, HL. Kirkbride to managers, 30 July 1866, Managers Papers: Correspondence with Superintendent of The Pennsylvania Hospital for the Insane, PH.

63 Kirkbride to William Awl, 24 July 1844, LP 1:326; Kirkbride to Dix, 18 August 1852, IPH.

64 MM 10:328–9; managers to Kirkbride, 26 December 1871, GC. Kirkbride evidently started at a salary of $3,000, but it was reduced to $2,500 in 1842 or 1843, apparently because the hospital was financially strapped. See Kirkbride to James Greeves, 22 February 1845, LP 1:40. A motion to raise his pay back to $3,000 was defeated in 1845 by a split vote (MM 9:260–1), but passed in 1846 (MM 9:291). The managers subsequently raised Kirkbride's salary to $4,000 in 1866 and $5,000 in 1871 (MM 10:217, 426). MM 9:531 records the managers' decision to pay his expenses for the AMSAII's annual meeting.

65 *AR* 1883, pp. 110, 58. The hospital's administrative structure was laid out in the Pennsylvania Hospital's by-laws, and in Kirkbride, *Code of Rules and Regulations for the Government of Those Employed in the Care of the Patients of the Pennsylvania Hospital for the Insane, Near Philadelphia*, first published in 1841 and revised in 1850.

66 Kirkbride to Edward Smith, 9 March 1862, outlines the assistant physician's duties quite succinctly. See also MM 9:349 for the hospital rules concerning assistants.

67 Kirkbride to managers, 30 June 1862, Managers Papers: Correspondence with Superintendent of the Pennsylvania Hospital for the Insane, PH; Kirkbride to managers, 23 December 1881, copy with Short Misc. Mss. See also "Proceedings," *AJI* 23 (1866):249. Ultimately, the managers decided not to take Kirkbride's advice, as we shall see in Chapter 7.

68 Mr. B, BB to Dr. Jones, 9 March 1861, PC; EDG, AWG, 9 September 1861, PC. See JB, JLS, 4 April 1860, PC: Kirkbride penciled a note on the back: "Dr. Jones will please write on this whether there is any change or prospect of change and return it to me." JC, ID, 23 June 1846, mentions Curwen but thanks only Kirkbride. In *AR* 1883, p. 108, Eliza Kirkbride states that her husband answered all the patrons' letters himself.

69 S. Preston Jones, 11 June 1870, GC; Edward A. Smith, GC [no date]; J. Edwards Lee, 16 October 1862, GC; Edward A. Smith, 21 September 1858, GC; William P. Moon, 13 June 1870, GC. See also William P. Moon, 7 June 1870, GC.

70 Miss V, Edward A. Smith, 20 December 1857, PC; S. Preston Jones, 13 December 1865, GC. The superintendent who came for treatment was Merrick Bemis of the Worcester State Hospital. His case is discussed more fully in Chapter 6.

71 "Proceedings," *AJI* 29 (1872):247. Salary information can be found in MM 9:193, 204, 323, 464, 622–3; 10:94, 186, 300, 314, 388, 445, 458, 481, 583.

72 MR, 23 November 1850; MM 10:313–14; Kirkbride to Edward A. Smith, 9 March 1862. See also MM 10:86 for the reference to Smith's resolve to take up private practice. Morton, *History*, p. 524, provides a convenient list of the assistant physicians and their length of service.

73 Dix to Kirkbride, 31 July [no year], IPH; Robert Given to Kirkbride, 18 May

1868, GC (this letter was written from the Woodbrook Retreat in Delaware County).

74 Curwen to Dix, 10 February 1849 and 19 June 1850, HL.

75 Lee to Charles Nichols, 27 June 1859, NA; MR, 28 November 1868. For facts concerning Lee's career, see Lee, 26 September 1858, 18 October 1858, 23 June 1859, 24 May 1860, 10 December 1860, GC. See also MR, 23 March 1861, PH; Kirkbride to managers [no date?], Managers Papers: Correspondence with Superintendent of Pennsylvania Hospital for the Insane. Kirkbride wrote to Pliny Earle that Lee had lost his place due to "political troubles...before the hospital was opened and as far as I can learn without any fault being found with him personally, further than it was his misfortune to have been appointed by a Board that was to be displaced." Kirkbride to Earle, 16 August 1860, AS. Kirkbride wrote a very personal memorial for Lee in the *AR* 1868, pp. 33–8.

76 Nichols, 20 July 1859, GC. As in Curwen's case a superior position facilitated Jones's plan to marry. "Hitherto," he wrote to Dix, "I have not been in a position to marry." Jones to Dix, 25 February 1858, HL. For references to the assistant physicians' service at other asylums see MM 9:423–4 (Lee at Utica); ibid., 551 (Smith at Worcester); Dix to Nichols, 29 March 1859, NA (Jones at Harrisburg).

77 Richard Gundry, 11 May 1879, GC. See also Kirkbride to managers, 26 May 1879, Managers Papers, for references to Moon's prior service.

78 In a letter to the absent Kirkbride, Smith urged him to stay away longer, writing, "You know how your assistant is wont to complain of nothing to do, etc....you can hardly give him a greater or more gratifying mark of confidence than by trusting him as long as other [matters?] besides the hospital will permit." Smith, 19 July 1869, GC.

79 Lee, 23 June 1859, 24 May 1860, and 10 December 1861, GC; Smith, 8 June 1858, GC.

80 See Andrew Abbott, "The Evolution of American Psychiatry, 1880–1930," Ph.D. dissertation, University of Chicago, 1982, esp. chap. 4, for a further discussion of this point.

81 MM 9:249. The steward's and matron's duties are outlined in the *Charter, Laws and Rules of the Pennsylvania Hospital* (Philadelphia, 1859), pp. 29–30. The steward's letters to Kirkbride during the latter's absences from the asylum suggest the broad scope of his responsibilites. See, for example, Jonathan Richards, 20 May 1852, GC; Joseph Jones, 12 June 1870, GC. During his superintendency, Kirkbride employed nine stewards and eight matrons, including four married couples. On the average, they served for nine years in the post, at a combined salary starting at $700.00 in the 1840s and rising to $1,200.00 in the 1870s.

82 Kirkbride to JM, 24 July 1842, LP 1:114.

83 Kirkbride, *Code of Rules*, 2nd ed., p. 15. Two of the wing supervisors' journals have survived: Diary, MD, 1873–7, and Logbook, FD, 1863.

84 WHC, 9 June 1870 [misfiled], GC.

85 "Proceedings," *AJI* 17 (1860):60; Kirkbride, *Code of Rules*, 2nd ed., p. 16; *AR* 1861, p. 31.

86 Rous Diary, July–September 1870. Quotations are from July 10, 22, 9, and 24 entries.

87 Lucy Rous to Eliza Kirkbride, 24 December 1879 and 15 February 1880, GC; Agnes Turner, 28 March 1878, GC.

88 Elizabeth Bennet, 28 July 1868 [misfiled], PC.

89 MR, 23 July 1864, PH; MS [no date], PC. See also Mrs. SAT, 21 February 1861, for a similar case. Elizabeth Bennet's letter to Kirkbride, 28 July 1868, PC, reveals her sense of religious mission. The Rous Diary mentions a relative in the Pennsylvania Hospital for the Insane.

90 Kirkbride, *Code of Rules*, 2nd ed., pp. 15–38.

91 Ibid., pp. 20, 21.

92 Ibid., pp. 19–20, 31, 23.

93 Ibid., p. 30. See also p. 31.

94 "List of Rules for Attendants," with subscript in Kirkbride's hand, "For at-

tendant's room," Short Misc. Mss. There is also a printed version of this list. The regulation concerning the signing of rulebooks was evidently enforced, for the hospital archives contain the copy of attendant Archibald Carson, complete with the initials of the steward or assistant physician for every week from 1854 to 1863.

95 Kirkbride, "Journal, 1841," entry for March 6, notes the firing of an attendant who would not give up tobacco.

96 I used the manuscript census schedules for Ward 24, District 5, 1860; Ward 24, District 78, 1870; and Ward 24, District 504, 1880.

97 Louisa Davis, 21 August 1865, GC; Joshua Worthington, 20 May 1853, GC; Emma Jack, 26 November [no year], GC; J. McDivit, 26 May 1862, GC. The superintendents' letters to one another frequently included references to (or warnings about) former employees. See, for example, Nichols to Edward Jarvis, 10 July 1858, CL.

98 Emily Browne, 10 May 1855, GC; Leo Hemien, 27 December 1854, GC; Garrible Miller, 27 June 1851, GC; Edward Jones, 17 December 1859 (he left the almshouse when his wages were lowered), GC.

99 Isaiah Hacker, 12 September 1849, GC; L. C. Davis, 27 November 1874, GC; Jane Filson, 29 August 1860, GC; Ella Cumming, 9 April 1879, GC; Eliza Smith, 5 March 1866, GC.

100 John Black, 2 March 1859, GC; Edwin Lawrence, 26 March 1859, GC; J. A. Scott, 22 March 1848, GC; Phoebe Stanley, 3 August 1859, GC; J. A. Scott, 11 March 1848, GC.

101 Phoebe Stanley, 3 August 1859, GC; Diary Begun 1870, MD; entries for 27 March 1870 and 8 July 1870.

102 Lee, 16 October 1862, GC; David Bright, 16 March 1857, GC; D. Andrews, 23 June 1857, [misfiled] PC.

103 Diary Begun 1870, MD; entry for 16 March 1870. Paris Brown, [no day] March 1847, GC; Kirkbride to Paris Brown, 27 March 1847, LP 2:355. Kirkbride refused Brown's request for money brusquely, saying that his wound would heal and that the patient's blow had not caused Brown's shoulder to abscess. From the tone of Kirkbride's reply, I suspect that the attendant had provoked the attack.

104 MR, 29 May 1869.

105 Ibid.

106 FF, WF, 12 May 1848, PC; Mr. E, AR, 9 August 1861, PC. Compare my account of asylum attendants with Mick Carpenter, "Asylum Nursing Before 1914," in *Rewriting Nursing History*, edited by Celia Davies, (Totowa, N.J., 1980), pp. 123–46.

CHAPTER 5. *A new kind of existence*

1 These parallels are suggested by Eugene Genovese's discussion of paternalism in *Roll, Jordan, Roll: The World the Slaves Made* (New York, 1974) and Gresham Sykes's account of a maximum-security prison in *The Society of Captives* (Princeton, N.J., 1958).

2 The calculations in the following section are based upon statistics given in *AR* 1883, pp. 11–19. The figure 8,852 represents the number of *cases* admitted to the asylum, including multiple readmissions for the same individual. The number of *individuals* admitted is given as 8,470 (p. 19). I have used the former figure in making my calculations here; when discussing cure rates, I use the latter figure.

3 See Tables A.1 to A.5 for more detailed information on the patient population. Kirkbride kept no record of the patients' race. I have come across only a few references to "colored" inmates.

4 To arrive at these figures, I used the coding scheme outlined by Theodore Hershberg et al., "Occupation and Ethnicity in Five Nineteenth Century Cities: A Collaborative Inquiry," *Historical Methods Newsletter* 7 (1973):174–216. When compared with the occupational structure for mid-nineteenth-century

Philadelphia, it becomes evident that the Pennsylvania Hospital for the Insane drew a disproportionate percentage of its clientele from the top two occupational categories. Using an 1860 sample of the adult male work force in Philadelphia, Hershberg found 5% in the high white-collar rank, 15% in the low white-collar rank, 46% in the artisan rank, and 32% in the unskilled categories (194). Considering its private status, the number of male patients from the artisan class is still impressive. I suspect that a good percentage of the working-class patients had their board paid by their employers. This would explain the relatively small number of coresident patients and securities I found in my sample from the manuscript census (see Chapter 3, note 4). A sizable number of securities whom I could not locate in the census gave what appeared to be business as opposed to home addresses, again suggesting that the patient might be an employee. In several cases, a working man's association or guild paid for a fellow worker's treatment. See, for example, Henry K. Strong for Order of Odd Fellows, 23 May 1869, PC, PH. However their care was financed, the presence of so many patients from the respectable working class must have reinforced Kirkbride's conception of his asylum as a multiclass institution.

5 More complex nosologies incorporating developmental characteristics of mental disorders were a major achievement of nineteenth-century German psychiatry. The work of Wilhelm Griesinger and Emil Kraepelin was particularly important in this regard. For a general survey of their significance for medical nosology, see Gregory Zilboorg, *A History of Medical Psychology* (New York, 1941), pp. 435–8, 450–64.

6 For example, Kirkbride identified a halting gait, difficulty in articulation, and confusion, or "mental weakness," as symptoms of organic mental disorder. See Kirkbride to JS, 18 February 1844, LP 1:225; Kirkbride to Dr. J. R. Riggs, 15 January 1845, LP 2:19. Like nineteenth-century physicians generally, he recognized general paralysis or paresis as a specific form of organic disease that always terminated in death, but did not understand its etiological relationship to syphilis. See Kirkbride to ET, 8 July 1845, LP 2:105. For Kirkbride's remarks on periodic insanity, see "Proceedings," *AJI* 12 (1855):65. In Kirkbride, *On the Construction, Organization and General Arrangements of Hospitals for the Insane*, 2nd ed. (Philadelphia, 1880), p. 23, he noted that untreated cases of mania and melancholia often sank into some form of dementia.

7 CB-OS 3:261; 2:141.

8 CB-OS 3:369, 145.

9 These percentages are based on statistics given in *AR* 1883, p. 18. I have excluded the small number of patients – twenty in the forty-two-year period – diagnosed as suffering from delirium. These patients had an acute illness that produced a severe mental disorientation, which was mistaken for insanity. They often died from the wearing effects of the journey to the asylum. Kirkbride warned against confusing the two conditions in *AR* 1843, p. 9.

Since Kirkbride disliked labeling patients as incurable, it is difficult to get a firm estimate on the asylum's chronically ill population. Kirkbride to managers, 20 May 1845, LP 2:81, stated that of 160 patients, 70 were under active medical treatment. Also, there is no way of determining how many nineteenth-century asylum patients suffered from mental disorders that we now know to be somatic in origin, such as general paresis, cerebral arteriosclerosis, senility, brain tumor, and the like. Gerald Grob estimates that at least one-third of all first admissions to state mental hospitals in the early twentieth century were suffering from these disorders. See Grob, "Abuse in American Mental Hospitals in Historical Perspective: Myth and Reality," *International Journal of Law and Psychiatry* 3 (1980):304–9.

10 Christopher Lasch, "The Origins of the Asylum," in *The World of Nations* (New York, 1973), pp. 16–17, uses the phrase "single standard of citizenship" to connote the values – chiefly "the duty of self-reliance and self-support" – promulgated in egalitarian societies to foster social order and cohesion. I would argue that Kirkbride had a well-defined, unitary notion of sanity closely akin to

this "single standard," but that his methods for fostering that standard implicitly recognized, indeed depended upon, class and sex differences.

11 Erving Goffman, *Asylums: Essays on the Social Situation of Mental Patients and Other Inmates* (New York, 1961), first laid out the concept of a "total institution": a "place of residence and work where a large number of like-situated individuals, cut off from the wider society for an appreciable period of time, together lead an enclosed, formally administered round of life" (p. xiii). Such an institution isolates its inhabitants from the outside world and forces them to undergo a ritual "mortification," or humiliation, so as to forge a new definition of self. The Pennsylvania Hospital for the Insane obviously conforms in some respects to Goffman's definition of a total institution; yet, as will be shown in the rest of this chapter, the degree of isolation from family and community, the rituals of humiliation, and the implied powerlessness of asylum patients were far less extreme than his "ideal type" suggests. Perhaps the degree of control Goffman associates with the total institution was simply not possible before the twentieth century. Nineteenth-century mental hospitals might best be thought of as prototypes of the institutions he describes. Cf. Charles Rosenberg, "And Heal the Sick: The Hospital and The Patient in Nineteenth-Century America," *JSH* 10 (1977):428–47, and "Inward Vision and Outward Glance: The Shaping of the American Hospital, 1880–1914," *BHM* (1979):346–91, for a similar argument for the nineteenth-century general hospital.

12 Modern observers might dispute the efficacy that nineteenth-century physicians attributed to their medical therapeutics. But their use of materia medica could be relied upon to produce certain predictable physiological effects: Soporifics induced drowsiness, emetics caused vomiting, and diaphoretics produced sweat. Even if exhibiting a drug could not alter the course of a particular disease, it still demonstrated some sort of mastery over the human body. This competency in itself could contribute, at least in some cases, to the healing process by reinforcing the patient's trust in the physician. So, for its placebo effect alone, Kirkbride's medical treatment has to be taken seriously. In addition, as the following discussion makes clear, he utilized certain drugs, particularly narcotics, in a fashion consistent with contemporary concepts of their physiological effect. Charles Rosenberg, "The Therapeutic Revolution," *Perspectives in Biology and Medicine* (Summer 1977):487–9, provides an excellent discussion of nineteenth-century therapeutics; his analysis has strongly shaped my own.

13 CB-FD 4:155. My estimates of morphine usage are based on a sample of fifty male and female patients admitted consecutively from August 1841 to January 1842, CB-OS 2:137–87, and twenty-five female patients admitted consecutively between March 1876 and December 1877, CB-FD 4:1–25. The Male Department casebooks cannot be used to calculate medication, since prescriptions were not entered for individual cases. The Prescription Book, MD, no. 1, 1859–80, gives an idea of the number of morphine prescriptions, but not the percentage of cases in which it was used. See also Prescription Book, FD, no. 1, 1863–76.

For Kirkbride's opinions on morphine, see "Proceedings," *AJI* 14 (1857):101, and *AJI* 36 (1879):212. For a general discussion of morphine's medical properties, as perceived in his time, see George B. Wood and Franklin Bache, *Dispensatory of the United States* (Philadelphia, 1833), p. 902. Eric Carlson and Meribeth Simpson, "Opium as a Tranquilizer," *American Journal of Psychiatry* 120 (1964):112–17, provide an overview of morphine use in psychiatric treatment.

Nineteenth-century physicians such as Kirkbride evidently had little fear of turning their patients into morphine addicts. David Musto, *The American Disease* (New Haven, Conn., 1973), shows that medical understanding of drug addiction was very limited in this period. Concern about the habit-forming properties of certain drugs did not appear until the 1870s. It should also be remembered that morphine taken by mouth is far less powerful than an injection directly into the bloodstream.

14 Wood and Bache, *Dispensatory*, pp. 247, 3; CB-OS 1:128. For Kirkbride's views on conium, see "Proceedings," *AJI* 14 (1857):101.

15 George B. Wood and Franklin Bache, *Dispensatory of the United States*, 12th ed. (Philadelphia, 1865), pp. 298, 1322. For Kirkbride's views on quinine's virtues as an "anti-periodic," see *AJI* 12 (1855):65.

16 Wood and Bache, *Dispensatory*, pp. 350, 951. Potassium bromide's value as an antiaphrodisiac was first noted in Wood and Bache, *Dispensatory*, 12th ed., p. 1293. At the Pennsylvania Hospital for the Insane, the drug was administered approximately eight times as often to male as to female patients, according to the Prescription Books, no. 1, MD and FD. Kirkbride discusses potassium bromide in "Proceedings," *AJI* 27 (1870):210.

17 George B. Wood and Franklin Bache, *Dispensatory of the United States*, 14th ed. (Philadelphia, 1878), p. 266; "Proceedings," *AJI* 27 (1870):210–11; "Proceedings," *AJI* 33 (1876):275. Kirkbride did not use ether or chloroform, drugs he thought of as very dangerous and not particularly efficacious. See "Proceedings," *AJI* 12(1855):67, and "Proceedings," *AJI* 22 (1865):60.

18 See, for example, CB-OS 2:133, 141 (mania); CB-OS 2:13, 137 (melancholia). The range of other drugs prescribed is indicated in the Prescription Books, MD and FD.

19 "Proceedings," *AJI* 14 (1857):101, and "Proceedings," *AJI* 27 (1870):210. Kirkbride noted of one chronic patient, who had resided in the hospital for thirty-five years, "He has of course long since ceased to be treated for insanity" (CB-OS 1:145). In a patient of only two years' residence with an apparently hereditary disorder, he "deemed it advisable not to put her on a regular course of treatment" (CB-OS 1:169).

On the whole, Kirkbride's medical treatment of insanity, as described in the previous section, corresponded to standard practice for the American specialty. He favored morphine more and chloral less than some of his fellow asylum doctors, but overall does not appear to have pursued an idiosyncratic course. Cf. Norman Dain, *Concepts of Insanity in the United States, 1789–1865* (New Brunswick, N.J., 1964), pp. 118–19; Gerald Grob, *The State and the Mentally Ill: A History of the Worcester State Hospital in Massachusetts, 1830–1920* (Chapel Hill, N.C., 1966), pp. 63–4; idem, *Mental Institutions in America: Social Policy to 1875* (New York, 1973), pp. 165–71.

20 CB-OS 3:329; Diary for 1870–1, MD, entry for October 1870. For examples of the use of seclusion, see Kirkbride, "Journal, 1841," entry for 31 January (the patient was also given opium); CB-OS 1:195. For other examples of the use of restraint, see CB-OS 2:9 (patient destructive, struck attendants); ibid., 2:78 (patient masturbating, injured self); ibid., 2:138 (patient scratched self badly). In the early 1840s, Kirkbride used the shower bath for violent and so-called filthy patients, but he eventually seems to have abandoned the practice. See Kirkbride to JB, 8 September 1843, LP 1:147; CB-OS 1:47, 169.

For a description of the restraining devices in use at the Pennsylvania Hospital for the Insane, see Kirkbride, *On the Construction*, 2nd ed., pp. 254–7.

In a letter to Pliny Earle (8 July 1845, AS), Kirkbride referred to the "bed apparatus" he had ordered, stating, "I like that term much better than 'straps' commonly employed and to which I have a great aversion." This comment points up the concern with language that runs through Kirkbride's asylum practice; by inventing less opprobrious terms for restraining devices, he hoped to make them less repulsive. The impulse revealed here was part of his larger effort to mask or conceal the asylum's repressive features, as discussed in Chapter 4.

21 Kirkbride to Dr. Thomas Smith, 23 October 1847, LP 2:370; "Proceedings," *AJI* 12 (1855):65. William Moon to Kirkbride, 12 June 1870, GC, recounts the story of the woman patient.

22 Diary for 1870–1, MD, entry for 25 May 1871.

23 "Proceedings," *AJI* 12 (1855):92. See John Bucknill, *Notes on Asylums for the Insane in America* (New York, 1973; reprint of 1876 ed.), esp. pp. 3–6. See also Kirkbride's statements on restraint in *AR* 1841, pp. 33–6, and Kirkbride, *On the Construction*, pp. 60–1. John Conolly, *The Treatment of the Insane Without Mechanical Restraints* (New York, 1973; reprint of 1856 ed.), outlined the nonrestraint system.

24 *AR* 1863, p. 24.
25 Ibid.
26 This reconstruction of the daily regimen is based upon Kirkbride, "A Hospital Day," in *AR* 1863, pp. 25–30; Rous Diary; and "Entertainment at Kirkbride's," *Press* 7 November 1871, Misc. Clippings. Details concerning the patients' diet are given in Kirkbride, "Memorandum Given to Matron...," LP 2:323.

Unlike some of his fellow superintendents, who limited their visits to once a week (or, in the case of John Gray, supposedly once a month), Kirkbride appears to have kept up his daily rounds throughout his long career. John Curwen, "Presidential Address," *Proceedings of the American Medico-Psychological Association* 1 (1885):35, makes this claim for his mentor.
27 The *Reports* chronicle the progress of the Pennsylvania Hospital's evening entertainments. George Layne, "The Kirkbride–Langenheim Collaboration," *PMHB* 105 (1981):182–202, shows that Kirkbride's use of slides represented both a psychiatric and a photographic innovation.
28 Kirkbride to IW, 17 May 1843, LP 1:82; Mrs. L, EL, 1 January 1866, PC. See also Patient Expense Book, MD, 1860-2.

Obviously, these practices do not suggest the concerted attempts to obliterate the inmate's identity that Goffman finds in his total institutions. Kirkbride's patients got to keep their "identity kits," to use Goffman's terms, i.e., their clothing, toiletries, and furnishings, which he sees as critical to the "management of the personal front." See Goffman, *Asylums*, esp. pp. 20–1.

A letter written by a woman patient in 1865 conveys the extent to which she expected to shape her own environment within the hospital. Asking permission to rent "some sort of a bureau to put all my smaller articles in," she continued:

I should like a towel horse, and permission to drive a few tacks in my room for some few pictures, and a little thing to keep the days of the week and month. I was told I could have flowers whenever I wanted, but don't care. Mrs. Lee has all my scissors but button-hole scissors, I should like them again sir?! I have a tooth which need filling and will be obliged for an opportunity to have it attended to. (See SH to Kirkbride, 12th. Sat. [no month] 1865, PC.)

29 See, for example, MR, 29 March 1851; Kirkbride to [illegible], 21 July 1844, LP 1:112. The *AR* 1883, pp. 119–20, states that after breakfast, the gardener "invited suitable patients," or those for whom such activity had been "prescribed," to work with him in the kitchen garden. The Rous Diary suggests the companion's efforts with lady patients.
30 I am not denying that Kirkbride's patients followed a routine, but rather want to make clear that it bore little resemblance to the lock-step precision supposedly being asked of nineteenth-century prisoners or even school children. Compare the hospital day with the prison routine described by W. David Lewis, *From Newgate to Dannemora* (Ithaca, N.Y., 1965) or the public schools described by David Tyack, *The One Best System* (Cambridge, 1974). The corporate asylum's inmates had neither a full nor a demanding schedule to follow; it included long blocks of time in which they were more or less left to their own devices. Kirkbride's inmates often complained that their regimen was too boring, rather than too harsh or inflexible.
31 The exact logic of the Pennsylvania Hospital for the Insane's classification scheme is difficult to reconstruct, because the ward rankings were an aspect of everyday knowledge that never got written down. My observations here are based on sporadic notations concerning ward assignments entered in the casebooks and ward diaries.

Of the two criteria bearing on ward assignments, social class and mental condition, the latter was apparently the more influential. Kirkbride often insisted that being rich did not entitle a troublesome individual to a room on the best corridor. Conversely, he pointed out to a patron angered over a relative's demotion to a lower ward, "The Lodge is not considered less respectable than any other division of the house, and some of its occupants belong to the finest families in Philadelphia." Kirkbride to Mrs. G, 27 March 1847, LP 2:357.

32 CB-MD 1:137. For an example of demotion due to furniture breakage, see Diary for 1870–1, MD, entry for 8 July 1871. The patients' acceptance of the ward hierarchy comes across most clearly in their complaints about being demoted from a more to a less desirable ward. See, for example, the letter cited in Note 31 above, and CPB to Kirkbride, 3 November 1865, PC. In the latter, an epileptic patient at the Bloomingdale asylum wrote that he wanted to move to an institution where the patients were "classified more strictly," to avoid the "profanity and smut" of lower-class attendants and patients, and to gain the "society of gentlemen and ladies." The fact that patients regarded taking tea with those of a higher ward as a privilege also suggests their acceptance of the asylum hierarchy.

33 Supervisor's Log Book, 1863 FD, entries for 10 August, 7 September, 17 September, 22 October.

34 Kirkbride to EE, 28 December 1843, LP 1:173; Kirkbride to IW, 14 October 1842, LP 1:13. For examples of the use of isolation see Kirkbride, "Journal 1841," entry for 31 January, and CB-OS 1:47. Diary 1870–1, MD, entry for 30 April 1871, notes punishment of a whole ward.

35 See, for example, Diary 1870–1, MD, entries for 30 October and 25 November 1870.

36 Kirkbride to EF, 16 February 1846, LP 2:257; Kirkbride to Mrs. G, 27 March 1847, LP 2:357.

37 SG, DG, 12 September 1851 (the patron is referring to Kirkbride's plan for a relative); CB-OS 1:173; CB-OS 2:367; AR 1852, p. 39. WL, HL, 5 June 1848, PC, mentions an attendant giving a patient a silver suspender buckle "for some little office" on the ward.

38 RA to Kirkbride, 26 October 1857, PC. Another female patient believed that Mrs. A was a "medium" who influenced her behavior. Her delusions may very well reflect the role Mrs. A was playing as a model patient. See HC, AC, 15 December 1857, PC.

39 John Curwen, 8 May 1848, GC; CB-OS 1:181; AR 1875, p. 18. Eliza Kirkbride states in the AR 1883, p. 66, that her husband always attended the tea parties and evening entertainments, so as to keep up patient interest in them. The most persuasive testimony for the strength of ward friendships comes from the letters patients wrote after leaving the hospital, in which they invariably sent messages to their special friends. One girl named friends from the First, Third, and Fourth wards, as well as the cottage, suggesting the range of contacts among the patients. It also belies the rigid classificatory scheme Kirkbride promised his patrons.

40 "Proceedings of the Second Annual Anniversary of the Light Gymnastics Class...1866," Misc. Material; MA [no day] March 1861, PC. For references to the family table, see AP, JEP, 28 November 1849, PC. The patients invited to the family table appear to have been wealthy or well-educated – for example, a "young man of large fortune," a clerk of the British Consul, and a clergyman with "talent and education." See CB-OS 1:159; CB-OS 2:86, 161. Kirkbride explained to a patron, "I ask gentlemen to the 'Family Table' occasionally, when I think they are likely to leave the hospital in a short time." Kirkbride to Mr. W, 9 August 1843, LP 1:127. For a reference to Mrs. Jones's dinner parties, see Diary Begun April 1871, MD, entry for 19 April 1873.

41 AR 1883, p. 72. Given the number of patients and the many demands on his time, Kirkbride obviously did not pursue his conversations with every individual every day. He appears to have confined his serious efforts to the most hopeful cases and utilized any occasion, including ward visits, parties, and chance encounters, to exercise his influence over them. As will be evident from the following description, Kirkbride's conversations resemble a primitive, unformulated type of psychotherapy. I suspect that Kirkbride did not give much thought to the methods he used in these encounters or discuss them at AMSAII meetings, not because he thought his influence was negligible, but because his paternal style of advice giving was second nature to him. It remained for a later generation,

and Sigmund Freud, to develop a more self-conscious approach to the physician–patient interaction.

42 Kirkbride's Letterpress volumes attest to the size and frequency of the superintendent's correspondence with the patrons. He wrote to the family only upon request. When relatives grew anxious for news, they wrote to him and asked for a report, rather than waiting for him to write. Kirkbride made it clear that he did not have the time for a frequent or lengthy exchange of letters. "The large number of patients in this house and the great amount of necessary correspondence makes this course necessary," he wrote to a patron (Kirkbride to WB, 9 March 1843, LP 1:47). After he stopped keeping Letterpress volumes in the mid-1850s, Kirkbride preserved only random copies of his letters to the patrons, but from references in their letters to him, it is evident that he continued an extensive correspondence until the very end of his career. See the discussion in Chapter 4, note 68. Citations to the Letterpress volumes give the recipients' initials and date of the letter; all letters were written by Kirkbride.

43 JM, 24 July 1842, LP 1:114.

44 IMW, 28 March 1844, LP 1:254; JY, 31 March 1843, LP 1:62. Barbara Rosenkrantz and Maris Vinovskis, "Sustaining the 'Flickering Flame of Life'," in *Health Care in America,* edited by Susan Reverby and David Rosner (Philadelphia, 1979), pp. 154–82, explore the problems asylum superintendents faced in accounting for patients' deaths. Obviously, an inmate's demise, whatever the cause, had to be carefully explained.

45 WB, 21 July 1845, LP 2:117; MC, 16 September 1845, LP 2:163. Kirkbride to B and CH, draft note on back of JH, B & CH, 20 August 1848, PC, records his response to patrons who wanted another physician to attend their brother in the asylum. Despite his reservations, Kirkbride did occasionally call in other doctors as consultants. He asked a woman physician to examine a female patient and make a supporter for her bladder and womb (see SB, 5 November 1860, GC). In another instance, he sought advice about a patient's "August cold," or hay fever (Mr. H, TB, 20 August 1848, PC).

46 JR, 31 December 1842, LP 1:36; DB, 7 September 1845, LP 2:149.

47 WM, 3 March 1843, LP 1:78; Dr. JA, 23 January 1846, LP 2:245; BC, 21 February 1844, LP 1:231; WM, 29 April 1844, LP 1:276.

48 Mrs. M, JM, 18 October 1865, PC; CD, 1 December 1845, LP 2:211; HR, 17 March 1843, LP 1:52.

49 WW, 12 October 1844, LP 1:376; TJL, 30 September 1845, LP 2:169; MG, RG, 2 August 1862, PC; CB-FD 4:156; TL, 9 August 1843, LP 1:125. Because he so frequently had difficulty in overcoming a patient's suspicions about hospital treatment, Kirkbride told the family preparing to commit a patient not to lie about what was going to happen. He told a patron's family doctor, "My own plan would be, to speak candidly to him, upon what was intended and why, and then to use force if necessary, but always if possible to avoid deception in intercourse with the Insane; it is rarely forgotten or forgiven and often does much harm" (TL, 26 March 1847, LP 2:355).

50 TL, 28 August 1843, LP 1:140; JG, 26 September 1843, LP 1:160; RN, 25 July 1844, LP 1:328; EB, C to EB, 29 December 1848, PC; Mrs. K, BFK, 2 October 1853, PC.

51 WM, 11 July 1843, LP 1:102; TH, 16 September 1845, LP 2:164.

52 CWD, 2 March 1846, LP 2:263; Mrs. TM, 20 October 1842, LP 1:16.

53 WS, 21 July 1844, LP 1:322; WC, 6 December 1844 and 15 February 1845, LP 2:3.

54 WW, 12 October 1844, LP 1:376; WN, 21 July 1845, LP 2:118; Mr.[?] Bumford, [7 August?] 1845, LP 2:134; WW, 26 November 1844 and 6 December 1844, LP 1:412, 414; JM, 21 November 1842, LP 2:26; Mrs. LS, LS, 6 September 1855, PC; JC, Kirkbride to Zachary Taylor (draft) [no date 1849], PC.

55 WL, 30 April 1845, LP 2:66; WL, 10 February 1845, LP 2:31; WS, 15 August 1844, LP 1:340; AK, 28 August 1844, LP 1:352; Mrs. JCT, JCT, 18 May 1853, PC.

56 WL, 23 May 1844, LP 1:291; JM, 2 April 1843, LP 1:64; CB-OS 2:122, 367; MB, MB 30 July 1848, PC.
57 DR, 20 June 1843, LP 1:97; HF, 10 January 1844, LP 1:217.
58 ED, ED, 30 October 1865, PC; DR, 20 June 1843, LP 1:97.
59 WS, 10 February 1847, LP 2:312; WM, 10 February, LP 2:32; ER, 24 March 1845, LP 2:53; CA, 15 August 1843, LP 1:132.
60 Mrs. S, 1 April 1845, LP 2:61; CB-OS 2:367; JB, 31 October 1844, LP 1:386; ID, 22 August 1844, LP 1:345; Mr. F, December 1843, LP 1:206.
61 CB-OS 3:32; HJM, JF, [no date], PC; EM, 14 February 1843, LP 1:44; WM, 10 June 1843, LP 1:94.
62 CB-OS 3:33–4; CB-OS 1:197.
63 AM, 22 November 1845, LP 2:205; "Memorandum given to JM," [October 1843], LP 1:180; RM, 30 September 1843, LP 1:167.
64 *AR* 1883, p. 72.
   Comparisons between religion and psychotherapy are commonplace in both popular and academic literature. William Sargant, *Battle for the Mind: A Physiology of Conversion and Brain Washing* (New York, 1957), and Jerome Frank, *Persuasion and Healing* (Baltimore, 1961), pursue the comparison, although in very different ways. Howard Feinstein, "The Prepared Heart: A Comparison of Puritan Theology and Psychoanalysis," *American Quarterly* 22 (1970):166–76, focuses more explicitly on the conversion process. But similarities between conversion and cure in pre-Freudian days have not been systematically explored. As an initial observation, I would suggest that Kirkbride's methods, and presumably those of his fellow superintendents as well, resembled the more gradual, intellectual process of conversion associated with Horace Bushnell and other nonevangelical Protestants. Given their conviction that religious revivals caused insanity, we would hardly expect asylum doctors to have copied the highly dramatic, emotional methods of the stump preachers of their time.
65 These figures are based on the table given in the 1883 *AR*, p. 19. The percentages were calculated using the number of *persons* rather than *cases* admitted to the Pennsylvania Hospital for the Insane, so as to eliminate readmissions from the count. Kirkbride claimed that he never discharged periodic cases as cured, only as improved. See Appendix 2 for further discussion of asylum cure rates.
   Kirkbride's cure rates were among the highest reported in the mid-nineteenth-century profession. See the chart prepared by Pliny Earle, *Annual Report of the Northampton State Hospital* (Northampton, Mass., 1885), p. 53, comparing cure rates for twenty hospitals. Of course, these rates must be viewed with some caution, since some doctors undoubtedly inflated their totals, whereas others did not have the administrative power that Kirkbride did to limit the admission of chronic patients.
66 Contemporary arguments over the effectiveness of psychotherapy in treating neuroses revolve around the possibility of spontaneous remission. Certain studies claim to show that treated and untreated patients improve at the same rate due to this phenomenon. For a review of this controversy, see A. E. Bergin and M.J. Lambert, "The Evaluation of Therapeutic Outcomes," in *Handbook of Psychotherapy and Behavior Change*, 2nd ed., edited by Sol L. Garfield and Allen E. Bergin (New York, 1978), pp.139-89.
67 EC, 8 January 1866, PC; BE, 20 February 1857, PC; SL, S to EL, [no date], PC; MS, 18 August 1848, PC; SL, S to EL, [no date], PC; *AR* 1883, p. 112.
68 GL, 3 April 1846, PC; *AR* 1883, p. 112; AL, 12 November 1857, PC.
69 MG, 16 October 1860, PC; MG, 1 January 1861, PC; JP, 21 April 1853, PC.
70 MG [no date 1855?], PC.
71 WS, 19 April 1856, PC; AF, TM, 22 February 1848, PC; Emma, 28 November 1865, GC; MC, 7 December 1853, PC; ZH, 13 November 1850, PC.
72 AL, 16 October 1858, PC; SR, 25 June 1859, PC. Numerous other patients mentioned having pictures of Kirkbride and the asylum in their homes. For letters asking for advice, see JG, 24 March 1851, PC; FH, 13 March 1865, PC.
73 MH, 26 February 1861, PC; MTW, 15 December 1856, PC; *AR* 1883, p. 113.

74 MTW, 15 December 1856, PC; MG, 1 January 1861, PC; MGJ, 25 February 1857, GC; Mrs. W, GWW, 11 May 1883, PC; CM, 23 October 1843, PC.

75 Women patients repeatedly referred to Kirkbride as a father figure. "You were indeed like a father and I shall never forget you," wrote Juliet [?], 22 July 1861, PC. Some of their letters had a flirtatious tone: "I cannot describe to you how much pain I felt in leaving you, I always knew I liked you, how much attached to Dr. Kirkbride I never knew until I left. . .I miss that sweet, 'Yes, you shall have it anything you want. . .it gives me great spiritual pleasure to write to the 'Beloved Physician' " (SR, 25 June 1859, PC). A tendency to form a crush on the superintendent did not affect patients alone; Kirkbride's correspondence includes one emotional letter from a woman companion who had developed a strong attachment to him (LP, 14 April 1879, GC). We would expect women's affections to be couched in spiritual rather than sensual terms, since women, at least of the upper classes, were being told (and many evidently believed) that they had no sexual instincts, but only religious or moral sensibilities. See Nancy Cott, "Passionlessness: An Interpretation of Victorian Sexual Ideology, 1790-1850," in *A Heritage of Her Own*, edited by Nancy Cott and Elizabeth Pleck (New York, 1979), pp. 162–81. Margaret Masson, "The Typology of the Female as a Model for the Regenerate: Puritan Preaching, 1690-1730," *Signs* 2 (1976):304–15, argues that the conversion process was essentially female in structure, because it required a total submission of body and will. Since Kirkbride's therapeutic methods resembled the conversion process, this might also explain his greater success with women patients.

The asylum doctors never publicly referred to the complexities involved in treating women patients, but I cannot help suspecting that they all experienced what the post-Freudian generation would term "transference problems." In this regard, it is interesting to note that Elizabeth Packard, the former patient who led a vigorous campaign for new commitment laws, wrote her doctor, Andrew McFarland (whom she later denounced), a love letter while in the asylum. See Myra Himelhoch and Arthur Shaffer, "Elizabeth Packard: Nineteenth Century Crusader for the Rights of Mental Patients," *Journal of American Studies* 13 (1979):355, 362–3. They claim that Packard wrote the letter only as a "last desperate attempt" to secure his cooperation in publishing her book on asylum conditions, and did not mean any of the statements she made in it. I find this argument unconvincing.

76 See David S. Muzzey, "Benjamin Franklin Butler," *Dictionary of American Biography*, edited by Allen Johnson, 11 vols. (New York, 1964), vol. 2, pp. 356–7. My discussion of the Butler household is based on family papers in the Firestone Library, Princeton University, which include correspondence, diaries, and books concerning several generations of Butlers. William A. Butler and Willard P. Butler, *Book of the Family and Lineal Descendants of Medad Butler* (New York, 1915), p. 8, provides a list of the Butler children. Eliza's brother, William Allen Butler, wrote an autobiography, *A Retrospect of Forty Years* (New York, 1911), which also has useful information on the family.

77 Benjamin Franklin Butler, 7 July 1858, GC.

78 Benjamin Franklin Butler, 29 June 1858, GC. A former patient observed to Kirkbride of her town, "We ladies are all very nervous here, having so little else to interest us we cultivate our nerves. I try to make mine as tough 'as a whip end'. . .but sometimes they rebel" (MG, 1 January 1861, PC). For a recent perspective on women's nervous diseases, see Carroll Smith-Rosenberg, "The Hysterical Woman: Sex Roles and Social Conflict in Nineteenth Century America," *Social Research* 39 (1972):652–78; and John Haller and Robin Haller, *The Physician and Sexuality in Victorian America* (New York, 1974).

79 Medical Register 2, entry for 13 January 1858; Benjamin Franklin Butler, 11 March, 17 March, 24 May 1858, GC. See also Benjamin Franklin Butler, 7 July 1858, GC.

80 Eliza Kirkbride to Dorothea Dix, 31 January 1882; *AR* 1883, p. 109; Edward A. Smith, 8 June 1858, GC. William Allen Butler, 20 August 1858, GC, mentions

Eliza's pledge not to harm herself. Eliza Butler's case interested Manager Samuel Welsh, who kept up with her progress after her discharge. See Welsh, 30 June 1859 and 6 January 1860, GC.

81 Benjamin Franklin Butler, 19 August, 30 August, 1858. GC.

82 Charlotte Brown to William Allen Butler, 8 November 1853, PL; Eliza Butler to "sister," 9 November 1858, PL. Butler, *Retrospect*, pp. 318–19, recounts the circumstances of his father's death.

83 Medical Register 2, entry for 13 November 1861. Margaret Crosby remained as a patient until December 1862, was readmitted in June 1863, and was discharged in May 1864. In the interval, she was treated at the Bloomingdale Asylum. EB Diary, 1862–3, TU, entry for 10 November 1863. I have deduced that Eliza was caring for Margaret's children by comparing the names she mentions in her diary with the list of the Crosby children in Butler, *Book of the Family*, p. 9.

84 EB Diary, entries for 7 July 1863, 6 September 1862, 6 November 1863, 31 December 1863, and 26 January 1864.

85 EB Diary, entries for 2 November 1863 and 22 December 1863.

86 James Bates, 21 May 1848, GC; Kirkbride to Jarvis, 20 October 1862, CL (Kirkbride describes Ann as "greatly afflicted for many years"); Eliza Kirkbride to Dorothea Dix, 1 April 1882, GC. Charles Nichols, 1 June 1858, GC; Harriet Collins, 8 June 1859; 17 and 25 May, 1862, GC, all mention the debilitating impact of Ann's illness. William Wade Hinshaw, *Encyclopedia of American Quaker Genealogy*, 6 vols. (Ann Arbor, Mich., 1938), vol. 2, p. 710, gives the birthdates of Ann and Joseph Kirkbride, children of Ann West and Thomas S. Kirkbride. Ann W. Kirkbride's death was recorded in the Philadelphia Monthly Meeting, Western District, Births and Burials 1814–83, p. 59, HC. She left her husband an estate valued at $40,000 in loans, railroad shares, and mortgages. The "Inventory and Appraisement of the Goods and Chattels...of Ann West Kirkbride," 29 April 1862, Will 1862, no. 396, in Account Book 7-48-83 P287-346-212, Registrar of Wills, PCA, lists them.

87 Eliza Kirkbride to Mary Butler, 29 November 1915, PL; EB Diary, entries for 21 May 1863[?], 15 and 17 October 1863. The entry for 20 October 1863 contains the cryptic sentence: "The happiest thing in all the world has come to me tonight." Perhaps Kirkbride returned to make his proposal on that day. Samuel Bettle, 15 October 1861, mentions receiving an "excellent" volume entitled "Comforting Promises." For references to visits between the two households, see Visitors' Register 2, entry for 20 October 1860; Benjamin Franklin Butler, Jr., 8 January 1861, GC; William Allen Butler, 8 February 1859, GC; Lydia Butler, 20 January 1860, GC.

88 Isaac Ray to Pliny Earle, 18 February 1872, AS; D.T. Brown, 12 December 1861 and 11 April 1864, GC (Prince married Kitty James, a cousin of Alice, Henry, and William James. Jean Strouse, *Alice James: A Biography* (New York, 1982), p. 73, discusses Kitty's illness); Charles Folsom to Earle, 15 May 1876, AS. The *New York Times*, 17 May 1866, carried a notice of the wedding.

For marrying out of meeting, Kirkbride faced expulsion from the Society of Friends. His daughter Ann was disowned in August 1862 for marrying a non-Quaker, Thomas G. Morton. (See Philadelphia Monthly Meeting, Western District Minutes 4:1, 3, 16 July and 20 August 1862, HC). Friends who married out of meeting could avoid disownment, however, by sending a formal apology to the meeting, expressing regret for their breach of the society's discipline. Kirkbride chose this latter course of action. The Minutes 4:139–40, 17 September and 16 December 1868, note that two representatives of the meeting, Samuel Bettle (the same man who admired Eliza's volume of Bible verses) and William Biddle (a Pennsylvania Hospital manager), visited Kirkbride to "treat" with him on the subject. According to their report, Kirkbride "expressed his esteem for the principles of our Religious Society, and his conviction of their truth and his desire to retain his right of membership." He sent a letter to the meeting "in which he expressed his regret for the violation of the discipline, and the attachment to our doctrine which he had for a long time cherished." The meeting decided to retain him as a member. Kirkbride belonged to the Twelfth Street Meeting, which pursued an independent line in most matters. Phillip S. Benjamin, *The Philadelphia Quakers in the Industrial Age 1865–1920* (Philadelphia, 1976), pp. 14–15, described it as a "bastion of Gurneyism," a brand of Quakerism that favored active reform over quietism. One can imagine the Twelfth Street Meeting's reluctance to part with so illustrious a figure as Kirkbride. Generally, this meeting had a low rate of disunions; also, the society as a whole saw a loosening of discipline in the late 1860s. See Benjamin, *The Philadelphia Quakers*, pp. 9, 20–1.

89 Eliza Kirkbride to Dorothea Dix, 24 August 1882, GC. Butler, *Book of the Family*, p. 53, gives the birthdates of Eliza and Thomas Story Kirkbride's children; Franklin Butler (born 1867) became a banker, and interested himself in institutions for the feebleminded; Thomas Story, Jr. (born 1869) was a promising young physician at the time of his death from typhoid fever in 1900; Elizabeth Butler (born 1872) became a prominent social worker in New York State; and Mary Butler (born 1874) became a physician specializing in bacteriology. Eliza Kirkbride's diaries for 1899 and 1903, TU, record her many philanthropic activities. She died on 17 November 1919. The *North American*, 18 November 1919, carried her obituary. See also the *Civic Club Bulletin* 13:3 (December 1919), 2–5, for tributes to her. As Jacques Quen pointed out to me, the marriage of a psychiatrist to a patient would not have had the same import in Kirkbride's era that it had for the post-Freudian generation, since physicians then understood so little about the transference process.

90 *AR* 1842, p. 29.

91 In "Proceedings," *AJI* 33 (1876):296, Kirkbride was reported to have said, "If in my hospital I thought any patients were made insane by being there, I should feel there was something the matter, either with the hospital or with me." Yet, modern studies of the mental hospital strongly suggest that certain facets of patient behavior, particularly regressive behavior such as feces smearing, are a reaction to the repressive features of institutional life. See Morris Schwartz, *The Mental Hospital: A Study of Institutional Participation in Psychiatric Illness and Treatment* (New York, 1954). Although the Male Department had a 250-bed capacity, the number of patients averaged only 150 in the 1860s and 200 in the 1870s. One ward remained totally unused until 1871. See Diary Begun in 1870, MD, entry for 19 June 1871.

92 RM, 16 August 1843, LP 1:132; William Moon, 9 June and 12 June, 1870, GC.

93 CB-FD 4:156; CB-OS 3:30.

94 AM, 29 May and 7 August, 1845, LP 2:84, 133.

95 CB-OS 2:122, 130. Kirkbride disliked using the term "moral insanity" because it caused so much controversy. See his statement in "Proceedings," *AJI* 20 (1863):103, 105–6, and *AJI* 23 (1866):143. But on occasion he did employ the term, as in this case record, and Mr. S and Mr. M, 2 September 1848, LP 2:373. He also admitted, "I have had patients under care whom I felt confident were insane, and in whom I could not *detect* delusions – but because I could not detect their delusions did not satisfy me, that they did not or had not existed." So, in practice, I think he did recognize the existence of moral insanity.

96 John B. Chapin, Scrapbook, Cornell University Archives, contains a clipping describing this incident. My thanks to Ellen Dwyer for drawing it to my attention.

97 1870–1 Diary, MD, entry for 21 November 1870; 1873 Diary, MD, entries for 2 and 3 May 1873; Mr. B, LP, [no date], PC.

98 Kirkbride, "Journal, 1841," entry for 14 April 1841.

99 Medical Register 1, entry for 22 February 1848; Wiley Williams, 17 February 1848, GC.

100 Testimony of Kirkbride, reprinted in the *Sun*, 15 December 1849, p. 1; testimony of Charles Stillwell, teacher, *Sun*, 17 December 1849, p. 1 (clippings in Wiley Williams Folder, GC); WW, CFM, 18 December 1848, PC.

101 Testimony of Kirkbride, *Sun*, 15 December 1849.

102 Trial testimony, *Sun*, 15 December and 17 December, 1849; Williams's name appears on a "List of Insane Criminals," dated 24 February 1873, in the Legal Affairs file, GC.

103 Testimony of William Bailey, supervisor, *Sun*, 17 December 1849; Wiley Williams, 26 May 1850, GC.

104 Kirkbride to Albert Williams, 28 October 1849 [copy], Kirkbride Misc. Letters; testimony of Kirkbride, *Sun*, 15 December 1849; Franklin Butler Kirkbride, "Reminiscences," unpublished memoir, IPH.

105 IW, 26 September 1843, LP 1:158.

106 JC, Dr. JC, [April?] 1846, AB, 24 April 1852, PC; CB-FD 4:156; BE, EE, 25 October 1855, PC; Mrs. H, CH, 11 August 1879, PC. VM, 20 October 1862, PC, expresses the suspicion that the attendants steal his belongings.

107 Mrs. M, JM, 18 October 1865, PC; MB, TB, 17 January 1860, PC; AB, WB, 31 August 1857, PC; Mrs. H, DM, 23 April 1852, PC; AG, EB, 20 December 1847, PC; Mrs. JW to "Willi," [no date]; PC.

108 EL, 8 October 1865 [misfiled], GC; JA, RJA, 7 August 1846, PC.

109 AG, EB, 20 December 1847, PC; ES, 19 October 1862, PC; A male patient complains about invalid life in JMW, 20 January 1848, PC, for example.

110 TL, [no date? 1860], PC; Mrs. EDM, 15 January 1845, LP 2:21. For complaints about being excluded from the family table, see Mr. W., 9 August 1843, LP 1:127. For the remark about the oil painting, see MR, 26 February 1853, PH.

111 SS to "Father," 7 October 1859, PC; JW, 29 March 1860, PC; JG, 3 July 1858, PC.

112 SH, CS, 23 February 1858, PC; MB, 1 August 1848, PC; S. Preston Jones, "Statement *Re* JM," in Lawsuits folder, Misc. Papers.

113 SS, "Mother," 29 April 1859, PC; WG, 29 December 1848, PC.

114 AB, 24 April 1852, PC; RA, 26 October 1857, PC.

115 DB, 5 November 1849, Misc. Kirkbride papers.

116 EG, JBB, 10 August 1861, PC.

117 *AR*, 1854, p. 9.

118 AF Sr., AF Jr., 31 May 1848, PC; JC, Dr. JC, [? April] 1846, PC.

119 SR, MR, 16 January 1857, PC; ER, 17 May 1845, LP 2:75.

120 Mr. L, 29 January 1845, LP 2:27.

121 I have compiled this list from materials in the Legal Affairs folder, Misc. papers. Compare my discussion here with Peter McCandless, "Liberty and Lunacy: The Victorians and Wrongful Confinement," JSH 11 (1978):366–86, on commitment controversies in Great Britain.

122 JM, 9 June 1844, LP 1:301. "Intemperance" was listed as the supposed cause of insanity in the Medical Register entries for four litigants. The Pennsylvania Hospital counsel, George Biddle, warned Kirkbride about keeping a "habitual drunkard" whose "unsound mind" was not evident; the hospital was not a "reformatory school," he concluded. George Biddle to Kirkbride, 30 January 1872.

123 My discussion of the Haskell case is based on Ebenezer Haskell, *The Trial of Ebenezer Haskell, in Lunacy, and His Acquittal Before Judge Brewster in November, 1868* (Philadelphia, 1869), and Earl D. Bond, *Dr. Kirkbride and His Mental Hospital* (Philadelphia, 1947), pp. 122–4, 128–9.

124 Haskell, *Trial*, pp. 5, 28–9. I have not been able to obtain any reliable accounts of the trial's outcome. Isaac Ray stated in a letter to Judge Charles Doe (7 August 1868, BH) that Brewster examined Haskell in the courtroom, thought him to be sane, and so discharged him.

125 "Opinion of Judge Allison in Case of LR," *Legal Gazette*, 25 March 1870, p. 91 (clipping in L. R. folder, GC). "Judge Paxson's Charge," *Times and Dispatch*, 18 November 1871, p. 2 (copy in AM file, GC). See clipping, "Another Haskell Habeas Corpus Case," *Evening Bulletin*, 21 May 1870 (clipping in Ebenezer Haskell file, GC). An editorial in *The Medical Times* (Philadelphia), 15 April 1871, criticized lawyers for their lack of scruples in bringing writs for patients who requested them. "Is it not equivalent to conferring on every lawyer in the

land a sort of roving commission to roam at will through the wards of our hospitals in search of fitting subjects for the writ?" (copy in Legal Affairs folder, GC). I suspect Isaac Ray may have written the editorial; the rhetoric sounds like his.

126 Isaac Ray to John Sawyer, 3 March 1876, BH. Judge Carroll Brewster, 3 August 1870, Patient Mistreatment folder, GC. See Mrs. ESW, 11 October 1865, Lawsuits folder, GC.

127 Ebenezer Haskell, *Trial*, pp. 42, 46–7, 45. Haskell supplies a humorous paragraph on "How Committees Examine the Pennsylvania Hospital for the Insane" (p. 47), in which he refers to a visit from a group of doctors; after a banquet of 2½ hours, Haskell claimed, some were "so full they had to be *conducted* from the table to their carriage." All left without seeing a single ward, "no wiser than they had come."

128 Ebenezer Haskell, 7 November 1871, GC; *Evening Star* (?), 11 March 1873, p. 1, clipping in Ebenezer Haskell file, GC. See also other clippings in this file.

129 See Frank Mott, *American Journalism, A History 1690–1960*, 3rd ed. (New York, 1962), esp. pp. 239–43, for a discussion of post-Civil War journalism.

130 [L. Clarke Davis ?], "A Modern 'Lettre de Cachet'," *Atlantic Monthly* 21 (1868):588–602. Quotations are from pp. 590, 597, 591, 596. In a letter to Edward Jarvis (28 March 1869, CL), Kirkbride referred to the "Atlantic man Davis," who had been "abusing us nearly every week since last May." Edward Jarvis, 28 May 1868, GC, refers to a Dr. Clarke at the *Atlantic;* I presume he meant Davis.

131 [Isaac Ray], "A Modern 'Lettre de Cachet' Reviewed," *Atlantic Monthly* 22 (August 1868):227–43.

132 *New York Tribune* 23 November [1869 or 1870?], clipping in miscellaneous folder, GC. *New York Tribune*, quoted in Haskell, *Trial*, p. 54. William Russell, *The New York Hospital: A History of the Psychiatric Service 1771–1936* (New York, 1945), pp. 269–83, discusses the *Tribune*'s investigations at the Bloomingdale Asylum.

133 *New York Tribune*, quoted in Haskell, *Trial*, p. 54.

134 *Sunday Transcript*, 26 December 1869, p. 2 (GD file, GC).

135 *Medical Times*, 15 April 1871, pp. 259–61. "The Hoyt Commission," *Evening Bulletin*, 19 March 1883, clipping in Hoyt Commission file, Miscellaneous Manuscripts, Kirkbride Memorabilia, IPH.

136 John Curwen et al., *Memoir of Thomas S. Kirkbride* (Warren, Pa., 1885), p. 33. J. A. Reed, 24 November 1870, GC.

137 *AR* 1883, p. 105.

CHAPTER 6: *The perils of asylum practice*

1 Frederick Wines, *Report on the Defective, Dependent, and Delinquent Classes of the Population of the United States, as Returned at the 10th Census (June 1, 1880)* (Washington, D.C., 1888), pp. 90–2, lists 139 mental institutions of various types. The "Proceedings" of the AMSAII, published each year in the AJI, list the members who attended. Henry M. Hurd, ed., *The Institutional Care of the Insane in the United States and Canada*, 4 vols. (Baltimore, 1916), vol. 1, p. 206, gives a list of states in which hospitals were built according to the Kirkbride plan: Alabama, California, Connecticut, District of Columbia, Georgia, Illinois, Iowa, Kansas, Kentucky, Louisiana, Maine, Maryland, Massachusetts, Michigan, Minnesota, Mississippi, Missouri, Nebraska, New Jersey, New York, North Carolina, Ohio, Tennessee, Texas, Utah, Virginia, West Virginia, and Wisconsin. In a study of architect Samuel Sloan, Harold Cooledge lists twenty-two hospitals that were probably based on the Kirkbride–Sloan plan; thirteen of these have been documented in the following towns: Tuscaloosa, Ala.; Hopkinsville, Ky.; Kalamazoo, Mich.; Trenton, N.J. (three additions); Indianapolis, Ind.; Middletown, Conn.; St. Peter, Minn.; Greystone, N.J.; Morganton, N.C.; Raleigh, N.C. (remodeling after 1875); Columbia, S.C. (center section); Philadelphia –

Pennsylvania Hospital for the Insane and Insane Department, Philadelphia General Hospital. See "The Kirkbride Plan: Architecture for a Treatment System That Changed," *Hospital and Community Psychiatry* 27 (1976):475.

2 See, for example, Deutsch, *The Mentally Ill in America*, 2nd ed. (New York, 1949), esp. chap. 10; Norman Dain, *Concepts of Insanity in the United States, 1789–1865* (New Brunswick, N.J., 1964), esp. pp. 139–44; David Rothman, *The Discovery of the Asylum*, (Boston, 1971), esp. chap. 6; and Gerald Grob, *Mental Institutions in America: Social Policy to 1875* (New York, 1973), esp. Chap. 4.

3 The asylum superintendents were by no means a monolithic group. There were serious disaffections among the southern and western physicians, and within the ranks of the dominant northerners, a long-standing antipathy existed between John Gray and his Utica Gang. When I discuss the brethren in this chapter, I refer only to the AMSAII's most active members. Although their viewpoints did not necessarily hold for the whole specialty, they were its most visible representatives. I would include among the brethren, circa 1840–75, Samuel Woodward, Amariah Brigham, Luther Bell, Isaac Ray, John S. Butler, William Awl, James Bates, Pliny Earle, John Curwen, Charles Nichols, H. A. Buttolph, Andrew McFarland, and D. T. Brown. By treating this group as a unified faction within the AMSAII, I by no means wish to suggest that they did not have serious differences of opinion on certain issues. See Charles Nichols to Dorothea Dix, 31 March 1867, HL, for a discussion of hospital plans.

4 D. T. Brown to Dix, 9 February 1857, HL. See Pliny Earle, "American Insane Hospital Reports: Bloomingdale Asylum," *AJMS* n.s. 32 (1856):439–42, for a very unfavorable review of the institution. For letters complaining about the Bloomingdale situation, see Nichols to Dix, 7 February 1852, HL; Pliny Earle, 18 August 1858, GC; and Brown to Nichols, 24 December 1859, NA. James MacDonald's Diary for 1836–7, NY, also contains numerous references to his difficulties while physician to the asylum.

5 S. Schulz to Dix, 9 February 1857, HL; H. A. Buttolph, 9 January 1847, GC.

6 Grob, *Mental Institutions*, p. 15.

7 See Appendix 3 for more information on paying patients in state hospitals.

8 Ray used the phrase "gross enormities" to describe the new North Carolina State Hospital. Ray to Dix, 3 November 1852, HL. Ray to Dix, 15 April 1854, HL, discusses the Taunton Asylum. For other examples of construction problems, see Dix to Nichols, 3 August 1858, NA; Nichols to Dix, 13 February 185[1?], HL; Ray to Dix, 24 March 1852, HL.

9 Curwen, 30 August 1852, GC; H. Stabb to Dix, 13 June 1855, HL.

10 Richard Patterson, 20 February 1852, GC. For remarks concerning the Irish as attendants, see "Proceedings," *AJI* 17 (1860):60.

11 E. Fisher, [no day] July 1855, GC. For another comment of Gray's role in Benedict's firing, see Brown, 4 September 1854, GC. For complaints about insubordinate employees, see for example, Schulz to Dix, 31 December 1879, HL; Ray to John Sawyer, [no day or month] 187[7?], BH.

12 Nichols, 30 March 1852, GC; Ray to Sawyer, BH. D. T. Brown wrote to Dix that the "large unwieldy" board at Bloomingdale was the "bane of this asylum, while at Trenton the concentration of wisdom (?) and power in one Governor has proved an equal obstacle." Brown to Dix, 9 February 1857, HL.

13 M. Ranney to Ray, 10 January 1875, BH. For two unflattering letters concerning Ranney, see Kirkbride to Earle, 19 October 1863, AS; Nichols to Dix, 18 March 1852, HL.

14 James Lawson, Secretary of the Interior, to L. A. Lamar, "Appointment Papers," NA. See Earle to Edward Jarvis, 2 August 1870, CL, for Earle's account of his own legal difficulties with a patient.

15 My discussion here is based upon Myra Himelhoch and Arthur Shaffer, "Elizabeth Packard: Nineteenth Century Crusader for the Rights of Mental Patients," *Journal of American Studies* 13 (1979), 343–75, a well-documented, if very one-sided, narrative of Packard's career.

16 Ibid., pp. 361–5.

17 McFarland to Jarvis, 12 August 1868, CL.

18 McFarland to Jarvis, 12 August 1868, CL. Patterson to Kirkbride, 20 February 1852, GC. Buttolph to Kirkbride, 12 April 1859, GC.

19 See, for example, Kirkbride to Board of Visitors, 10 December 1869, Papers Relating to Nichols Investigation, NA. Of all the many state superintendents Dix corresponded with, she seemed most attached to Nichols. Some of their letters border on the romantic; see, for example, Nichols to Dix, 28 November 1853 and n.d. [185?].

20 Nichols to Dix, 30 July 1869, and 22 December 1869, HL. Even Nichols's handwriting deteriorated; the strain he felt can be seen in its increasingly disjointed, erratic character. Details of the Nichols investigations can be found in the Minutes of the Board of Visitors, pp. 201–12, "Hearings Before The Committee of Investigations Concerning Charges Against Supt. C. H. Nichols, 1869," and "Papers Relative to Charges vs. C. H. Nichols, 1876." NA Nichols also gives many details of the 1869 investigation in his letters to Dix. Francis Hamlin to Earle, 8 January 1878, AS, reported that Nichols was having problems at Bloomingdale: "A cloud of difficulties and mishaps seems to follow Dr. Nichols wherever he may go," he concluded.

21 Henry Landon to Nichols, 18 August 1876, NA; H. Stabb to Dix, 3 March 1859, HL; J. A. Reed to Nichols, 18 August 1876, NA; Reed to Kirkbride, 24 November 1870, GC; Nichols to Dix, 4 July 1869, HL.

22 Curwen to Jarvis, 15 March 1860, CL. Kirkbride to Dix, 2 March 1856, HL (Kirkbride was referring to the investigations of Curwen, which he hoped had taught the young doctor a lesson); T. M. Franklin to Earle, 15 May 1881, AS. For reference to Benedict, see Brown, 4 September 1854, GC.

23 Luther Bell to Earle, 24 December 1857, AS. Francis Stribling, 23 September 1850, GC, uses the phrase "victims" to describe Amariah Brigham. George Chandler made a similar comment concerning Woodward in "On the Proper Number of Patients in an Institution . . .," an unpublished paper read at the AMSAII meeting, Mss. in Chandler Collection, AS. See also Ray to trustees of Butler Hospital, 17 January 1866, JB. As an added worry, the superintendents had to consider the impact of asylum life on their wives and children. Henry Stabb confided to Dix of his wife, "She has never been wholly reconciled to living in the Institution in consequence of the Centre building in which we live being anything but impervious to the sounds issuing from the wards – and this with young children and infants is not quite agreeable – especially when after childbirth, Fanny is in a nervous state" (Stabb to Dix, 3 March 1859, HL).

24 J. Bates, 22 October 1849, GC; Brown, 3 February 1858, GC. See also F. Stribling, 23 September 1850, GC. *JNMD* 3 (1876):500 records the death of George Cook. *AJI* 38 (1882):466–8 mentions the assault on John Gray. The man who attacked him was not a patient. Gray died several years later, never having recovered from a gunshot wound to the face.

25 M. Bemis, C. Bemis, 12 December 1865, PC; Jarvis, 8 February 1866, GC. Himelhoch and Shaffer, "Elizabeth Packard," 366, note 88, mention McFarland's suicide. William Russell, *The New York Hospital: A History of the Psychiatric Service 1771–1936* (New York, 1945), pp. 284–8, discusses Brown's tragic death. Dr. Peticolas of the Eastern State Hospital in Virginia also committed suicide. See Nichols to Dix, 3 December 1868, NA.

26 Eugene Genovese, *Roll, Jordan, Roll: The World the Slaves Made* (New York, 1974), esp. pp. 3–7, provides a forceful elucidation of the slaveholders' paternalistic ideology.

27 "Proceedings," *AJI* 8 (1851):86–7, and *AJI* 10 (1853):86, record the passage of the propositions. The propositions themselves were reprinted in the same volumes, pp. 79–81 and 67–9, respectively.

28 See Grob, *Mental Institutions*, esp. chap. 5. My argument here differs little from his.

29 Andrew Scull, *Museums of Madness* (New York, 1979), esp. pp. 164–5, discusses the private–public distinction in the English specialty.

30 Ray to Robert Ives, 8 January and 21 May 1844, JB. The custom of providing paying patients with more genteel employments and accommodations appears to have been commonplace in most state hospitals. Nichols explained the practice at the Government Asylum: "We give him a costly furnished room, more delicacies, and more personal attendance than is strictly required for his most advantageous treatment." Patients were classified, he continued, "according to their education and social and official position, but we do not annoy the quiet with excited and noisy patients, regardless of pay." Nichols, to Eugene Grissom, 2 October 1869, NA.

31 For elucidations of this dominant social philosophy, see William McLoughlin, *The Meaning of Henry Ward Beecher* (New York, 1970) and Stephen Thernstrom, *Poverty and Progress* (Cambridge, Mass., 1964).

32 John Galt, "The Farm of St. Anne," *AJI* 11 (1855):352–7. The quotation is from p. 354. See Grob, *Mental Institutions*, pp. 325–36, for a discussion of Gheel.

33 Brown, 5 May 1855, GC; "Proceedings," *AJI* 12 (1855):43; Pliny Earle, "Reports of American Institutions for the Insane," *AJMS* n.s. 29 (1855):449. Kirkbride also received letters from Buttolph, 27 April 1855, and Nichols, 8 July 1855, GC, expressing indignation about Galt's paper. Kirkbride himself gave vent to some angry remarks about Galt in a letter to Dix: "He never comes to the meetings, makes no improvements himself, but sits in his armchair criticizing whatever is done by his more active brethren, and publishing what he writes at home and abroad." Kirkbride to Dix, 22 July 1855, GC. These are easily the most negative comments the normally good-natured Kirkbride ever made about a fellow superintendent; his tone demonstrates how close to home Galt's remarks had struck. Nichols, 8 July 1855, GC, accused Gray of rewriting the proceedings of the AMSAII. In another letter, 9 July 1855, GC, Nichols describes Gray as "intoxicated" with his power as editor of the *AJI*.

34 At times, R. Hills, Benjamin Workman, E. H. Van Deusen, and W. S. Chipley joined the dissidents, as did C. A. Lee, a physician in private practice who wrote occasionally for the *AJI*. The Canadian asylum doctors, including Henry Landor and Workman, tended to be critical of AMSAII policies. See, for example, Landor to Jarvis, 3 February 1872, CL.

35 George Cook, "Provision for the Insane Poor in the State of New York," *AJI* 23 (1866):45–75. The quotation is from p. 73. See also John Chapin, "On Provision for the Chronic Insane Poor," *AJI* 24 (1867):29–42; and Edward Jarvis, "On the Proper Functions of Private Institutions or Homes for the Insane," *AJI* 17 (1860):19–31. These reformers all felt that the American specialty would benefit by emulating European trends in asylum medicine. As Jarvis wrote to Kirkbride after a trip abroad, "There are many things to be learned there." Jarvis, 20 September 1860, GC.

36 Grob, *The State and the Mentally Ill: A History of the Worcester State Hospital in Massachusetts, 1830–1920* (Chapel Hill, N.C., 1966), pp. 209–17, discusses Bemis's plan. Grob, *Mental Institutions*, pp. 309–14, 327–8. Note that in 1854, Brown was already questioning the expense of regular state hospitals. Brown to Jarvis, 19 December 1854, CL.

37 "Proceedings," *AJI* 23 (1866):168–250.

38 Grob, *The State and the Mentally Ill*, pp. 217–28; Russell, *The New York Hospital*, p. 264, quotes Brown as saying that Kirkbride had talked him out of the cottage plan. The private correspondence of the principals involved in the Willard controversy reveals the highly personal dimension of their disagreements. See, for example, John Gray to Dix, 10 January 1869, HL; C. A. Lee to Earle, 18 January 1872, AS; J. B. Chapin to Dix, 28 February 1867, HL.

39 Kirkbride to Earle, 3 March 1873, AS; Earle to Jarvis, 8 December 1860, CL. For the orthodox superintendents' views on employment, see "Proceedings," *AJI* 19 (1862):57–9, esp. remarks by Ray and Curwen. See ibid., pp. 57–71, for other superintendents' views of employment. John Gray, "The Willard Asylum," *AJI* 22 (1865):210, stated his willingness to consider a "wise eclecticism" in hospital architecture. See "Proceedings," *AJI* 23 (1866):168–251, on the mod-

erates' support for the modified propositions. Gray's speech, pp. 174–90, was particularly vehement in its opposition to separate asylums for the chronic insane.

40 "Proceedings," *AJI* 24 (1868):317 (these are not the official proceedings, which were published separately that year, to protest Gray's tinkering with the transcripts; this is his account of the debate); "Proceedings," *AJI* 28 (1871):321–2.

41 Brown to Jarvis, 13 May 1862, CL; "Proceedings," *AJI* 12 (1855):43.

42 Brown to Dix, 31 March 1866, HL.

43 Ray to Dix, 8 December 1851, HL.

44 See Grob, *Mental Institutions*, pp. 270–302, for background on the development of the State Boards of Charities.

45 Quoted in "Proceedings of the Neurological Society," *JNMD* 3 (1876):495. For general works on American neurology, see references in Chapter 3, note 40.

46 Edward Spitzka, "Reform in the Scientific Study of Psychiatry," *JNMD* 5 (1878):215. The *JNMD* kept up a running fire of articles, reviews, and editorials excoriating the superintendents. This article is an excellent example of the neurologists' critique of asylum medicine.

47 Himelhoch and Shaffer, "Elizabeth Packard," 366–74, give details of her public crusade. Charles Reade, *Hard Cash: A Matter of Fact Romance* (New York, n.d.), first appeared as a serial in Charles Dickens's magazine, *All the Year Round*, and subsequently went through many editions. [Adeline Lunt], *Behind the Bars* (New York, 1871). There were many other patient exposés published in this period. Gerald Grob has found at least fifty in his research. See Grob, "Abuse in American Mental Hospitals in Historical Perspective: Myth and Reality," *International Journal of Law and Psychiatry* 3 (1980), 301, note 16. See also Walter Alvarez, *Minds That Came Back* (New York, 1961), for a bibliography of patient accounts.

48 Sawyer to Ray, 18 February 1875, BH. See Kathleen Jones, *A History of the Mental Health Services* (Boston, 1972), esp. pp. 101–49, for a history of the Lunacy Commission.

49 To judge from their correspondence, Ray and Kirkbride had established their friendship as young superintendents. When Ray retired from the Butler Hospital in 1867, he chose Philadelphia as his new home, partly to be near his good friend. Until his death, he made a practice of spending every other Sunday afternoon at the Pennsylvania Hospital. See Franklin B. Kirkbride, "Reminiscences," unpublished memoir, IPH. The two men worked together closely, collaborating on professional and political matters of all sorts.

50 Pliny Earle, *Annual Report of the Northampton State Hospital* (Northampton, Mass., 1877). Earle later expanded his critique and published it as a book, *The Curability of Insanity* (Philadelphia, 1887). In this book, Earle described Kirkbride as a "moderate" in the cult of curability (see pp. 37–8). The two men appear to have been close friends in the 1840s and 1850s. Despite the 1877 *Annual Report*, Kirkbride wrote to Earle in 1880 that their many years of professional comradeship had "only increased the respect and regard, with which I subscribe myself, as always, thy Friend." See Kirkbride to Earle, 1 December 1880. For more on Earle's critique, see Appendix 2.

51 John Chapin to Earle, 1 May 1877, AS; Franklin B. Sanborn, *Memoirs of Pliny Earle, M.D.* (New York, 1973; reprint of 1898 ed.), p. 267; John Yale to Earle, 20 January 1877, AS; J. Bodine to Earle, 12 January 1877, AS. Francis Wells to Earle, 13 February 1877, AS, refers to the propositions as the "cast-iron creed of some excellent Superintendents." In the same letter, Wells professed his admiration for Earle's regime at Northampton because "you manage your hospital for nothing and save money every year."

52 Isaac Ray, "Recoveries from Mental Disease," *Transactions of the College of Physicians of Philadelphia* 3rd series 4 (1880):217–30. After his son's death in December 1879, Ray began to fail rapidly, and died only a year and a half later. See Kirkbride, "Memoir of Isaac Ray, M.D., L.L.D.," *Transactions of the College of Physicians* 3rd series 5 (1881):clvii–clxxiii. Kirkbride's last years will be discussed in the Conclusion.

53 *Appeal to the People of Pennsylvania on the Subject of an Asylum for the Insane Poor*

of the Commonwealth (Philadelphia, 1838), p. 3; *Second Appeal to the People of Pennsylvania on the Subject of an Asylum for the Insane Poor of the Commonwealth* (Philadelphia, 1841), p. 6. See also Dorothea Dix, *Memorial Soliciting a State Hospital for the Insane, Submitted to the Legislature of Pennsylvania, February 3, 1845* (Harrisburg, 1845).

54 John Curwen et al., *Memoirs of Thomas Story Kirkbride* (Warren, Pa., 1885), p. 19, notes his service on the Harrisburg board of trustees. Brown to Dix, 28 October and 27 December 1850, HL, mentions other competitors for Curwen's post.

55 Kirkbride, *On the Construction, Organization, and General Arrangements of Hospitals for the Insane*, 2nd ed. (Philadelphia, 1880), p. 249. See also p. 47 of the second edition; pp. 1–2 of the first edition.

56 Nichols to Dix, 19 December 1852, HL.

57 Curwen to Dix, 26 January 1852, HL.

58 Curwen frequently referred to his financial problems in his letters to Kirkbride. See, for example, Curwen, 15 June 1859 and 10 December 1861, GC.

59 Curwen to Kirkbride, 9 May 1865, GC. For figures on paying patients, see PSLA *AR* 1855, p. 7, and *AR* 1875–6, p. 33.

60 The Pennsylvania Legislature, *LR*, for each year listed the annual appropriation for the Harrisburg Hospital in the section entitled "Reports of Appropriation Bills."

61 *LR* 1863 no. 77, p. 611.

62 *LR* 1868 no. 121, pp. 962–3; *LR* 1877 no. 176, p. 1404; Curwen, 10 December 1861, GC.

63 *LR* 1862 no. 85, p. 679; *LR* 1862 no. 85, p. 679.

64 PSBC *AR*, vol. 6, p. xi.

65 Kirkbride was hostile to the concept of a State Board of Charities long before one was established in Pennsylvania. He wrote to Dix in 1864 that he wanted to confer with her on the "prospect of having a *hired* agent of the state to visit all institutions, (a man probably who has no knowledge of this subject) and aid patients who are dissatisfied in their efforts to get away. Such a theory is really advocated in Boston and elsewhere." Kirkbride to Dix, 19 August 1864, HL.

66 PSBC, *Addenda to a Plea for the Insane in the Prisons and Poorhouses of Pennsylvania: Paying Patients in the State Lunatic Hospitals* (Philadelphia, 1873), p. 14; PSBC, *A Plea for the Insane in the Prisons and Poorhouses of Pennsylvania* (Philadelphia, 1873), p. 22; PSBC, *Addenda*, p. 12.

67 PSBC, *Addenda*, p. 15; PSBC, *Plea*, pp. 24–5.

68 PSBC, *Addenda*, p. 6; PSBC, *Plea*, pp. 26, 97–8.

69 See PSBC, *Plea*, pp. 75–9; PSBC, 5th *AR* (1874–5), pp. 52–9, for a discussion of their proposals. See also George Harrison, 27 February 1873, GC.

70 "Memorial on Insane Criminals," presented to the House and Senate of Pennsylvania, 19 February 1874, copy in Misc. Papers. The memorial was signed by Kirkbride, Ray, Curwen, J.A. Reed of Dixmont, S. S. Schulz of the Danville State Hospital, and Joshua Worthington of the Friends Retreat. See also "Proceedings," *AJI* 30 (1873):213–38. In response to a letter from George Harrison on the PSBC, the superintendents passed a set of resolutions outlining the ideal treatment of the criminal insane in an asylum attached to a state prison.

71 PSLA *AR* 1861, p. 6.

72 For letters referring to the superintendents' lobbying efforts, see Ray to Sawyer [15?] February 1873, BH; and George Harrison, 27 February 1873, GC. Kirkbride was a Whig until the Civil War and a Republican thereafter (*AR* 1883 p. 118). Presumably, the degree of influence he had in Harrisburg depended on which party was in office.

73 PSBC, *Compilation of the Laws Relating to the Board of Public Charities...* (Harrisburg, 1916), pp. 47, 122; *LR* 1876 no. 249, p. 1987.

74 PSBC, *Plea*, pp. 75, 74; Curwen, 27 May 1874, 22 January 1876, GC.

75 PSBC, *Plea*, p. 23. See Curwen, 12 March 1878, for the charge concerning Dixmont.

76 Hiram Corson to Earle, 10 March 1877, AS. For Corson's charges against Curwen, see also Corson to Earle [no date; ans. 25 January 1879] and 1 July 1877,

AS; and Hiram Corson, *A Brief History of Proceedings in the Medical Society of Pennsylvania to Procure the Recognition of Women Physicians by the Medical Profession of the State* (Norristown, Pa., 1894). John Gray referred to Corson as "preeminent" among the "disturbing elements and blatherskites" active in asylum reform. See Gray, 11 March 1881, GC. Constance McGovern, "Doctors or Ladies? Women Physicians in Psychiatric Institutions, 1872–1900," *BHM* 55 (1981):93–5, discusses the Pennsylvania debate. Although the controversy over appointing a woman doctor was a major factor in Curwen's dismissal, it was also part of an ongoing battle over the superintendent's autonomy.

77 Curwen to Dix, 31 December 1880 and 6 December 1880, HL; Kirkbride to Dix, 7 January 1881, GC. See also Schulz to Dix, 21 January 1881, HL. Schulz told Dix that Curwen's foes wanted to "make the medical authority subordinate to the Steward." At first glance, it might seem puzzling that Curwen, having just been fired at one state hospital, easily found a job at another. But the choice of superintendent was left entirely to the Warren trustees; the PSBC had no control over the hiring process there, or at any other state institution. Curwen did find that the same parties who troubled him at Harrisburg tried to block state appropriations to Warren. See Curwen, 25 September 1882, GC.

78 "Report of the Commission to Examine into the Present System for the Care of the Insane of the State...," 1883, copy in Misc. Papers. For Mitchell's views on asylum reform, see his controversial paper, "Address Before the 50th Annual Meeting of the American Medico-Psychological Association," *JNMD* 21 (1894):413–37. Curwen, 27 May 1874, GC, refers to L. Clark Davis's articles in the *Inquirer*. Reed to Earle, 12 October 1877, AS, expresses his agreement with Earle's statements in the 1877 *AR*. Reed was the PSBC's favorite among the asylum doctors.

79 "Kirkbride to the Joint Committee of the Senate and House on the Bill in Reference to the Care of the Insane," 20 February 1883, copy in Hoyt Commission file, Misc. Papers. He also wrote individual letters to W. A. Wallace, Eckley B. Coxe, and John Reyburn.

80 "The Law Regulating Insane Hospitals," unidentified clipping in State Legislature file, Misc. Papers; "Review of Commission on Lunacy, PSBC, 1st Annual Report," *JNMD* 11 (1884):675.

81 See Section 3 of Appendixes for more on paying patients in state hospitals. "Editorial," *JNMD* 4 (1877):799, refers to Utica as a mixed asylum, i.e., one "where both public and private patients are treated." Henry Burdett, *Hospitals and Asylums of the World*, 5 vols. (London, 1891), vol. 1, p. 529, wrote that in New York State, the private patient issue came to a head after passage of the State Care Act in 1890, which required all pauper lunatics to be transferred from poorhouses to state hospitals. On 1 October 1890, the State Commission on Lunacy issued an order stating that henceforth, no private patients were to be admitted to state institutions except in strict conformity to the statute, and then only when vacancies existed; and that no differences would be allowed in "scale of care and accommodations" provided for private and public patients. The Danvers hospital was widely criticized as "wasteful" by Kirkbride's critics, for example, *JNMD* 4 (1877):799. Kirkbride's advocates, on the other hand, thought it was a fine state hospital. See, for example, Ray to Sawyer, [no day] November 1875 and 8 September 1877, BH.

82 *AJI* 35 (1878):102; and *AJI* 30 (1873):187.

83 Ray to Dix, 29 December 1869, HL.

Conclusion: A generous sympathy

1 [Eliza Butler Kirkbride], "Memorial of Thomas Story Kirkbride," *AR* 1883, p. 133. I compared the two editions of Kirkbride's book, *On the Construction, Organization, and General Arrangements of Hospitals for the Insane*, and found pp. 17–18 and 36–223 of the 1880 edition to be substantially unchanged from the 1854 text. The new edition of Kirkbride's treatise did little to still the growing

revolt against his principles of asylum design. In his review for the *Journal of Mental Science* 27 (1881–2):66, the English alienist Thomas S. Clouston paid respectful tribute to it as a "landmark...showing the state at which asylum construction and management had arrived in the lifetime and experience of one man." Although praising Kirkbride's achievements, however, Clouston took issue with the most cherished tenets of his asylum philosophy: the curability of insanity; the desirability of regular state hospitals; the need for "expensive precautionary arrangements" to restrain the patients without creating an oppressive atmosphere; and the value of uniformity and regularity in asylum design. The whole tenor of Clouston's review suggests that Kirkbride was a man who had outlived his usefulness.

2 Henry M. Hurd, ed., *The Institutional Care of the Insane in the United States and Canada*, 4 vols. (Baltimore, 1916), vol. I, p. 221; D. H. Tuke, 27 December 1880, GC. Hurd does not mention anyone by name in his passage concerning the tension between the older and younger members, but it is obvious from the context that Kirkbride and Ray were the "elderly men" to whom he referred.

3 See Chapter 6, note 52.

4 *AR* 1883, pp. 136. Ibid., pp. 137–41, recounts Kirkbride's physical decline and death. Many obituary notices incorrectly stated that he died on 17 December at around 1 a.m., but Eliza Kirkbride's account gives the time as 11:45 p.m., 16 December 1883, as does the Petition for Probate of his Will, PCA. The *Evening Bulletin*, 20 December 1883, carried a lengthy description of Kirkbride's funeral. He was buried in the Laurel Hill Cemetery, next to the grave of his first wife, Ann West Kirkbride. The Probate Petition estimated the value of his estate as between $20,000 and $50,000. An "Inventory and Appraisement of the Goods and Chattels...of Thomas Story Kirkbride," 12 January 1884, listed bonds and stocks from several railroad companies, worth around $85,000; miscellaneous mortgages, valued at around $19,000; and about $10,000 in cash and life insurance. The total value of the estate was set at $122,405. Kirkbride had inherited a substantial amount from his wife Ann, whose father, Joseph R. Jenks, had been very wealthy. He could hardly have amassed an estate of this size from his superintendent's salary. Under the terms of his will, Eliza Kirkbride inherited one-third of the estate, and the rest was divided among his six children. See Account Book 55, p. 152 (1883 no. 124), Registrar of Wills, PCA.

5 *AR* 1883, pp. 114, 77.

6 "Proceedings," *AJI* 41 (1884):47. John Curwen et al., *Memoir of Thomas Story Kirkbride* (Warren, Pa., 1885), reprinted the AMSAII proceedings relative to Kirkbride's death, along with a biographical sketch.

7 "Proceedings," *AJI* 41 (1884):47.

8 "Proceedings," *AJI* 45 (1888):137, 141.

9 Ibid., 142, 134. Earle did not attend the meeting, but sent Godding a letter stating his views on the propositions.

10 Richard S. Dewey, "Present and Prospective Management of the Insane," *JNMD* 5 (1878):60–94; idem, "Differentiation in Institutions for the Insane," *AJI* 39 (1882):1–21, provide a good example of late-nineteenth-century views on asylum architecture. Barbara Sicherman, *The Quest for Mental Health in America, 1880–1917* (New York, 1980), esp. chaps. 1–3, gives a good overview of the specialty.

11 *Buffalo Express*, 8 August 1884, clipping in Harriet Chapin's Scrapbook, p. 66. This scrapbook is in the possession of Miss Dorothy Bodine, Chapin's granddaughter.

12 The day after Kirkbride's death, his son-in-law, Thomas G. Morton, handed the managers a memo the superintendent had dictated during his 1880 illness, which presented his argument for the two-doctor plan. The managers at first voted to follow Kirkbride's advice. They received a number of applicants for the two posts, but none impressed them as much as Chapin. According to Chapin's daughter, Frances, they took a trip by private railroad car to see Willard, and were "much astonished" by its beauty and good order (Frances Gilbert, 12 October 1951, private letter in the possession of Dorothy Bodine). Chapin agreed to come to the Pennsylvania Hospital only if he would be chief physician of

both departments. The managers finally agreed to his terms. See MM 11:205, 213, 232–4. Chapin, MR 29 September 1884, PH, states that he took over the hospital on the first of the month.

13 My remarks on Chapin's administration are based on the *Annual Reports*, the Monthly Reports, Chapin's Letterpress volumes, and the Case Records.

14 The Medical Journals contain a count of patients under restraint or in seclusion, as well as an explanation for their confinement, i.e., "hit attendant," "mutilated self," and the like. Chapin's correspondence contains numerous letters concerning the proper filing of commitment papers. See, for example, Chapin to Governor Stockley, 9 February 1885, LP 1:128. There are no references to or notations by Chapin in the Casebooks. Letters to the patrons were written by the assistants, who signed them "J.B. Chapin per Brush," etc. On Progressive era institutions, see David Rothman, *Conscience and Convenience: The Asylum and Its Alternatives in Progressive America* (Boston, 1980).

15 See, for example, *AR* 1891, p. 17.

16 John Curwen, "Presidential Address," *Proceedings of the American Medico-Psychological Association* 1 (1895):32–100; G. Alder Blumer, "A Half-Century of American Medico-Psychological Literature," *AJI* 51 (1895):40–50; Hurd, ed., *Institutional Care*, vol. 1, p. 221. See also Henry Hurd, "The Alienists of the Past Half-Century," in *Proceedings*, (1885):167–71; and William A. White, "Presidential Address," *American Journal of Psychiatry* 82 (1925):1–20, esp. 2–4.

17 Hurd, ed., *Institutional Care*, vol. 1, p. 221; Norman Dain, *Concepts of Insanity in the United States, 1789–1865* (New Brunswick, N.J., 1964); Gerald Grob, *Mental Institutions in America: Social Policy to 1875* (New York, 1973); J. Sanbourne Bockoven, *Moral Treatment in American Psychiatry* (New York, 1963); Eric Carlson and Norman Dain, "The Psychotherapy That Was Moral Treatment," *American Journal of Psychiatry* 117 (1960):519–24; idem, "Milieu Therapy in the Nineteenth Century," *JNMD* 131 (1960):277–90.

18 See, for example, Albert Deutsch, *The Mentally Ill in America*, 2nd ed. (New York, 1949), esp. Ch. 10.

19 See Andrew Abbott, "Status and Status Strain in the Professions," *American Journal of Sociology* 86 (1981):819–35, for a provocative discussion of professional attitudes toward the value of service vs. research.

20 "Dr. Thomas Story Kirkbride," *Evening Bulletin* 17 December 1883, clipping in Obituary File, Miscellaneous Manuscripts, Kirkbride Memorabilia, IPH. Jarvis to Sir James Clark, 28 January 1868, Jarvis Letterpress 1867–9, p. 87, CL, explicitly compared Kirkbride to Conolly.

21 Bucknill, 30 March 1879, GC.

Appendixes

1 William Malin, *Some Account of the Pennsylvania Hospital* (Philadelphia, 1828).

2 In fact, the elderly were disproportionately underrepresented in the mid-nineteenth-century asylum population, as Barbara Rosenkrantz and Maris Vinovskis have shown in "The Invisible Lunatics: Old Age and Insanity in Mid-19th Century Massachusetts," in *Aging and the Elderly*, edited by Stuart Spicker (Totowa, N.J., 1978), pp. 95–125.

3 Pliny Earle, *Annual Report of the Northampton State Hospital in 1877*, and *The Curability of Insanity* (Philadelphia, 1887).

4 J. Sanbourne Bockoven, *Moral Treatment in American Psychiatry* (New York, 1963), p. 61.

5 Norman Dain, *Disordered Minds: The First Century of Eastern State Hospital in Williamsburg, Virginia 1766–1866* (Williamsburg, Va. 1971), pp. 45–46.

6 *AR* 1870, p. 24.

7 23rd *AR*, p. 15.

8 Commission on Lunacy, PSBC, 1st *AR* (Harrisburg, Pa., 1884), pp. 85–90.

MANUSCRIPT SOURCES

This study has been based primarily on the extensive manuscript collections of the Pennsylvania Hospital and the Institute of the Pennsylvania Hospital. Both archives have been recently inventoried through projects funded by the American Philosophical Society and the National Library of Medicine. The Pennsylvania Hospital Archives, located in the Pine Building at the Eighth Street Hospital, contain records relating to the early treatment of the insane and the general management of the asylum. The Institute of the Pennsylvania Hospital Archives, located in the Kirkbride Building at the 49th Street institution, contains the majority of records concerning the asylum's daily administration. In citing individual documents, I have followed the form used in the "Checklist to the Archives of the Pennsylvania Hospital" prepared by Bonnie Blustein and Caroline Morris in 1978. I have included the item numbers assigned the various records on the checklist to facilitate their identification and location.

Pennsylvania Hospital Archives – Eighth Street Hospital

Series 1: Board of Managers and contributors
Board of Managers' Minutes, vols. 1–11, 1751–1884   *item* 2–11, 238
Board of Managers, Miscellaneous Papers, 2 boxes, 1751–1860   50, 50a

Series 3: Administration
Steward and Matron. Ledgers, vols. A–I, 1781–1880   96–103, 269

Series 4: Medical staff
General Material, Loose Papers, 1 box, 1752–1858   155
Material on Individual Physicians, 3 boxes, ca. 1773–1859   156–8

Series 5: Patients
Book of Patients, 2 vols., 1781–8, 1791–6   159–60
Admissions and Discharges, 9 vols., 1804–40   161–9
Brief Summary of Each Admission, 2 vols., 1811–52   175–6
Accounts of House of Employment and Overseers of the Poor with Hospital, 1 vol., 1784–9   189
Collection of Cases (also labeled "Hospital Cases"), two vols., 1803–34   193,–
Miscellaneous General Material, 1 box, 1752–1858   195b
Miscellaneous Papers Relating to Individual Patients, four boxes, 1763–1860   196–9

Note: Samuel Coates's memorandum book, "Cases of Several Lunatics in the Pennsylvania Hospital," is kept in the rare book collection of the hospital library, although it does not appear on the "Checklist."

Institute of the Pennsylvania Hospital Archives – Forty-ninth Street Hospital

Note that upon the opening of the new hospital, or Male Department, at 49th and Market streets in 1859, the original asylum at 44th and Haverford streets became the Female Department. The asylum's administrative records reflect this division in its services. Up to 1859, they covered the operation of the 44th Street institution, which included both the men's and women's wards. After 1859, the original record series reverted to the Female Department, and a new set of books was begun for the Male Department.

Note: Lucy Rous's manuscript, Diary of a Companion, 1870, is included among Kirkbride's miscellaneous documents.

INDEX

University of Pennsylvania Press
STUDIES IN HEALTH, ILLNESS, AND CAREGIVING
Joan E. Lynaugh, General Editor

Barbara Bates. *Bargaining for Life: A Social History of Tuberculosis, 1876–1938.* 1992

Michael D. Calabria and Janet Macrae, editors. Suggestions for Thought *by Florence Nightingale: Selections and Commentaries.* 1994

Janet Golden and Charles Rosenberg. *Pictures of Health: A Photographic History of Health Care in Philadelphia.* 1991

Anne Hudson Jones. *Images of Nurses: Perspectives from History, Art, and Literature.* 1987

June S. Lowenberg. *Caring and Responsibility: The Crossroads Between Holistic Practice and Traditional Medicine.* 1989

Peggy McGarrahan. *Transcending AIDS: Nurses and HIV Patients in New York City.* 1994

Elizabeth Norman. *Women at War: The Story of Fifty Military Nurses Who Served in Vietnam.* 1990

Anne Opie. *There's Nobody There: Community Care of Confused Older People.* 1992

Elizabeth Brown Pryor. *Clara Barton, Professional Angel.* 1987

Margarete Sandelowski. *With Child in Mind: Studies of the Personal Encounter with Infertility.* 1993

Nancy Tomes. *The Art of Asylum-Keeping: Thomas Story Kirkbride and the Origins of American Psychiatry.* 1994

Zane Robinson Wolf. *Nurses' Work, The Sacred and The Profane.* 1988

Jacqueline Zalumas. *Caring in Crisis: An Oral History of Critical Care Nursing.* 1994